Current Techniques in Ophthalmic Laser Surgery

CURRENT TECHNIQUES IN

Ophthalmic Laser Surgery

Third Edition

EDITED BY

Lawrence J. Singerman, MD
Retina Associates of Cleveland
Clinical Professor
Department of Ophthalmology
Case Western Reserve School of Medicine
Cleveland, Ohio, USA

Gabriel Coscas
Professor of Clinical Ophthalmology
Department of Ophthalmology
University of Paris XII
Professor of Clinical Ophthalmology
Eye University of Créteil
Créteil, France

With 26 contributors

BUTTERWORTH
HEINEMANN

BOSTON OXFORD JOHANNESBURG MELBOURNE NEW DELHI SINGAPORE

Developed by Current Medicine, Inc.
Philadelphia

Current Medicine

Director of product development: **Lori J. Bainbridge**
Developmental editor: **Jennifer Wood**
Design and layout: **Christine Keller-Quirk**
Illustrator: **Lisa Weischedel**
Art director: **Paul Fennessy**
Illustration director: **Ann Saydlowski**
Production: **Lori Holland and Amy Watts**
Index: **Holly Lukens**

Special discounts on bulk orders of this book are available.
For information, please contact:

Manager of Special Sales
Butterworth-Heinemann
225 Wildwood Avenue
Woburn, MA 01801-2041
Tel: 781-904-2500
Fax: 781-904-2620
For information on all B-H medical publications available, contact our World Wide Web home page at: http://www.bh.com

ISBN: 0-7506-7032-0
ISSN: 1062-4813

Printed in Hong Kong by Paramount
5 4 3 2 1
Distributed worldwide by Butterworth-Heinemann.

Contents

Contributors

Gavin G. Bahadur, MD
Cataract Service
The Sinskey Eye Institute
Santa Monica, California, USA

Jack M. Dodick, MD
Clinical Professor of Ophthalmology
Department of Ophthalmology
Columbia University College of Physicians and Surgeons
Chairman
Department of Ophthalmology
Manhattan Eye, Ear, and Throat Hospital
New York, New York, USA

Daniel A. Ebroon, MD
Clinical Instructor
Department of Ophthalmology
Northwestern University
Clinical Practice Director
Department of Ophthalmology
Northwestern Medical Faculty Foundation
Chicago, Illinois, USA

Gregory A. Eippert, MD
Senior Clinical Instructor
Department of Ophthalmology
Case Western Reserve University
Cleveland, Ohio, USA;
Glaucoma Specialist
Ophthalmic Consultants and Surgeons of Cleveland
South Euclid, Ohio, USA

Daniel Finkelstein, MD
Professor of Ophthalmology
Wilmer Eye Institute
John Hopkins University School of Medicine
Baltimore, Maryland, USA

Evangelos S. Gragoudas, MD
Professor
Department of Ophthalmology
Harvard Medical School
Surgeon
Massachusetts Eye and Ear Infirmary
Boston, Massachusetts, USA

David R. Guyer, MD
Director of Residency Training
Department of Ophthalmology
Manhattan Eye, Ear, and Throat Hospital
Clinical Associate Professor
Cornell University Medical Center
New York, New York, USA

Albert Hornblass, MD
Clinical Professor
Department of Ophthalmology
State University of New York
Brooklyn, New York, USA;
Director of Ophthalmic Plastic, Orbital, and Reconstructive Surgery
Manhattan Eye, Ear, and Throat Hospital
Lenox Hill Hospital
New York, New York, USA

Matthew R. Jones, MD
Fellow
Cornea/External Disease
Wills Eye Hospital
Philadelphia, Pennsylvania, USA;
Heed Ophthalmic Foundation
Cleveland, Ohio, USA

Joel M. Krauss, MD
Research Fellow
Manhattan Eye, Ear, and Throat Hospital
New York, New York, USA

Peter R. Laibson, MD
Professor
Jefferson Medical College of Thomas Jefferson University
Director, Cornea Service
Wills Eye Hospital
Philadelphia, Pennsylvania, USA

Kathleen A. Lamping, MD
Associate Clinical Professor
Department of Ophthalmology
Case Western Reserve University
Cleveland, Ohio, USA

Jeffrey Liebmann, MD
Clinical Associate Professor
Department of Ophthalmology
New York Medical College
Valhalla, New York, USA;
New York Eye and Ear Infirmary
New York, New York, USA

Joan W. Miller, MD
Associate Professor
Department of Ophthalmology
Harvard Medical School
Associate Surgeon
Massachusetts Eye and Ear Infirmary
Boston, Massachusetts, USA

Robert P. Murphy, MD
Glaser Murphy Retina Treatment Centers
Baltimore, Maryland, USA

John H. Niffenegger, MD
Director, Retinal-Vitreous
Eye Centers of Ohio, Inc.
Canton, Ohio, USA

Michael A. Novak, MD
Retina Associates of Cleveland
Cleveland, Ohio, USA

Scott D. Pendergast, MD
Retina Associates of Cleveland
Cleveland, Ohio, USA

Christopher J. Rapuano, MD
Associate Professor
Jefferson Medical College of Thomas Jefferson University
Associate Surgeon, Cornea Service
Wills Eye Hospital
Philadelphia, Pennsylvania, USA

Douglas J. Ripkin, MD
Assistant Clinical Professor
Department of Ophthalmology
Case Western Reserve University
Director of Glaucoma Service
St. Luke's Hospital of Case Western Reserve University
Cleveland, Ohio, USA;
Glaucoma Consultant
Northeast Ohio Eye Surgeons
Kent, Ohio, USA

Robert Ritch, MD
Professor of Clinical Ophthalmology
Department of Ophthalmology
New York Medical College
Valhalla, New York, USA;
New York Eye and Ear Infirmary
New York, New York, USA

Paul N. Schacknow, MD
Chief of Glaucoma Services
Visual Health and Surgical Center
Lakeworth, Florida, USA

Gisèle Soubrane, MD, PhD
Professor
Department of Ophthalmology
University of Paris XII
Hospital of Créteil
Créteil, France

Z. Nicholas Zakov, MD
Retina Associates of Cleveland
Cleveland, Ohio, USA

Hernando Zegarra, MD
Retina Associates of Cleveland
Cleveland, Ohio, USA

Leonidas Zografos, MD
Professor of Ophthalmology
Department of Medicine
Université de Lausanne
Chairman
Hôpital Ophtalmique Jules Gonin
Lausanne, Switzerland

Preface

Ophthalmology was the first specialty to use lasers in medicine, more than 30 years ago. It remains the leading specialty using this modality, because we have continuously developed new instruments and new indications for the use of lasers in ophthalmic diseases. Several experts in laser therapy for various ophthalmic diseases have generously contributed their extensive clinical and research experience to this book. They present the latest lasers, which offer increasingly efficacious options for treating diseases affecting almost every tissue in the eye and adnexa.

Lasers in cataract surgery offer exciting promise for refinement of surgical technique. A chapter by Dr. Jack Dodick, developer of the first laser lens ablation method, describes in detail the evolution of new laser technologies for cataract surgery and the ongoing studies of these exciting new modalities. The state of the art in laser therapy is presented authoritatively, providing a reference that allows ophthalmologists to discuss with their patients the most recent advances in this area.

New options for corneal treatment introduced with the advent of the excimer laser have greatly expanded the uses of lasers in ophthalmology beyond the traditional pathologies to encompass the large percentage of the population interested in having refractive errors corrected without glasses or contact lenses. The remarkable rapidity of advances in phototherapeutic keratectomy (PTK), photorefractive keratectomy (PRK), photoastigmatic refractive keratectomy (PARK), and laser-assisted in situ keratomileusis (LASIK) for refractive surgery have enhanced the precision and safety of these procedures. Chapter 2 clarifies the areas of controversy in refractive surgery, thereby helping the ophthalmologist choose the optimum approach in a given patient.

Lasers have become an important tool in the practice of the oculoplastic surgeon who uses laser therapy directed at many different tissues. The CO_2 laser, in particular, has enabled many advances in oculoplastic surgery. The hemostatic properties are very important. Because of the high degree of effectiveness, the resurfacing capabilities may allow this modality to reach a larger population. These technologies require excellent training for optimum results, and Chapter 3 provides a good introduction that may stimulate many ophthalmologists to further study in this area.

The devastating complications of proliferative diabetic retinopathy (PDR) inspired the development of photocoagulation by Dr. Gerd Meyer-Schwickerath and the classic studies on laser therapy for PDR by Dr. Lloyd Aiello in the late 1960s. The Diabetic Retinopathy Study, performed in the early 1970s and first published in 1976, proved the dramatic benefits of laser therapy for PDR and set a standard for clinical trials, not just in retina and in ophthalmology, but also in other branches of medicine. Many of the lasers we use in other ophthalmic disorders have now been proven effective by similar randomized clinical trials. Notable among these is the Early Treatment Diabetic Retinopathy Study, which is discussed in detail in Chapter 5.

Similar studies by the Branch Vein Occlusion Study group, chaired by Dr. Daniel Finkelstein, coauthor of Chapter 6, demonstrated the efficacy of grid laser photocoagulation for macular edema in branch retinal vein occlusion. Thus, many ophthalmologists were beginning to believe that lasers might be effective in all of the retinal diseases in which they were used. However, the Central Retinal Vein Occlusion Study group demonstrated that prophylactic panretinal scatter laser therapy is not necessary and does not always prevent the development of iris or angle neovascularization. Furthermore, grid laser therapy for macular edema, although effective in branch vein occlusion, did not improve visual acuity in central vein occlusion.

Over a period of 15 years, the American Macular Photocoagulation Studies and the French and other studies of laser therapy for choroidal neovascularization (CNV) in age-related macular degeneration have shown the benefits of such treatment, particularly for extrafoveal and juxtafoveal vessels. Even some subfoveal vessels can be treated effectively with standard laser techniques. However, due to the damage to retinal tissue by heat, newer modalities are being studied.

Photodynamic therapy (PDT), using 1/1000 the power of standard lasers, can avoid much of the damage the latter create. The rationale and experimental studies leading to current clinical trials of PDT for subfoveal classic and occult CNV are presented clearly in Chapter 7. The development of new photosensitizers and the improved understanding of the mechanism of the efficacy of this modality have led to its resurgence. In addition to treating CNV, PDT can be efficacious in treating selected ocular tumors. Other laser techniques useful in the treatment of pigmented tumors are also discussed in the text.

Endolaser photocoagulation is now an integral part of vitreoretinal surgery. It has greatly enhanced the safety and efficacy of vitrectomy for proliferative retinopathies and complicated retinal detachments.

Various lasers have been shown to be very effective in the management of different types and stages of glaucoma. The Glaucoma Laser Trial and the Glaucoma Laser Trial Follow-up Study have clarified the role of argon laser trabeculoplasty in the armamentarium of the ophthalmologist. The Advanced Glaucoma Intervention Study promises to elucidate this role further. The types and mechanisms of glaucoma that respond to laser iridotomy and peripheral iridoplasty are discussed in detail in Chapter 15. The indications, techniques, and complications in these procedures are clearly outlined.

It appears that lasers are replacing cyclocryotherapy as the cyclodestructive procedure of choice. Lasers allow better titration of therapeutic effect and minimize complications. The increased safety of cyclodestruction with lasers may allow expansion of the indications to eyes with potential for useful vision.

The tunable dye laser and other lasers allowed sophisticated refinements in laser techniques for the treatment of CNV, retinal vascular diseases, and other abnormalities. Many of these instruments, however, were large and costly, thus limiting their use to large institutions and group practices. Diode laser technology is allowing smaller, less expensive, and more versatile units, which do not require water-cooling. As the technology is refined, it is possible that, instead of a large, multifunction apparatus, the ophthalmologist will use several smaller units that have fewer functions each but are more accessible, both economically and geographically. Lower-cost units are particularly important and welcome in the current socioeconomic medical environment. Cost-effective, accessible instrumentation will allow laser treatment to be more readily available to people who need it.

This book emphasizes the practical laser treatment parameters that are clinically important for ophthalmologists. It provides a comprehensive review of current literature and precise analyses of the various lasers used in each ophthalmic subspecialty. The indications, results, and complications are clearly presented. The most important and current literature is cited and discussed. All this is enhanced with excellent illustrations. The text will be very valuable to every ophthalmologist, from the beginning resident to the experienced clinician, who is interested in learning new laser procedures.

Lawrence J. Singerman, MD
Gabriel Coscas, MD

Acknowledgments

We are indebted to Arnall Patz, who, by setting an example, inspired our interest in clinical trials of laser therapy. This provided to us the privilege of participating in many clinical trials that have proven the benefits of therapies for leading causes of blindness.

We want particularly to thank Joan Hornik, the editor at Retina Associates of Cleveland, for her outstanding efforts on this volume.

We appreciate the help and professionalism of Jennifer Wood, editor at Current Medicine.

We are grateful to our wives, Margaret S. and Gisèle C., and to our children, Stacy and Seth, and Florence and Brigitte, who have graciously accepted our sacrificing many family activities to support our academic efforts.

CHAPTER 1

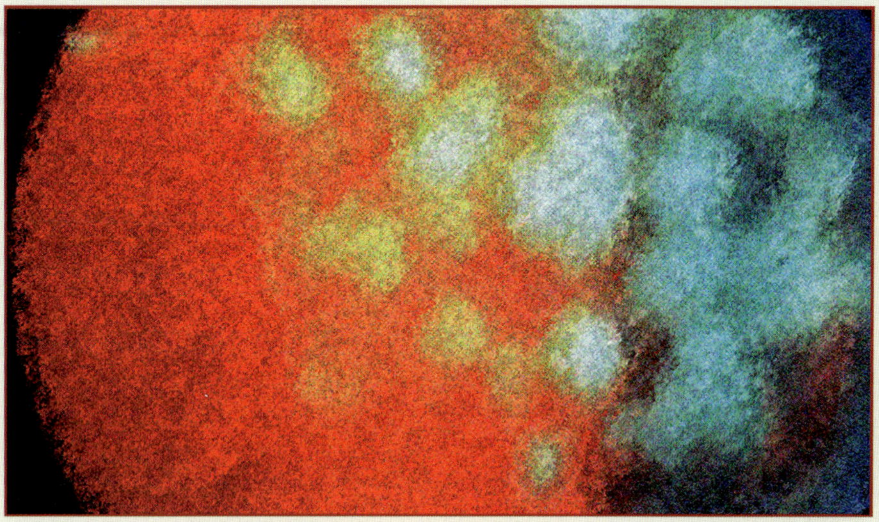

Lasers in Cataract Surgery

JACK M. DODICK
GAVIN G. BAHADUR

Cataract surgery has undergone numerous technologic advances during the past several decades. Although current small-incision phacoemulsification techniques provide safe and effective treatment for cataracts, they require considerable skill and can result in trauma to the corneal endothelium, iris, and posterior capsule. Several laser technologies—including the neodymium:yttrium-aluminum-garnet (Nd:YAG) and erbium:yttrium-aluminum-garnet (Er:YAG) wavelength lasers—have been developed recently to create a safer, easier, and more economical alternative to phacoemulsification.

Since the development of phacoemulsification by Charles Kelman in 1967 [1], cataract surgery has experienced many technologic innovations and has now become one of the safest and most effective of surgical procedures. When compared with nuclear expression, small-incision phacoemulsification cataract surgery induces less astigmatism and produces quicker rehabilitation and fewer wound complications [2]. Although small-incision phacoemulsification cataract surgery is clearly an effective procedure with a low complication rate, further refinements need to be made.

Phacoemulsification cataract surgery is associated with a considerable learning curve. The vibrating ultrasonic phacoemulsification needle can open the posterior capsule in mere seconds. Furthermore, total ultrasound energy used in the eye has been shown to have a detrimental effect on endothelial pump function. It can also result in corneal edema and, secondarily, in reduced visual acuity [3]. Heat produced by the vibrating phacoemulsification tip can result in collateral thermal damage to the cornea or sclera, which may cause large astigmatic effects with or without attendant tissue defects [4]. The new generation of laser-based cataract extraction systems currently in development may help shorten the learning curve and provide a procedure with a lower overall complication rate.

LASER-BASED SYSTEMS

Unlike the ultrasound frequency vibrations created by conventional phacoemulsification probes, laser-based systems rely on shock waves generated by Nd:YAG or Er:YAG lasers to disrupt the nucleus.

Laser systems do not dissipate any appreciable amount of thermal energy, which makes them ideal for small, watertight, clear corneal incisions without the risk of corneal burns. A laser probe's temperature is also largely independent of flow rate, unlike that of a conventional phacoemulsification probe, which relies heavily on adequate irrigation to prevent corneal burns [5]. A truly watertight seal between probe and incision may be used with laser systems, resulting in a stable anterior chamber and decreased requirement for volume of irrigation solution. Ultimately, designers of laser-based cataract systems hope to lower the complication rate of cataract surgery significantly and also to lower the costs of surgery.

DODICK LASER LENS LYSIS

I described the earliest approach to laser lens ablation, Dodick laser lens lysis [6,7]. This method uses a pulsed

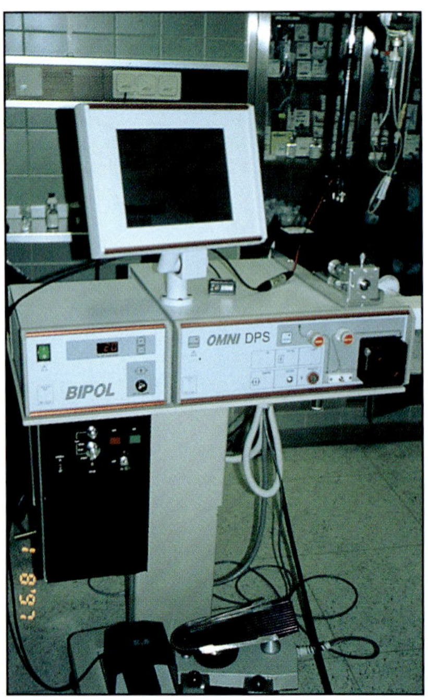

FIGURE 1-1. Neodymium:yttrium-aluminum-garnet laser lysis unit shown under the console of a phacoemulsification unit. The laser lysis unit uses the fluidics of this system.

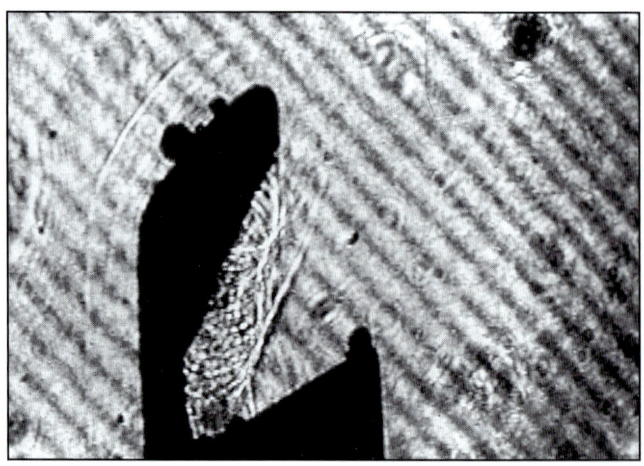

FIGURE 1-2. High-speed photograph of shock wave produced on the surface of the target of a laser lysis probe. The shock wave is produced when pulsed 1064-nm neodymium:yttrium-aluminum-garnet laser energy is directed onto the titanium target, creating optical breakdown and plasma formation.

Q-switched Nd:YAG laser similar to capsulotomy lasers (Fig. 1-1). The laser energy pulses onto a titanium target contained in an irrigation–aspiration probe. This event ignites a plasma on the surface of the titanium target, producing shock waves (Fig. 1-2). These shock waves collect at the mouth of the aspiration port, where they are used to disrupt and aspirate the cataract (Fig. 1-3).

This technology is currently under development by A.R.C. Laser in Eckental-Forth, Germany. I am working under an investigational device exemption (IDE) from the US Food and Drug Administration and to date have performed 26 procedures. In addition, seven surgical research sites have been established in Europe: in Bonn, Friedberg, Bad Hersfeld, and Nümberg, Germany; in Salzburg, Austria; in Athens, Greece; and in Teufen, Switzerland. Plans have been drawn up to establish an additional 20 sites in Europe by the end of 1998.

This technology claims several advantages over conventional ultrasound. The light handpiece is, in essence, an irrigation–aspiration probe containing a quartz laser fiber and titanium target (Fig. 1-4). It can be manufactured in disposable plastic or reusable stainless steel. In the latter version, the only disposable element is the titanium tip, which promises to reduce the cost of small incision surgery.

In vitro studies of Dodick laser phacolysis by Alzner and Grabner [8] have demonstrated that this technology, unlike ultrasound, produces no clinically significant heat (Figs. 1-5 and 1-6). Thermal measurements have been taken comparing the Nd:YAG (1064 nm) laser, set at 10 mJ with a pulse duration of 14 nanoseconds, with the conventional ultrasound handpiece of the Sonocat (Ortli, Switzerland). In a dry artificial anterior chamber, the laser tip was shown to generate an increased heat difference of up to 3.4°C, whereas the temperature of the ultrasonic probes reached up to 55.3°C. This temperature differential was smaller under balanced salt solution (maximal difference 0.3°C for the laser, 12°C for ultrasound), underscoring the critical role of water cooling in conventional ultrasound technology [8]. As a result, corneal burns are not possible.

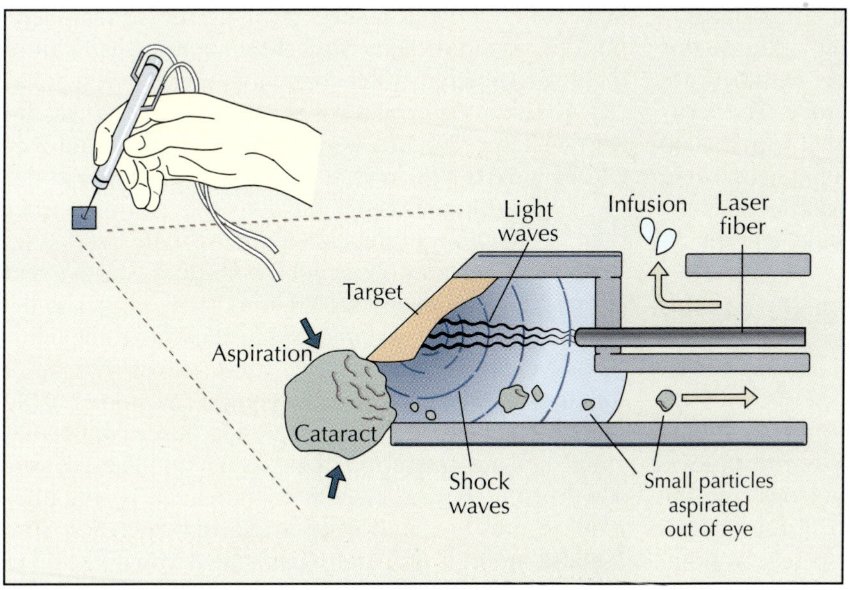

FIGURE 1-3. Schematic of laser lysis probe. The neodymium:yttrium-aluminum-garnet laser is delivered by a quartz fiber in the infusion port. The laser energy strikes the titanium target, producing plasma formation and shock waves. The shock waves are collected at the mouth of the infusion port where the cataract is held by aspiration (*short arrows*) and lysed.

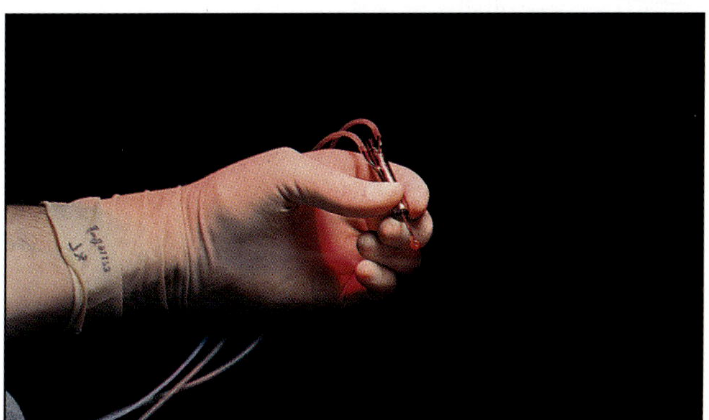

FIGURE 1-4. Photograph of the probe illustrating its size in relation to the surgeon's hand.

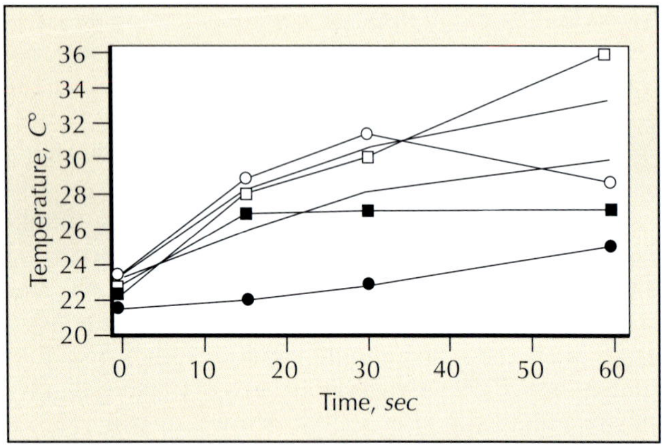

FIGURE 1-5. Temperature profile of conventional ultrasound. (*Adapted from* Alzner and Grabner [8]; with permission.)

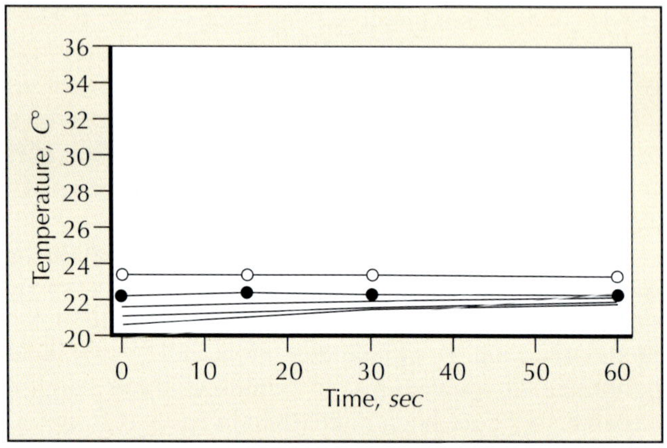

FIGURE 1-6. Temperature profile of laser system. (*Adapted from* Alzner and Grabner [8]; with permission).

Because water cooling is unnecessary, infusion can be introduced through a separate port, reducing incision size and making cataract surgery through two 1-mm corneal incisions possible (Fig. 1-7). Incisions may be as tight as desired, and irrigation can be slowed or even discontinued without the risk of incision burns.

Unlike other laser approaches using erbium, this technique does not expose the eye to laser light because all laser light is contained within the probe. The technology operates at 1 to 5 Hz and, compared with 24,000 to 40,000 Hz for a standard ultrasound handpiece, could conceivably result in increased safety to nontargeted tissues, such as the endothelium, lens capsule, and iris.

ERBIUM:YTTRIUM-ALUMINUM-GARNET LASERS

Premier Laser Systems

Premier Laser Systems of Irvine, California, currently has an approved IDE for its Er:YAG laser for the removal of cataracts. As in the 1064-nm wavelength of the Nd:YAG laser, the 2.94-nm wavelength of the Er:YAG laser lies in the infrared spectrum and has several properties that make it particularly useful for lens ablation in the eye. The laser delivers nonultraviolet radiation and for this reason limits potential mutagenicity and toxicity to the corneal endothelium and retina [9].

The Er:YAG wavelength has the capacity to ablate high water-content tissues, such as the human lens nucleus, without pigmented chromophores. It is more highly absorbed in water than any other tissue type; in fact, it has a water absorption 1000 times that of the Nd:YAG laser. The Er:YAG laser is a solid-state unit that excites a YAG host crystal to produce energy and the element within the crystal, the dopant, is erbium (rather than neodymium in the case of the Nd:YAG laser) [9].

The Er:YAG laser operates on both photoablative and photoacoustic phenomena. Erbium tends to vaporize tissue as it emulsifies. Cataract removal occurs using energy delivered from the acoustic shock waves. The tip of the Er:YAG laser probe emits a conical cavitation bubble that implodes, generating a photoacoustic wave that emulsifies the cataractous lens tissue [9]. The acoustic wave of the Er:YAG laser is characterized by impulse-induced pressure and by laser-induced cavitation. The impulse-induced pressure is generated when the laser

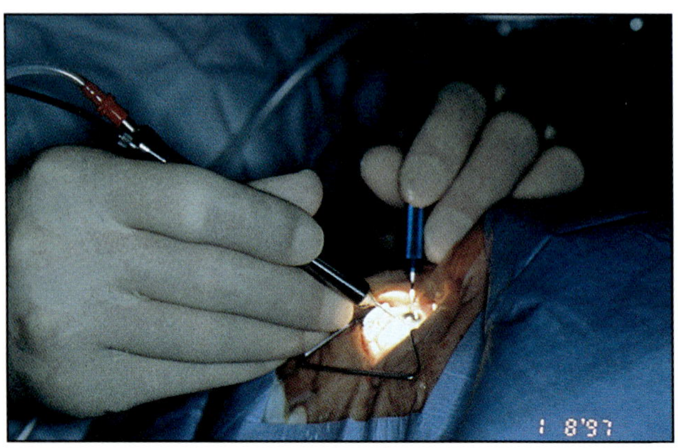

FIGURE 1-7. Bimanual laser lysis of the nucleus. Because this technology produces no clinically significant heat, infusion and aspiration can be split and introduced through two paracentesis ports of 1-mm width each. This dramatically reduces the incision size compared with that currently possible using ultrasound technology.

pulse removes a volume of target tissue. Collapse of an Er:YAG laser pulse-induced bubble causes cavitation-induced pressure [9,10]. The emulsified cataract tissue consists of tiny flakes of nucleus that are held in suspension and then subsequently aspirated. For lens emulsification, the repetition rate is 10 to 15 Hz at energy levels of 20 to 60 mJ and a 400- to 800-μm spot size [9].

Unlike the equipment used in ultrasonic phacoemulsification, the erbium handpiece is light weight, approximately the weight of a pencil, making it easier to hold and manipulate. Furthermore, the tip of the fiber is smooth, spherical, and without points and sharp edges.

The cataract removal procedure with the Er:YAG laser initially consisted of a two-handed technique, whereby a laser probe was introduced through one incision and an irrigation–aspiration tip was introduced through a paracentesis. More recently, the laser probe has been redesigned to a coaxial configuration incorporating irrigation and aspiration within the same laser probe. This probe can enter through a 3-mm incision. Er:YAG energy is delivered through a 600-μm fiber, through which laser light converges at a focal point 0.5 mm from the fiber tip [11]. According to Premier, the coaxial design increases the laser's efficiency significantly and has been reported to reduce total laser time to approximately 3 to 5 minutes from the 8 to 12 minutes of the bimanual technique.

Energy levels below the photoablation threshold result in localized thermal reactions [12]. By adjusting delivered energy to just above the ablation threshold, the laser can be used effectively to perform anterior capsulotomy by inscribing a circle on the surface of the anterior capsule with a relatively high repetition rate using primarily photoablative properties [9]. The capsulotomy probe employs an erbium fiberoptic delivery system, which has a modified clear silica top with a 45° wedge-shaped cylinder. This tip angle allows for internal reflection of laser energy so that the longitudinal laser beam is redirected at a 90° angle at the tip and laser energy is focused directly at the anterior capsule. The clear tip allows visualization of the capsule and direct observation of the lasing action [9].

Capsulotomy is easily carried out by inscribing a circle with the probe. The capsule can even be lased under the iris. A repetition rate of 10 Hz with energy of 12 to 15 mJ and a spot size of 800 μm is used for anterior capsulotomies [9]. Because the laser emits repetitive pulses rather than a continuous wave, the tip of the probe must be moved in a slow, controlled fashion to achieve a continuous capsulotomy margin.

The effect of laser energy on endothelial cell counts is currently being studied in Phase II trials; preliminary results suggest an endothelial cell count drop-out rate of 10% or lower. Furthermore, although the laser probe generates acoustic shock waves and cavitation bubbles, it does not appear to break the posterior capsule in animal studies conducted to date. Moreover, no ruptures in the posterior capsule secondary to the laser probe itself have been found in the preliminary study of human eyes (60). Firing the laser directly at the posterior capsule results in only a pinprick hole.

Although every laser has some thermal component, the Er:YAG laser has minimal dispersion of thermal energy because of the wavelength's high degree of water absorption. The erbium laser is a solid-state unit, approximately the size of a suitcase (Figs. 1-8 and 1-9), that can run on standard wall electricity and requires no replacement gases or specially trained engineers. These factors could make it fairly competitive in pricing compared with current phacoemulsification units [9].

Designing fibers that can carry the erbium wavelength reliably and inexpensively remain a technologic challenge. Fibers composed of high water-content zirconium–fluoride can themselves absorb the erbium energy and be easily damaged.

Premier Laser Systems is currently conducting a Phase II FDA study involving 100 patients enrolled across four sites. The company also has 510K-approval for Er:YAG laser anterior capsulorhexis, as well as an IDE for internal and external sclerotomies.

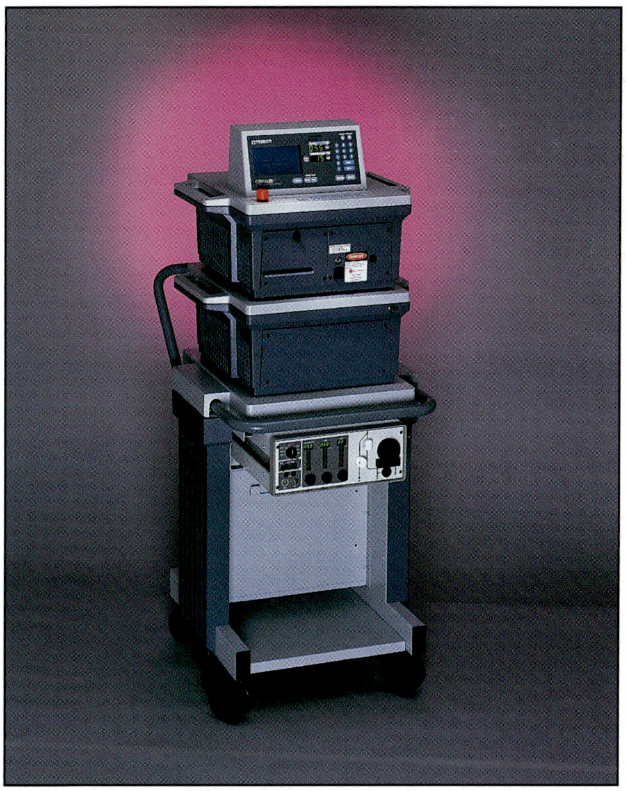

FIGURE 1-8. Premier Laser System's (Irvine, CA) Centauri erbium:yttrium-aluminum-garnet laser unit.

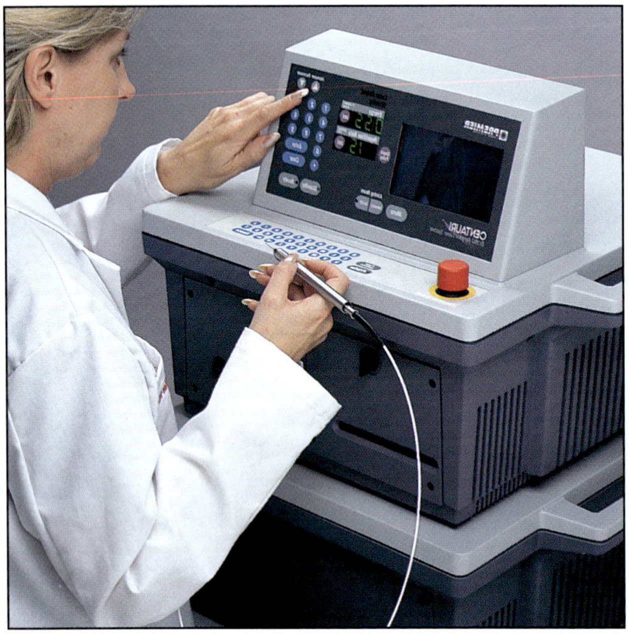

FIGURE 1-9. Centauri console.

Aesculap-Meditec

Aesculap-Meditec's (Jena, Germany) MCL 29 Phaco-Lase system also employs an Er:YAG 2.94-µm wavelength laser. According to Aesculap-Meditec, an initial trial with the MCL 29 on 10 patients demonstrated that this system was at least as effective as a conventional phacoemulsification unit. In this procedure, a capsulorhexis is performed in the conventional fashion, as is hydrodissection, and the laser probe is inserted through a 3.5-mm incision. The nucleus is removed using a standard divide-and-conquer technique. It has been demonstrated that even the MCL 29 tip can rupture the posterior capsule [13]. The most recent prototype of the MCL 29 uses a 1.1-mm tip with a repetition rate of 60 Hz. In situations with a 3+ cataract with a hard nucleus, the MCL 29 is often ineffective and surgeons must switch to conventional ultrasound.

The MCL 29 is currently in clinical trial in Italy, Germany, and Spain and its price is estimated to be in the same range as that of ultrasound systems [13]. As with Premier's Er:YAG approach, the current drawback to this approach appears to be the expensive, easily damaged fiber technology. Sapphire fiber technology is being evaluated but this also damages easily and is, at present, extremely expensive.

Other companies exploring erbium:yttrium-aluminum-garnet lasers

At the present time, Coherent, of Palo Alto, CA, and Light Wave, a German laser company, are conducting evaluations of the erbium approach.

PARADIGM'S NEODYMIUM:YTTRIUM-ALUMINUM-GARNET LASER

Paradigm's (Salt Lake City, UT) Nd:YAG laser was invented by Daniel Eichenbaum, who started work on the project in 1983 [14].

In the Photon system, a quartz fiberoptic cable transmits 1064-nm Nd:YAG laser energy across an area called the *photofragmentation zone* within a probe. The laser penetrates deeper than erbium wavelength systems. The prototype probe inserts through a 1.9-mm incision; however, production models may fit through an incision as small as 1.6 mm [14].

In this system, a single coaxial probe is used for both laser irrigation and aspiration. The probe does not heat collateral tissue by more than 5°C. The seal between the probe and the incision can be watertight, because no significant heat is generated to create thermal burns in the surrounding tissue. This tight seal at the incision allows stable depth maintenance of the interior chamber. The disposable laser probes are discarded before any probe material is eroded and has been lost into the eye. According to Eichenbaum, the laser cataract system can remove a nucleus with 3+ density in approximately 3 minutes [14].

The Paradigm probe is similar in appearance to an ultrasonic phacoemulsification probe, but the 1.8-mm diameter tip, shaped like the end of a ski, lases cataracts with a 1064-nm Nd:YAG laser. The probe has a rounded zone beneath the cannula, which is 0.9 mm in diameter. It is under this "photovaporization chamber" that laser energy reduces the cataract to the consistency of plasma. The collimated laser beam terminates in a metal backstop [15]. The thermal acoustic effects of Nd:YAG wavelength may help to expedite the emulsification, relative to those of erbium-based systems. Paradigm's system uses a three-position foot pedal, giving control over irrigation, aspiration, and laser firing. After being softened to plasma form, the emulsate is aspirated with a port located at the base of the photovaporization chamber. A computer drives the laser at variable repetition rates of 10 to 50 Hz, and changes in computer software can be used to modify the laser's output. According to Eichenbaum, the probe is actually most efficient on thick cataracts, because the higher protein level and pigmentation allow for greater energy absorption by the tissue.

The claimed advantages of Paradigm's system include energy containment within the probe and greater reliability. The collimated laser beam is confined within the metal tube of the probe tip. The action of the laser is limited solely to the photovaporization chamber, unlike conventional ultrasound, in which tissue damage from shock waves can occur in tissues that are not in direct contact with the probe itself [16].

Because the solid-state laser has no moving parts, the device is not as subject to wear and tear as ultrasound systems are. The aspiration tube and laser fiber, which are most prone to wear during use, are designed to be disposable components.

Paradigm claims that their system is also capable of performing an anterior capsulorhexis.

According to Paradigm, the laser probe is so safe that it can be rubbed against the posterior capsule with no effect. The current 1.8-mm diameter probe is reusable, is approximately 20% of the weight of a conventional phacoemulsification handpiece, and can fit through a 1.9-mm incision. The system will retail for $120,000 in the United States. Paradigm's Precisionist 30,000 phacoemulsification unit can now be converted to the Nd:YAG laser probe for between $10,000 and $16,000 [17].

REFERENCES AND RECOMMEND READING

Recently published papers of particular interest have been highlighted as:

- Of interest

•• Of outstanding interest

1. Kelman CD: Phaco-emulsification and aspiration: a new technique of cataract removal, a preliminary report. *Am J Ophthalmol* 1967, 64:23–35.

2. Leaming DV: Practice styles and preferences of ASCRS members—1987 survey. *J Cataract Refract Surg* 1988, 14:552–559.

3. Hayashi K, Hayashi H, Nakao F, Hayashi F: Risk factors for corneal endothelial injury during phacoemulsification. *J Cataract Refract Surg* 1996, 22:63–71.

4. Hwang DG, Smith RE: Corneal complications of cataract surgery. *Refract Corneal Surg* 1991, 7:77–80.

5. Berger JW, Talamo JH, LaManche KJ: Temperature measurements during phacoemulsification and erbium:YAG laser phacoablation in model systems. *Cataract Refract Surg* 1996, 22:372–378.

6. Dodick JM, Sperber LTD: Can cataracts be removed using laser technology? *Ophthalmol Clin North Am* 1991, 4:355–364.

7. Dodick JM, Lally JM, Sperber LTD: Lasers in cataract surgery. *Curr Opin Ophthalmol* 1993, 4:107–109.

8. Alzner E, Grabner G: Dodick laser phacolysis—thermal effects. *J Cataract Refract Surg,* 1998: in press.

9. Colvard MD, Kratz RP: Cataract surgery utilizing the erbium laser. *Phacoemulsification New Technology and Clinical Applications.* Edited by Fine IH. Thorofare, NJ: Slack, 1995:155–158.

10. Cozean C: *Er:YAG Phacoemulsification with Fiber.* Irvine, CA: Premier Laser Systems.

11. Stevens G Jr, Long B, Hamann JM, *et al.*: Erbium-YAG laser assisted cataract surgery. *Ophthalmic Surg Lasers* 1988, in press.

12. Boulnois JL: *Laser in Medical Science.* London: Balliere-Tindall; 1986.

13. Singer HW: Laser phaco makers aiming for safety improvements, shorter learning curve. *Ocular Surg News.* 1997, 15:20–26.

14. DuBosar R: Laser cataract system vies for domestic, international market. *Ocular Surg News* 1997, 15:27.

15. Bethke W: Cataract extraction at the speed of light. *Rev Ophthalmol* May 1996:149.

16. Eichenbaum DM: Paradigm system: A laser probe for cataract removal. In *Phacoemulsification New Technology and Clinical Application.* Edited by Fine IH. Thorofare, NJ: Slack, 1995:155–158.

17. Gluck R: Laser-driven cataract surgery probe readies for US market. *EyeWorld* 1997, 2:24.

CHAPTER 2

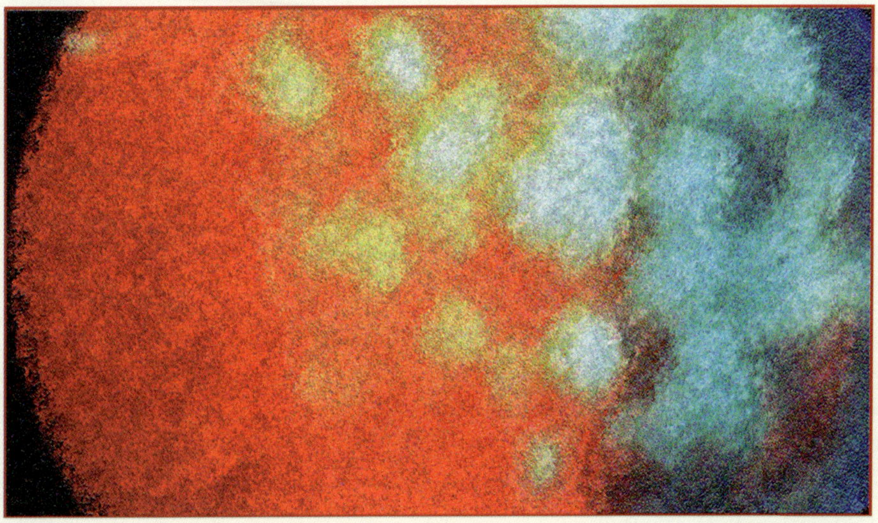

Lasers in Corneal Surgery

CHRISTOPHER J. RAPUANO
MATTHEW R. JONES
PETER R. LAIBSON

Just as the 1980s were frequently called the "decade of vitreoretinal surgery" in ophthalmologic circles, the 1990s are often dubbed the "decade of the cornea." Although various surgical techniques have previously been available for treatment of superficial corneal opacities and refractive errors, the recent advent of the excimer laser has made available exciting new options for treating the cornea. Superficial corneal opacities, previously requiring lamellar or penetrating keratoplasty, now in many cases can be treated with phototherapeutic keratectomy (PTK). Photorefractive keratectomy (PRK), photoastigmatic refractive keratectomy (PARK), and laser-assisted in situ keratomileusis (LASIK) use excimer technology to reshape the cornea and correct various degrees of myopia and astigmatism. LASIK, PRK, and the holmium:yttrium-aluminum-garnet (Ho:YAG) laser are being intensively studied for correction of hyperopia. Advances in corneal topography, laser, and microkeratome technology hold promise for making refractive surgery safer and more precise.

EXCIMER LASER

The excimer (*exci*ted di*mer*) laser uses an argon-fluoride gas combination to create a high-powered ultraviolet beam. The resulting 193-nm laser pulses break organic molecular bonds, removing tissue in the area of application with very little adjacent thermal damage. The

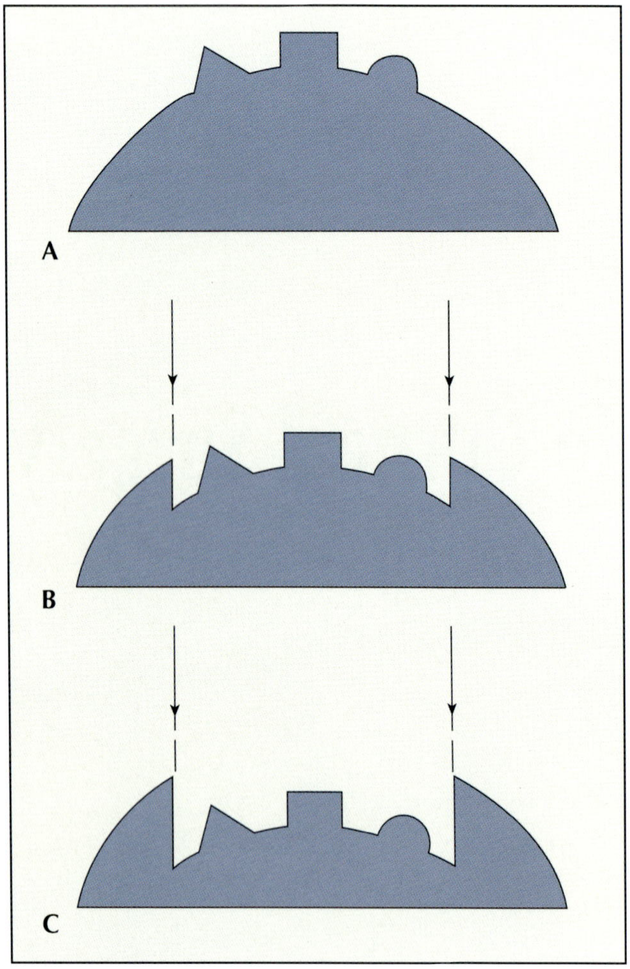

FIGURE 2-1. The effect of excimer laser photoablation on an unmasked irregular surface. **A,** The original irregular surface. **B** and **C,** As the excimer laser removes a uniform amount of tissue over the entire ablation zone, the irregularity is perpetuated deeper and deeper into the material. (*Adapted from* Gartry *et al.* [1]; with permission.)

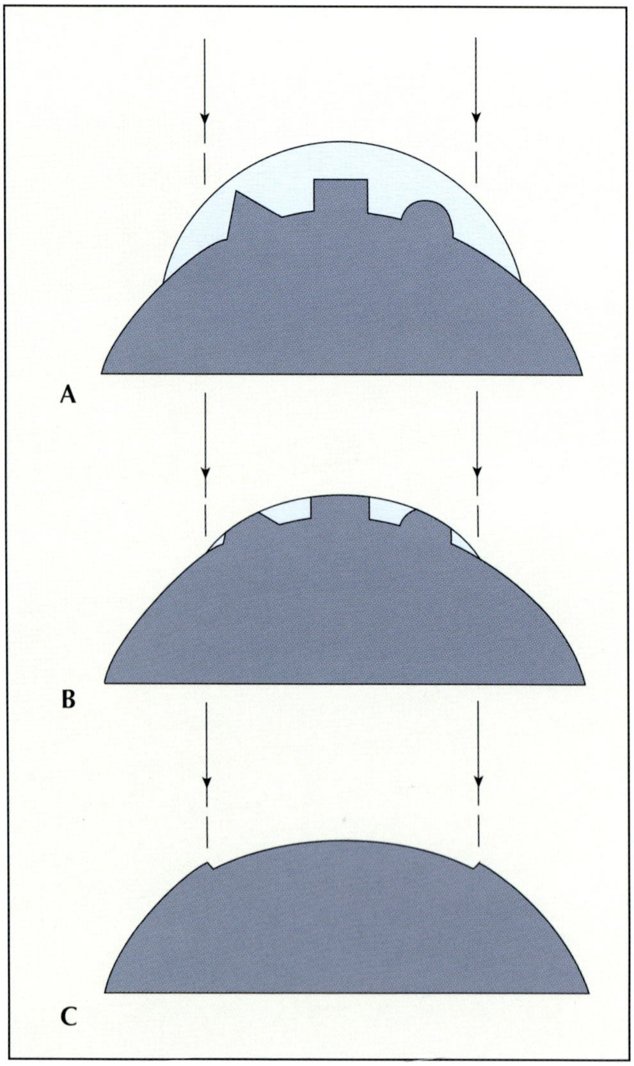

FIGURE 2-2. The effect of a masking agent placed on an irregular corneal surface. **A,** A masking agent placed on the surface irregularity. **B** and **C,** If the masking agent ablates at the same rate as the underlying material, the result will be a smooth surface for the excimer laser to ablate. (*Adapted from* Gartry *et al.* [1]; with permission.)

precision of this process makes the excimer laser ideal for removing and reshaping corneal tissue.

Early animal studies demonstrated that the excimer laser was capable of reproducible corneal flattening without significant haze formation [2–5]. In the 1980s, blind-eye studies confirmed this effect in human corneas [6,7]. With these early studies, the era of phototherapeutic and photorefractive corneal surgery was born. Within the last decade, this field has continued to grow as one of the most exciting and promising areas of surgical ophthalmology.

PHOTOTHERAPEUTIC KERATECTOMY

In 1995, PTK became the first US Food and Drug Administration (FDA)-approved excimer laser procedure when the excimer lasers of both Summit Technology (Waltham, MA) and VISX (Santa Clara, CA) were approved for removal of superficial corneal dystrophies, epithelial basement membrane dystrophy, irregular corneal surfaces (*eg*, nodular scars), and other anterior stromal opacities of the cornea (*eg*, scarring secondary to infection). Used in clinical trials since the late 1980s, PTK has provided a less invasive and often superior method for treating these anterior corneal pathologies previously treated primarily by lamellar or penetrating keratoplasty. The relative speed of the procedure, along with the ability to titrate the extent of treatment intraoperatively, offers significant advantages over previous techniques.

General principles

Indications for PTK can be divided into three broad categories: 1) removal of visually significant central anterior corneal opacities; 2) smoothing of an irregular surface; and 3) treatment of recurrent erosions not amenable to less invasive or expensive options. Central anterior opacities may be intrastromal, such as with the stromal dystrophies, or subepithelial, such as with keratoconus nodules or Salzmann's nodular degeneration. These lesions can affect vision by the opacity itself or by an irregular surface created by an uneven opacity. Various corneal disorders such as posttraumatic lesions, anterior basement membrane dystrophy, anterior stromal dystrophies, and bullous keratopathy can give rise to painful erosions. Excimer laser PTK can be useful in these disorders in creating a smooth surface for re-epithelialization when traditional medical or surgical options fail.

If a patient is to be considered a candidate for PTK, the bulk of the visually significant opacity must be anterior, that is, within the anterior one third of the stroma. It is generally agreed that a *minimum* of 250 µm of corneal thickness should be left after PTK; however, best results are obtained when the opacity is within the most superficial (*ie*, 10% to 20%) layers of the stroma. The goal of treatment should be the ablation of anterior confluent opacities with the minimal amount of tissue removal, not the eradication of all pathology. Deeper ablations risk significant hyperopic shift and possible ectasia.

Most types of anterior corneal pathology are unevenly distributed in the x, y, and z planes and may create an irregular corneal surface. Furthermore, pathologic opacity tends to ablate at a different rate than the normal corneal stroma. As such, simple ablation of such corneas may result in significant surface irregularities with associated healing problems and irregular astigmatism. The use of mildly to moderately viscous fluids as "masking agents" during ablation can help produce smoother, more homogeneous surfaces. These fluids fill in the microdepressions that are created by uneven tissue ablation, protecting the normal corneal stroma while allowing elevated areas to be ablated preferentially (Figs. 2-1 and 2-2).

Many substances including hydroxymethylcellulose 2%, hydroxypropylcellulose, tetracaine 0.5%, dextran 0.1%, and saline have been used as masking agents with variable results. The use of a type I collagen derivative that is liquid at 45°C but solidifies on cooling has been used with a hard contact lens template to produce a smooth surface for subsequent ablation in the Biomask system (Maverick Technologies, Pinellas Park, FL) (Fig. 2-3) [8,9].

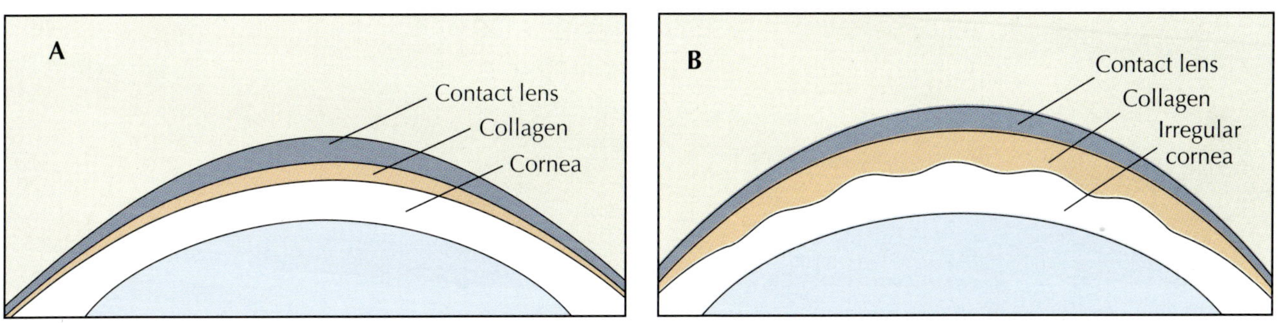

FIGURE 2-3. **A,** The relationship among the cornea, collagen gel, and rigid contact lens. **B,** The collagen gel molds to an irregular collagen surface, creating a smooth "template" for subsequent ablation. (*Adapted from* Englanoff *et al.* [8].)

Clinical results

Phototherapeutic keratectomy has been used to treat corneal opacities secondary to corneal dystrophies, degenerations, and scars. The opacities most amenable to treatment are those that are most anterior. As such, granular, lattice, and Reis-Buckler's dystrophies are among the most successfully treated, often producing marked improvements in visual acuity [10] (Fig. 2-4). Success, as defined by improvement in visual acuity or comfort, has also been reported for Meesmann's [11], gelatinous drop-like [12], macular [13,14], and Avellino dystrophies [15]. Schnyder's dystrophy has also been treated with more modest results [11,16,17].

Corneal degenerations affecting the superficial cornea, including Salzmann's nodular degeneration, band keratopathy, and the smooth variant of climatic droplet keratopathy, can be good candidates for PTK. Many cases of Salzmann's may be simply treated with mechanical superficial keratectomy if a smooth plane exists between the nodule and underlying stroma. If an irregular base remains after manual dissection of the nodule, the excimer laser can be used to smooth the surface (Fig. 2-5). Maloney [18••] used this technique on 41 eyes with Salzmann's nodular degeneration and reported a mean improvement of 1.6 lines of best spectacle-corrected visual acuity.

Excimer PTK, with or without mechanical debulking, has been used to treat visual loss and ocular discomfort associated with band keratopathy. O'Brart *et al.* [19] reported the results of 122 eyes with a mean follow-up of 12.3 months. Improvement in visual acuity was reported in 88% of eyes, and ocular discomfort was reduced in 95%. Maloney [18••], however, noted a mean improvement of only 0.1 lines of best spectacle-corrected visual acuity in 14 eyes with band keratopathy treated with PTK and attributed this lack of improvement to coexisting ocular disease. Because the density of calcium deposition in band keratopathy is

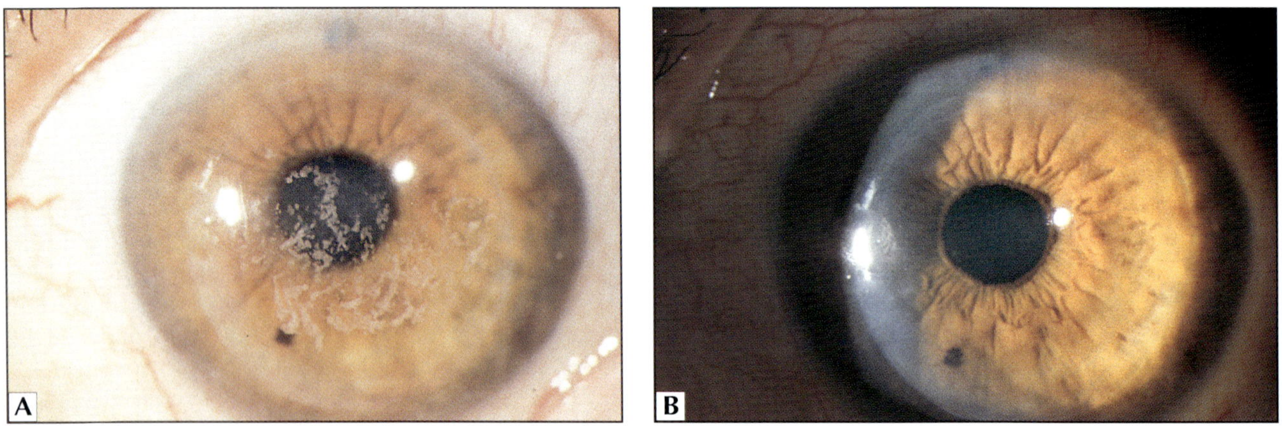

FIGURE 2-4. A, Patient with recurrent granular dystrophy within the graft 17 years after penetrating keratoplasty. Best corrected visual acuity is 20/200. **B,** Same patient 2 months after excimer phototherapeutic keratoplasty. Corrected visual acuity is 20/30.

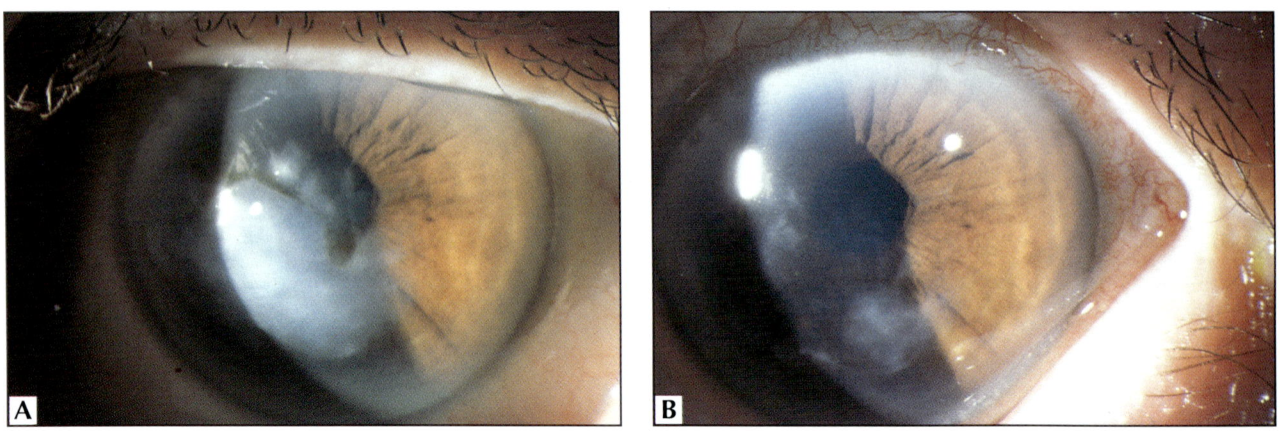

FIGURE 2-5. A, Salzmann's nodular degeneration before phototherapeutic keratoplasty (PTK). **B,** Same patient 11 days after excimer PTK.

typically not uniform, excimer PTK can leave an irregular base after treatment [20]. As such, EDTA chelation continues to be the best option for the treatment of band keratopathy in most patients.

Badr *et al.* [21•] reported reduced corneal opacification in 98% of 55 eyes with smooth climatic droplet keratopathy and 80% of 20 eyes with irregular climatic droplet keratopathy. Improvement in best corrected visual acuity was 61.8% in the former and 21.2% in the latter group. However, in the irregular climatic droplet keratopathy group, delayed re-epithelialization defined as greater than 14 days was 21%, and incidence of microbial keratitis was 10%, warranting caution in treating eyes with this subset of climatic droplet keratopathy [21•].

Scarring secondary to varicella zoster virus (VZV), herpes simplex virus (HSV), bacterial infection, adenoviral infection, vernal keratitis, keratoconus, and trauma have been treated with PTK [10,22–28, 29•]. It is difficult to make generalizations regarding treatment of corneal scars with PTK because no two scars share identical clinical features. Again, depth of scarring determines which patients will have the greatest chance of success. As with Salzmann's nodular degeneration, some keratoconus nodules are easily removed through mechanical superficial keratectomy with a blade. In those cases in which a smooth plane cannot be obtained during mechanical removal, excimer PTK with a small ablation zone can be used with a masking agent to remove residual nodular material and smooth the surface [20]. Treatment of scarring after herpetic keratitis deserves special mention because recurrences of HSV infection after PTK have been reported [24,30–32]. Use of prophylactic oral acyclovir is recommended to reduce the risk of this complication [24,31].

The issue of potential patient-to-surgeon transmission of HSV, HIV, or other infectious viruses has been investigated by several authors [33•–35•]. Although Moreira *et al.* [33•] demonstrated that HSV and adenovirus could be transmitted from one culture plate to another during excimer laser ablation of an infected plate, Hagen *et al.* [34•] reported not detecting transmission of pseudorabies virus (a porcine-enveloped herpes virus similar in structure and life cycle to HIV and HSV) in a similar experiment. Taravella *et al.* [35•] collected plume material during the ablation of VZV-infected fibroblasts. Although the authors detected VZV particles by polymerase chain reaction, viral cultures of the plume material were negative.

Recurrent erosions, such as those seen in association with anterior basement membrane dystrophy, can be treated with excimer PTK. The most appropriate candidates are those who have failed medical and other surgical therapies including lubricants, bandage soft contact lenses, epithelial debridement (with or without diamond burring), and anterior stromal puncture. In addition, those patients whose erosions occur centrally may be more appropriately treated with PTK as opposed to anterior stromal puncture, because the latter treatment may cause fine scarring over the visual axis. By performing a superficial (*eg*, 5 µm) "Bomanectomy" after manual epithelial removal over the area of the erosion, the resulting smooth surface allows for even re-epithelialization, potentially allowing stronger and more stable epithelial adhesions.

Complications

The greatest problem with PTK is induced refractive effect, especially hyperopia, but astigmatism in asymmetric ablations and myopia in peripheral ablations also occur. Ideally, PTK either smoothes elevated areas to the level of the rest of the cornea or removes a plano disc of tissue, or both. In theory, neither of these procedures should change refractive error. However, PTK, especially removal of central corneal stromal abnormalities, tends to flatten the central cornea and induce hyperopia. The deeper the ablation, the more extensive the corneal flattening becomes. Several theories exist regarding the etiology of this hyperopic shift. Subsequent epithelial hyperplasia may be greater at the peripheral edge of the ablation, where drop-off is significant and less prominent centrally, creating a flatter central cornea [36] (Fig. 2-6). Liu [36] also suggested that masking agents may creep up the wall of deeper central ablations while the laser is firing, thus causing a deeper ablation centrally and subsequent corneal flattening. Due to the curvature of the cornea, ablation may be less effective peripherally because the excimer laser is interacting with the cornea at an

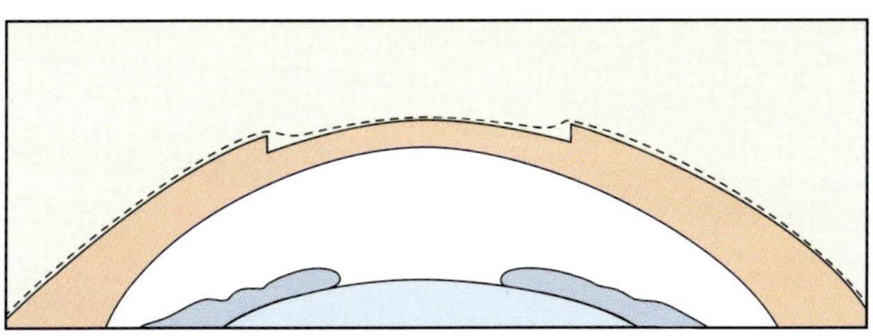

FIGURE 2-6. Epithelial hyperplasia may occur in the periphery of an excimer phototherapeutic keratectomy, which will result in central corneal flattening and induced hyperopia.

oblique angle in the periphery, and not perpendicular to the cornea as it does centrally. This nonperpendicular peripheral ablation will not be as deep toward the center of the eye as the perpendicular central ablation (Fig. 2-7). Gartry *et al.* [1,37] proposed that corneal lamellae could undergo centrifugal differential contraction with central flattening. To combat this induced corneal flattening, Stark *et al.* [38] performed a modified taper in an attempt to correct hyperopia. After the central ablation of corneal pathologic tissue, they used a circular ablation 2.0 mm in diameter to treat the circumference of the original ablation. This additional ablation straddles the original treatment to taper the edge of unablated tissue and create a deeper ablation in the periphery of the original treatment zone (Fig. 2-8). Theoretically, this modification would tend to steepen the cornea and induce less peripheral epithelial hyperplasia, but the exact amount of antihyperopia treatment has not been established. Use of a secondary hyperopic ablation, as described by Sher *et al.* [39], may become a more reproducible and useful option as hyperopic PRK technology continues to develop.

Other complications of PTK include scarring, bacterial keratitis, induced regular and irregular astigmatism, and delayed re-epithelialization. Recurrence of anterior corneal pathology (*eg,* the stromal dystrophies) is encountered after PTK as it is after penetrating keratoplasty. Any of these complications can lead to loss of best spectacle-corrected visual acuity.

Development of PTK represents a tremendous advance in the treatment of anterior corneal pathology. Judicious patient selection and a conservative, "less is more" surgical approach help maximize beneficial outcomes and limit complications. Perhaps more than any other excimer technique, PTK requires practicing the "art of medicine" as an integral part of the procedure.

PHOTOREFRACTIVE KERATECTOMY AND PHOTOASTIGMATIC KERATECTOMY

Photorefractive keratectomy involves reshaping the anterior surface of the cornea by using the excimer laser to ablate tissue at the submicron level. A single pulse of the laser removes about 0.25 µm of tissue, allowing for extremely precise ablations. In myopic PRK, a "plus" lenticule is removed by ablating more tissue centrally than peripherally. This effect is achieved most commonly by the use of an expanding circular diaphragm, whereby initial pulses have a small diameter and subsequent pulses increase in diameter. By combining the expanding diaphragm with a simultaneously narrowing slit (as with the Model B and STAR excimer lasers by VISX), elliptical ablations can be created for the correction of astigmatism.

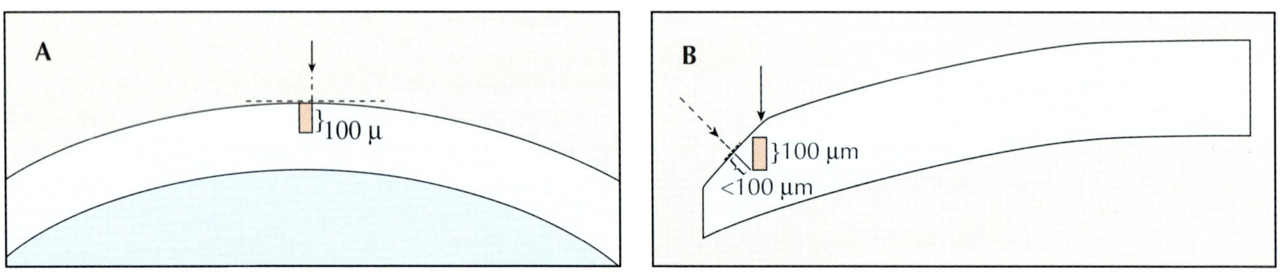

FIGURE 2-7. A, Central perpendicular excimer laser photoablations penetrate deeper into the corneal stroma. **B,** Peripheral excimer laser photoablations remove tissue at an oblique angle, resulting in a shallower ablation. Deeper central and shallower peripheral ablations tend to cause corneal flattening and induced hyperopia.

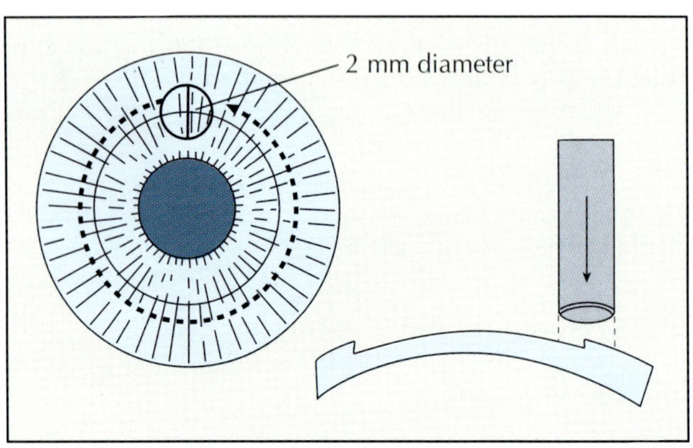

FIGURE 2-8. Modified peripheral excimer laser taper after phototherapeutic keratoplasty (PTK). After the central PTK ablation, a circular ablation 2.0 mm in diameter is used to treat the circumference of the original ablation in an attempt to correct hyperopia.

Other methods of delivering excimer laser energy to the corneal surface are being actively studied. To overcome uneven ablations produced by inconsistencies in beam homogeneity, second generation lasers such as the Nidek (Fremont, CA) EC 5000 combine a small-diameter continuously moving beam (*scanning spot*) with a rotating slit to produce theoretically smoother ablations. Third generation systems such as Autonomous Technology's (Orlando, FL) LADARVision (formerly T-PRK) employ sophisticated eye-tracking software in conjunction with scanning spot technology to produce precise custom-made ablations. Eventually, by coupling such systems to intraoperative real time topographic analysis, the hope is that in addition to increasingly precise myopic, hyperopic, and regular astigmatic ablations, *irregular* astigmatism could be treated in a way never before possible.

Clinical results

Although numerous articles appeared in the peer-reviewed literature in the late 1980s and early 1990s reporting results of excimer PRK, various lasers and techniques were employed, making comparisons of outcomes difficult. However, results were generally good, and in October 1995, the FDA approved Summit Technology's excimer laser for the treatment of myopia between -1.50 diopters (D) and -7.00 D (with ≤1.50 D of astigmatism) at the corneal plane in patients aged 21 years and older. About 5 months later, VISX received approval for the treatment of -1.00 D to -6.00 D of myopia (with ≤1.00 D of astigmatism) at the corneal plane in patients aged 18 years and older.

Summit's FDA approval was based on the results of 398 eyes treated with a 6.0-mm diameter ablation zone and observed in follow-up for 1 year. Uncorrected visual acuity (UCVA) was 20/20 or better in 65% of eyes at 6 months and 81% of eyes at 1 year. UCVA of 20/40 or better was achieved by 95% and 99% of eyes at 6 and 12 months, respectively. At 6 months, loss of best spectacle-corrected visual acuity (BSCVA) of two lines or more occurred in 6.8% of eyes (including 2.1% losing three to five lines). At 1 year, however, only 1.2% had lost two lines, and none had lost more than two lines of BSCVA. Paralleling this loss of BSCVA was the incidence of stromal haze, with 2.3% of eyes having 2+ haze at 6 months, decreasing to 0% at 12 months. 5.6% of eyes were overcorrected by greater than 1.00 D at 1 year.

VISX received FDA approval in March 1996 for excimer PRK with a 6-mm diameter ablation zone based on results in 480 eyes with at least 2 years follow-up. At 6 months, UCVA of 20/20 or better was achieved in 56% of eyes, and 20/40 or better was achieved in 93%. At 1 year, 20/20 or better and 20/40 or better was achieved by 64% and 95% of eyes, respectively. At 2 years, 58% of eyes achieved 20/20 or better vision, and 94% achieved 20/40 or better. At 2 years, overcorrection of greater than 1.00 D occurred in 1.3% of eyes, and only one eye (0.3%) lost two lines of BSCVA, which was secondary to scarring. No eyes lost more than two lines of BSCVA at 2 years.

In April 1997, the FDA approved VISX's excimer laser system for the treatment of myopia and astigmatism. Treatment parameters include myopia of up to -6.00 D and astigmatism from 0.75 D to 4.00 D of minus cylinder at the spectacle plane. In contrast to VISX's PRK approval, PARK is approved for patients 21 years and older. The VISX Model B and STAR lasers correct myopic astigmatism by creating an elliptical ablation using the simultaneous expansion of an iris diaphragm and closure of slit blades during ablation. This creates a deeper and wider ablation (and thus a more pronounced flattening) in the axis of the slit blades, which correspond with the steepest axis of the cornea.

Photoastigmatic refractive keratectomy with the VISX lasers produces somewhat less favorable results than PRK. FDA approval was based on the prospective evaluation of 641 eyes at three centers in the United States, Canada, and England. In the US study, 40% of eyes achieved 20/20 or better, 82% achieved 20/30 or better, and 91% achieved 20/40 or better at the final visit. Mean cylinder after treatment was -0.55 D, a reduction of 69%. Loss of two or more lines of BSCVA at the final visit occurred in four eyes (4.8%); however, two of these eyes dropped from 20/10 or 20/12.5 to 20/20. Worsening photophobia (15.5%) and night vision difficulties (22.6%) were the most frequent complications. The relatively large percentage of patients with night vision difficulties can be explained by the small minor axis diameter (as small as 4.5 mm in some ablations), which can cause visually significant aberrations when the pupil expands beyond the junction of the treated and untreated cornea.

Complications

The most common complications of PRK and PARK are related to the normal wound healing response. Some patients will be overcorrected or undercorrected to some degree regardless of how refined treatment algorithms become, because individual variation in wound healing response can lead to different refractive outcomes in two different eyes receiving exactly the same ablation. Of course, variation in hydration of the cornea during the procedure, beam homogeneity, and surgical technique can all affect the refractive outcome.

Increased fibroblastic activity after excimer laser treatment results in the laying down of collagen in an irregular fashion, as opposed to the regular, evenly spaced collagen lamella that are present in the normal cornea. This irregular collagen manifests clinically as "haze," which can lead to decreased BSCVA, decreased contrast sensitivity, and increased complaints of glare (Fig. 2-9). This scarring most commonly appears at about 1 month, increases over 2 to 3 months, and then fades. A second, much rarer, type of corneal haze appears late, 4 to 12 months after PRK [40,41•], and is associated with decreased visual acuity and refractive regression.

Fortunately, permanent haze that affects visual function is uncommon. Topical corticosteroids are commonly used in the postoperative period to reduce development of haze and limit regression. Newer ablation techniques, such as those that use multizone, multipass, or scanning systems to produce smoother ablated surfaces and blend the periphery to prevent a "step" at the edge of the ablation, have been developed to reduce the incidence of haze. Tsubota *et al.* [42] reported decreased haze in eyes receiving balanced salt solution chilled to 4°C when compared with contralateral eyes not receiving chilled balanced salt solution, stating that thermal damage during PRK leads to haze formation.

Glare, halos, and night vision difficulties can result when smaller optical zones (*eg*, 5 mm) are used, especially when coupled with larger mesopic/scotopic pupil size (not uncommon in younger patients). These complications have led to a minimum 6.0-mm optical zone as the standard [43•,44,45].

Central areas of steeper corneal curvature greater than 2.00 D, or central islands, are thought to result from decreased absorption of laser energy by the central cornea from central pooling of fluid with ongoing ablation and/or partial absorption of laser energy by the central plume (Fig. 2-10). Central islands have become much less common as newer treatment algorithms have been built into laser software. Alternatively, the surgeon may pretreat the central cornea with several small-diameter pulses before the refractive ablation. Central islands, if they do occur, tend to resolve with time. A trial of topical steroids or re-treatment with a small-diameter ablation over the island can be used to address persistent, visually significant islands.

Decentration can occur secondary to problems with patient fixation, beam homogeneity, or surgeon error (Fig. 2-11). Proper calibration of the excimer laser preoperatively and monitoring of patient fixation during the procedure is of obvious importance. In addition, it is helpful to explain the concept of centration to the patient before the procedure and remind the patient to maintain fixation during the procedure. Currently, visually significant decentrations are difficult to treat. Occasionally, asymmetric corneal healing can make an ablation appear decentered months after PRK, whereas early postoperative topographic analyses demonstrated excellent ablation centration. Newer eye tracking systems promise to reduce or eliminate this complication.

The necessary formation of an epithelial defect during PRK can lead to various complications. Although most defects heal within 2 to 5 days, persistent defects lasting 1 week or longer can occur, increasing chances of corneal haze. Microbial keratitis, fortunately rare, is perhaps the most dreaded complication of PRK, with resultant scarring and potential marked loss of visual acuity. As such, a broad-spectrum topical antibiotic is an important part of the postoperative regimen. Reactivation of HSV keratitis has been reported but is rare [30–32].

Monitoring intraocular pressure (IOP) in the postoperative period deserves special attention for two reasons. First, increased IOP in patients taking topical steroids can and does occur post-PRK, often necessitating a change in the type or frequency of steroid admin-

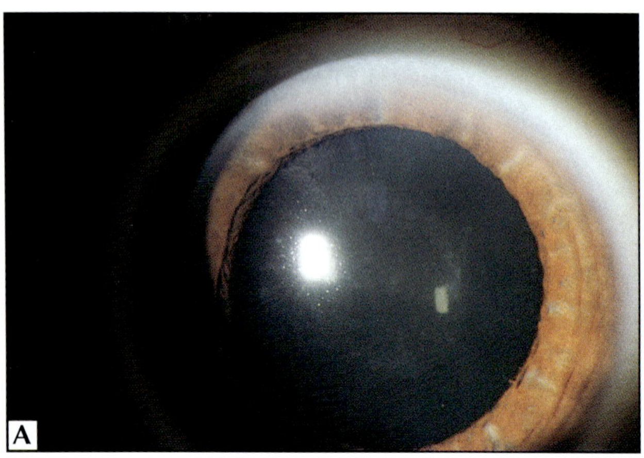

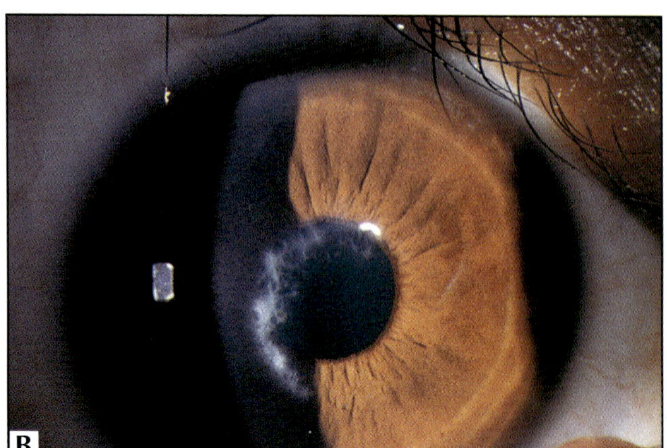

FIGURE 2-9. Anterior stromal "haze" after excimer photorefractive keratectomy (PRK). **A**, Three months after PRK. **B**, Different patient 9 months after PRK. Uncorrected visual acuity is 20/25, correcting to 20/20.

istration. Second, the thinning of the cornea by PRK can result in artifactually low IOP measurements, potentially leading to underdiagnosis and undertreatment of harmful IOP elevations [46–48].

Surgical technique and postoperative management

After checking laser calibration and centration, the surgeon has three main concerns: 1) properly positioning the patient; 2) rapidly, effectively, and atraumatically removing the epithelium; and 3) maintaining centration of the laser during the treatment. If astigmatism is being corrected, the 3- and 9-o'clock axes need to be marked on the cornea at the slit lamp before surgery to check for any cyclotorsion that could significantly decrease effectiveness of the astigmatism correction. If significant cyclotorsion is found after the patient is under the laser, it should be corrected for by tilting the patient's head to the right or left to line up the corneal marks with the reticle in the microscope. The patient's head should be level to the ground before centering the operative eye under the laser. Epithelial removal can be performed mechanically with a blunt blade, sharp blade, or epithelial "scrubber." Before epithelial removal, an epithelial softening agent such as 4% lidocaine or alcohol can be placed on the central 6 mm to ease removal. After the central 6 mm of epithelium has been cleared, the ablation is performed, making certain that the patient maintains excellent fixation throughout the entire procedure.

Postoperatively, topical antibiotics are prescribed until re-epithelialization is complete. Topical nonsteroidal anti-inflammatory drops are often used for several days for pain control. Although controversial, frequently applied dilute proparacaine (0.5%) distributed in small amounts (*eg*, 0.5 mL) is used by some surgeons to provide pain relief during the first several days after PRK. At this concentration, proparacaine is reportedly nonanesthetic and nontoxic [49•]. A bandage soft contact lens or pressure patch is also often used to decrease painful symptoms and aid in re-epithelialization. Use of topical steroids after PRK is controversial [50–54] but is frequently done for several months to decrease the chance of haze and regression.

LASER-ASSISTED IN SITU KERATOMILEUSIS

Laser-assisted in situ keratomileusis (LASIK) involves creating a hinged flap of anterior corneal tissue with a microkeratome, reflecting the flap, performing excimer laser ablation upon the stromal bed, and repositioning the flap without sutures. Although lamellar procedures have been used since 1949 [55], older techniques involving manual excision of a stromal lenticule and even with an automated keratome (vis-à-vis automated lamellar keratoplasty [ALK]), have produced less-than-precise results and less-than-enthusiastic acceptance of these procedures by most ophthalmologists. Development of the excimer laser has brought with it the ability to perform precise reshaping of the corneal stroma, improving the predictability and safety of lamellar procedures for the correction of refractive error. Furthermore, LASIK is associated with less discomfort and faster healing, causes essentially no haze, and allows a wider range of myopic treatment when compared with PRK. Refinements in ablation algorithms and microkeratome technology are continually improving the outcomes of patients treated with this exciting procedure.

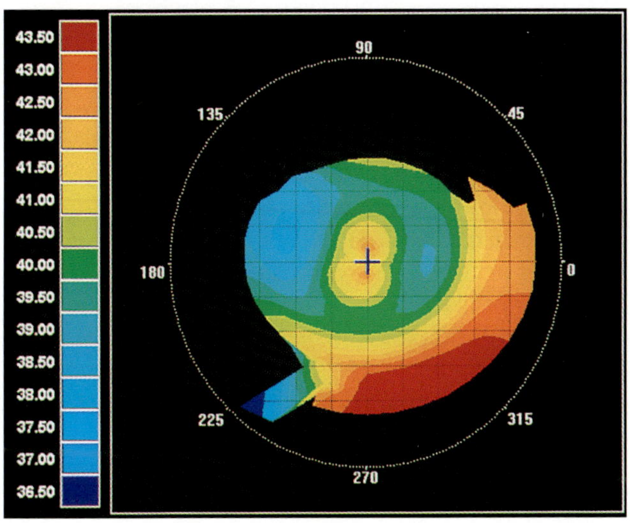

FIGURE 2-10. Corneal topography showing central island 1 month after excimer photorefractive keratectomy.

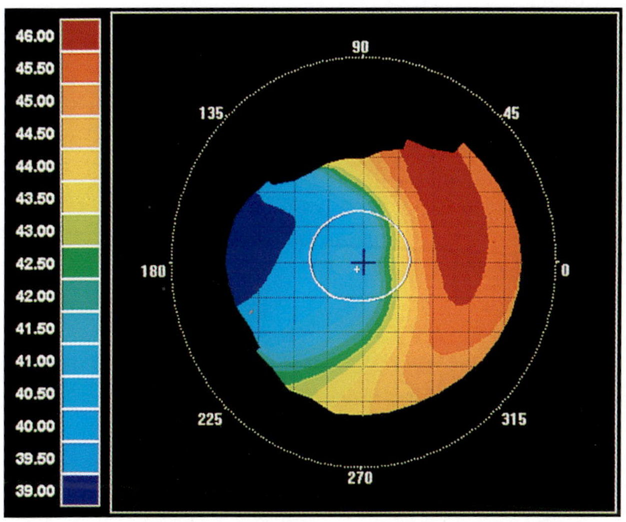

FIGURE 2-11. Corneal topography showing decentered ablation.

Clinical results

The range of myopia that is appropriate for LASIK is controversial. Some surgeons feel that lower myopia (*eg*, up to -6.00 to -7.00 D) is best treated with PRK, where predictability is high, permanent significant haze is rare, and the risks of microkeratome-related complications are absent. Other surgeons feel that after proficiency with the microkeratome has been achieved, the benefits of rapid healing, little or no haze formation, early visual rehabilitation, and patient comfort make LASIK generally preferable to PRK, and that no lower limit of myopia need apply. The upper limit of myopia has also not been established. Most surgeons feel it is between -12.00 and -15.00 D, but others feel LASIK is appropriate for much higher degrees of myopia.

Salah *et al.* [56•] retrospectively evaluated 88 eyes receiving LASIK with the Chiron (Claremont, CA) Automated Corneal Shaper and the Summit Omnimed laser. Preoperative refractive error ranged from -2.00 to -20.00 D and mean follow-up was 5.2 months. Refractive errors within 1.00 D of emmetropia were achieved in 93% of eyes within the low myopia group (-2.00 to -6.00 D), 65% of eyes within the moderate myopia group (-6.12 to -12.00 D), and 43% of eyes within the high myopia group (-12.10 to -20.00 D). Overall, UCVA was 20/20 or better in 36% of eyes and 20/40 or better in 71% of eyes. Three eyes (3.6%) lost two lines or more of BSCVA.

Perez-Santonja *et al.* [57••] prospectively evaluated their LASIK results in 143 eyes with between -8.00 and -20.00 D myopia using the Chiron Automated Corneal Shaper and the VISX Model B laser with a multizone profile. At 6 months, 46.4% of eyes saw 20/40 or better uncorrected. Refractive error within 1.00 D of emmetropia was achieved by 60% of all eyes, 72.4% of eyes with preoperative myopia of -8.00 to -11.92 D, 46% of eyes with preoperative myopia -12.00 to -15.97, and 50% of eyes with preoperative myopia of -16.00 to -20.00 D. The authors concluded that LASIK was effective and predictable for high myopia but most accurate for myopia up to -12.00 D.

Pirzada and Kalaawry [58•] reported their results of LASIK for low myopia (-1.00 to -3.50 D). Eighty-five eyes underwent LASIK using the Chiron microkeratome and the Nidek EC 5000, a "second generation" scanning laser. UCVA was 20/30 or better in 80% of eyes at 1 month and 93% of eyes at 6 months. One eye was complicated by corneal abscess formation with subsequent scarring and visual acuity of 20/100. The authors concluded that LASIK is safe and effective for low myopia.

In the past 2 years, unique developments have occurred with regards to LASIK and FDA approval. First, in 1996 the FDA approved a LASIK Investigational Device Exemption (IDE) to the private ophthalmologist-owned corporation called Comprehensive Refractive Surgery-USA (CRS-USA, Scottsdale, AZ). Under the IDE, private ophthalmologists from various centers are performing LASIK and pooling their results, using the Chiron microkeratome and the Summit or VISX lasers. Second, in the summer of 1997, the FDA approved an IDE for Emory University's LASIK procedure using the Chiron microkeratome and Summit's excimer laser. The IDE requires additional data on refractive stability, complications, and patient satisfaction at the 6-month mark. These investigations should provide essential data on the safety and efficacy of LASIK and help further define the role of this procedure in correcting refractive error.

Complications

Although LASIK offers certain advantages over PRK, use of the microkeratome introduces a surgical component that can result in visually significant complications. The most feared complication is entry of the blade into the anterior chamber and damage to the anterior segment, which can occur when the depth plate is inadvertently omitted during preoperative assembly of the microkeratome. Meticulous preoperative and intraoperative inspection of the microkeratome equipment by a qualified technician and the surgeon is imperative to avoid this and other intraoperative complications. Newer microkeratome designs may safeguard against assembly errors; for example, in the One system from Microtech/Moria (Doylestown, PA), the microkeratome is designed to cut at a single depth and thus has eliminated the need for interchangeable depth plates. LaserSight Technologies (Orlando, FL) has introduced the Automated Disposable Keratome, a preassembled, presterilized disposable microkeratome for single use.

Complications may occur during creation of the flap. Incomplete flaps may occur if the microkeratome or gear assembly is blocked before full passage has occurred. As such, it is imperative that the microkeratome path is clear of redundant skin, lids, and lid speculum, and that the microkeratome is thoroughly cleaned between uses to prevent debris from accumulating in the gear assembly. Thin flaps or "free caps" (complete separation of the flap from the rest of the cornea) can occur if suction is lost or inadequate during the microkeratome passage. Marking the corneal epithelium at the margins of the intended flap before its creation helps facilitate reorientation in the case of a free cap.

During laser ablation, complications such as decentration, central islands, and over- and undercorrections can occur in LASIK as they do in PRK. A consistent approach to the timing of ablation after flap creation and attention to the hydration status of the stromal bed are important to ensure reproducible results for a given surgeon's technique. As such, ablation nomograms need to be modified for each laser and even each individual surgeon.

Flap wrinkles or folds (seen especially with thin flaps and sutured flaps) can lead to irregular astigmatism and loss of BSCVA. Epithelial cells or debris within the flap–bed interface can also lead to irregularity of the flap surface and, thus, astigmatism. If significant, epithelial cells in the interface need to be removed by lifting the flap. Rarely, the corneal flap may become dislocated in the early postoperative period, requiring repositioning with or without sutures.

Microbial keratitis, although rare, has been reported [59–61]. Treatment consists of frequent topical antibiotics and consideration of performing washout of the interface. Needless to say, maintaining sterile technique is extremely important in preventing such devastating complications.

Surgical technique and postoperative care

Laser calibration, centration, and patient preparation and positioning are similar to those in PRK. In addition, the suction ring and microkeratome equipment must be assembled, inspected, or both by the surgeon before use. A lid speculum is placed to open the palpebral fissure widely to decrease the chance of the lids interfering with the microkeratome cut. The epithelium is marked in several locations with one of many available epithelial markers. These marks are made where the microkeratome will initiate its cut, so a free flap can be replaced in its original position. The suction ring is placed slightly nasally decentered to keep the flap hinge away from the ablation zone. After adequate suction has been achieved and confirmed, the microkeratome is placed in the suction ring apparatus and moved either manually or with an automated device across the cornea and back. The flap is then gently lifted toward the hinge and off the central cornea. Excess fluid is removed from the corneal stromal bed, the laser is centered on the pupil, and the ablation is performed. The flap is then gently replaced in its original position. The interface is irrigated to remove all debris and epithelial cells. The flap is left to air dry for several minutes until it is felt to have adhered to the stromal bed. This can be confirmed by the "striae test," in which indentation of the peripheral cornea with a cellulose sponge produces continuous striae in the cap. The lid speculum is then removed, taking extreme care not to dislodge the flap. Postoperative medications include topical antibiotics and steroids for several days.

HYPEROPIA

The ideal procedure for correcting hyperopia has not yet been perfected. Unlike in myopic correction with PRK or LASIK, in which removal of tissue from the central cornea results in central flattening, hyperopic correction requires steepening of the central cornea, which is more difficult to achieve and maintain in a controlled fashion. The three modalities under most intense study at present are hyperopic PRK, hyperopic LASIK, and Ho:YAG laser thermokeratoplasty (LTK).

Hyperopic PRK involves creating a relative steepening of the central cornea by ablating, and thus flattening, surrounding peripheral tissue. Wound healing responses tend to fill in this peripheral furrow, causing regression of the refractive effect. In addition, this deeper peripheral ablation necessitates an adjacent transition zone to smooth the interface of the treated and untreated cornea. As such, for the same total treatment diameter, hyperopic PRK produces a smaller optical zone than myopic PRK. For example, a total treatment diameter of 6 to 7 mm is required to produce an optical zone of 4 mm in hyperopic PRK. Smaller optical zones such as this are more sensitive to decentration, and increase the risk of postoperative complaints such as haloes and glare. Consequently, larger ablation zones are generally used.

Pietila *et al.* [62] did follow-up on 34 eyes for 1 year after hyperopic PRK with an Aesculap-Meditec (Jena, Germany) excimer laser. Only 40% of eyes with preoperative refractive error of +1.50 D to +6.00 D were within 1.00 D of emmetropia at 1 year, and only 17% of eyes with preoperative refractive error of +6.25 D to +9.75 D achieved ±1.00 D of emmetropia. Regression in the high hyperopia group continued past 6 months.

Other authors have reported better results with hyperopic PRK. Dausch *et al.* [63] used an enlarged treatment zone of 9.0 mm using a Aesculap-Meditec laser to treat 68 hyperopic eyes (range +2.00 D to +8.25 D). At 1 year, 81% of eyes were within 1.00 D of the target correction, with 97% of eyes 20/40 or better and 40% at 20/20 or better. Two percent of eyes lost two or more lines of BSCVA. Daya *et al.* [64•] treated 45 consecutive hyperopic eyes (with and without astigmatism) of up to +6.50 D spherical equivalent with the Chiron Keracor 116 excimer laser. At 6 months, 88% of PRK and 85% of PARK eyes were within 1.00 D of emmetropia. UCVA was 20/40 or better in 93% and 20/20 or better in 38% of all eyes. Loss of two lines of BSCVA occurred in 6.7% of eyes, and no eye lost more than two lines of BSCVA. Thirteen percent of eyes gained two or more lines of BSCVA.

Jackson *et al.* [65] assessed PRK with the VISX STAR excimer laser to correct low hyperopia in 25 eyes with refractive errors of +1.00 D to +4.00 D and ≤1.00 D of astigmatism. UCVA of 20/25 or better was achieved by 80% of eyes at 6 months. By 6 months, all patients were within one line of their preoperative BSCVA. Eighty-four percent gained two to seven lines of near UCVA, with one patient (4%) losing more than one line. Eighty percent were within ± 0.50 D, and 88% were within ±1.00 D of emmetropia. The authors conclude that PRK appears to be safe and effective for treatment of low hyperopia, noting that longer follow-up is needed.

Laser-assisted in situ keratomileusis has shown some early promise for hyperopic correction. Suarez *et al.* [66•] reported the results of LASIK on 326 eyes of 178 patients with or without astigmatism, using the Chiron Automated Corneal Shaper and the Coherent/Schwind (Santa Clara, CA) Keratom II excimer laser. Preoperative hyperopia ranged from +1.00 D to +8.50 D with astigmatism <0.75 D (group 1) or +1.00 D to +6.50 D (group 2). At 3 months, UCVA of 20/40 or better was achieved in 72% of eyes in group 1 and 58% of eyes in group 2. Astigmatism in group 2 was <1.50 D in 71% postoperatively, compared with only 37% before surgery. The authors conclude that hyperopia with or without astigmatism can be successfully treated by LASIK, although long-term stability is unknown.

Laser thermokeratoplasty utilizes the Ho:YAG laser to reshape the central cornea by placing one or two symmetric rings of burns in the peripheral cornea. These rings can be placed sequentially, via a hand-held fiberoptic/focusing probe (contact), or simultaneously, through a slit lamp delivery system (noncontact). This treatment causes shrinkage of stromal collagen with local midperipheral flattening and concomitant steepening of the central cornea.

Koch *et al.* [67••] reported the results of an FDA Phase IIA clinical study of noncontact Ho:YAG LTK. Twenty-eight eyes were treated to correct low to moderate (up to +3.88 D) hyperopia and observed for 2 years. Treatments consisted of one (6-mm diameter) or two (6- and 7-mm diameter) symmetric octagonal rings of eight spots per ring. At 2 years, the mean change in manifest refraction spherical equivalent was -0.53 D for the one-ring group, and -1.48 D for the two-ring group. Unfortunately, a permanent refractive effect (liberally defined as >±0.25 D) was not achieved in the one-ring group in 41% of eyes at 1 year and 29% of eyes at 2 years. All eyes in the two-ring group had some lasting effect, although the effect was generally small (-0.38 D to -2.25 D). No eye lost two or more lines of BSCVA.

Unfortunately, regression with LTK may limit the usefulness of this technique in the correction of naturally occurring hyperopia. However, early reports with contact [68] and noncontact [69] LTK in the setting of hyperopia after myopic PRK have produced more encouraging results, with stability of up to 82% of eyes at 1 year [68]. Larger studies with longer follow-up are necessary to determine what role LTK will ultimately play in correcting hyperopia.

Future developments

Picosecond laser

The neodymium:yttrium lithium fluoride (Nd:YLF) laser may have a future role in refractive surgery. This laser uses extremely short duration (picosecond) and extremely small focal point laser bursts to create optical tissue breakdown with very little energy. Using computer-driven control mechanisms, series of laser spots spaced 20 to 30 μm apart can be applied in various patterns (*eg*, an expanding spiral) to create lamellar dissections in the cornea. Based on early animal studies, the picosecond laser was initially envisioned as a true intrastromal ablating device, with tissue removal causing collapse of the corneal layers and flattening of the cornea [70]. Subsequent investigations have shown that the laser does not produce corneal thinning and flattening in a clinically applicable manner [71,72], and the picosecond laser is now being investigated as a cutting, rather than ablating, tool. Although the laser can create a hinged flap like a microkeratome [73•], its ultimate refractive application may involve intrastromal lenticule formation with removal of the lenticule through a small peripheral "cut-down."

New microkeratome designs are directed toward producing an anterior stromal flap more safely and reproducibly. As previously mentioned, simpler designs and the development of single-use disposable microkeratomes should decrease or eliminate complications arising from improper assembly. A side-cutting microkeratome developed by Chiron Vision creates a superior hinge, which may be more stable and less subject to displacement from blinking. Waterjet keratomes use a very thin stream of water at high velocity to create a smooth lamellar corneal incision [74]. Time will tell which of these designs will produce the most consistently precise and safe flap.

Within the last decade, treatment of the cornea (more than any other ocular tissue) has undergone revolutionary changes in surgical options involving lasers. Refractive techniques that 10 or 15 years ago were science fiction are now readily available to the general public. Exciting new procedures and technologies are now being introduced into mainstream clinical practice with others just on the horizon. With the advent of any new surgical modality, a compromise must be achieved between conservatism and progress, so that reliable, safe surgical options can be made available to patients at an appropriate stage of the procedure's development. As the decade comes to a close, the use of lasers in corneal surgery continues to increase, with future advances likely to outpace even the rapid evolution of recent years.

ACKNOWLEDGEMENTS

The authors would like to acknowledge and thank Kimberly S. Jones for her assistance in the preparation of the manuscript.

REFERENCES AND RECOMMENDED READING

Recently published papers of particular interest have been highlighted as:
- • Of interest
- •• Of outstanding interest

1. Gartry D, Kerr Muir M, Marshall J: Excimer laser treatment of corneal surface pathology: a laboratory and clinical study. *Br J Ophthalmol* 1991, 75:258–269.
2. Goodman GL, Trokel SL, Stark WJ, *et al.*: Corneal healing following laser refractive keratectomy. *Arch Ophthalmol* 1989, 107:1799–1803.
3. Fantes FE, Hanna KD, Waring GO III, *et al.*: Wound healing after excimer laser keratomileusis (photorefractive keratectomy) in monkeys. *Arch Ophthalmol* 1990, 108:665–675.
4. Hanna KD, Pouliquen TM, Savoldelli M, *et al.*: Corneal wound healing in monkeys 18 months after excimer laser photorefractive keratectomy. *Refract Corneal Surg* 1990, 6:340–345.
5. Del Pero RA, Gigstad JE, Roberts AD, *et al.*: A refractive and histopathologic study of excimer laser keratectomy in primates. *Am J Ophthalmol* 1990, 109:419–429.
6. McDonald MB, Kaufman HE, Frantz JM, *et al.*: Excimer laser ablation in a human eye: case report. *Arch Ophthalmol* 1989, 107:641–642.
7. McDonald MB, Frantz JM, Klyce SD, *et al.*: Central photorefractive keratectomy for myopia: the blind eye study. *Arch Ophthalmol* 1990, 108:799–808.
8. Englanoff JS, Kolahdouz-Isfahani AH, Moreira H, *et al.*: In situ collagen gel mold as an aid in excimer laser superficial keratectomy. *Ophthalmology* 1992, 99:1201–1208.
9. Stevens SX, Bowyer BL: Corneal modulators and their use in excimer laser phototherapeutic keratectomy. *Int Ophthalmol Clin* 1996, 36:119–125.
10. Rapuano CJ: Excimer laser phototherapeutic keratectomy: long-term results and practical considerations. *Cornea* 1997, 16:151–157.
11. Orndahl M, Fagerholm P, Fitzsimmons T, *et al.*: Treatment of corneal dystrophies with excimer laser. *Acta Ophthalmol* 1994, 72:235–240.
12. John ME, Martines E, Cvintal T, *et al.*: Excimer laser photoablation of primary familial amyloidosis of the cornea. *Refract Corneal Surg* 1993, 9(Suppl):138–141.
13. Niesen U, Thomann U, Schipper I: Phototherapeutic keratectomy. *Klin Monatsbl Augenheilkd* 1994, 205:187–195.
14. Droutsas DD, Tsioulias GE, Kotsiras JE, *et al.*: Phototherapeutic keratectomy in macular corneal dystrophy with recurrent erosions. *J Refract Surg* 1996, 12:S293–S294.
15. Cennamo G, Rosa N, Rosenwasser GO, *et al.*: Phototherapeutic keratectomy in the treatment of Avellino dystrophy. *Ophthalmologica* 1994, 208:198–200.
16. Rapuano CJ, Laibson PR: Excimer laser phototherapeutic keratectomy. *CLAO J* 1993, 19:235–240.
17. Rapuano CJ, Laibson PR: Excimer laser phototherapeutic keratectomy for anterior corneal pathology. *CLAO J* 1994, 20:253–257.
18. •• Maloney RK, Thompson V, Ghiselli G, *et al.*: A prospective multicenter trial of excimer laser phototherapeutic keratectomy for corneal vision loss. The Summit Phototherapeutic Keratectomy Study Group. *Am J Ophthalmol* 1996, 122:149–160.

This multicenter trial evaluated PTK for various types of anterior corneal vision loss in 232 eyes of 211 patients. At 12 months, BSCVA improved in 45% of eyes and worsened in 9%. Mean refractive shift was 0.87 D toward hyperopia.

19. O'Brart DP, Gartry DS, Lohmann CP, *et al.*: Treatment of band keratopathy by excimer laser phototherapeutic keratectomy: surgical techniques and long term follow up. *Br J Ophthalmol* 1993, 77:702–708.
20. Rapuano CJ: Excimer laser phototherapeutic keratectomy. *Int Ophthalmol Clin* 1996, 36:127–136.
21. • Badr IA, al-Rajhi A, Wagoner MD, *et al.*: Phototherapeutic keratectomy for climatic droplet keratopathy, KKESH Excimer Laser Study Group. King Khaled Eye Specialist Hospital. *J Refract Surg* 1996, 12:114–122.

Reduced corneal opacification was achieved in 98% of 55 eyes with smooth climatic droplet keratopathy and 80% of 20 eyes with irregular climatic droplet keratopathy. Improvement in best corrected visual acuity was 61.8% in the former group and 21.2% in the latter.

22. Forster W, Grewe S, Busse H: Clinical use of the excimer laser in treatment of surface corneal opacities: therapeutic strategy and case reports. *Klin Monatsbl Augenheilkd* 1993, 202:126–129.
23. Campos M, Nielsen S, Szerenyi K, *et al.*: Clinical follow-up of phototherapeutic keratectomy for treatment of corneal opacities. *Am J Ophthalmol* 1993, 115:433–440.

24. Vrabec MP, Anderson JA, Rock ME, *et al.*: Electron microscopic findings in a cornea with recurrence of herpes simplex keratitis after excimer laser phototherapeutic keratectomy. *CLAO J* 1994, 20:41–44.

25. Poirier L, Coulon P, Williamson W, *et al.*: Results of therapeutic photokeratectomy using the excimer laser. Apropos of 12 cases. *J Fr Ophtalmol* 1994, 17:262–270.

26. Binder PS, Anderson JA, Rock ME, *et al.*: Human excimer laser keratectomy. Clinical and histopathologic correlations. *Ophthalmology* 1994, 101:979–989.

27. Cameron JA, Antonios SR, Badr IA: Excimer laser phototherapeutic keratectomy for shield ulcers and corneal plaques in vernal keratoconjunctivitis. *J Refract Surg* 1995, 11:31–35.

28. Ward MA, Artunduaga G, Thompson KP, *et al.*: Phototherapeutic keratectomy for the treatment of nodular subepithelial corneal scars in patients with keratoconus who are contact lens intolerant. *CLAO J* 1995, 21:130–132.

29.• Forster W, Atzler U, Ratkay I, *et al.*: Therapeutic use of the 193-nm excimer laser in corneal pathologies. *Graefes Arch Clin Exp Ophthalmol* 1997, 235:296–305.

Phototherapeutic keratectomy was performed in 252 eyes of 216 patients suffering from pain or decreased visual acuity from various pathologies. Of these eyes, 91% with recurrent erosions were erosion-free after treatment. No beneficial effect was seen after alkali burns or in a patient with corneal protuberance.

30. Starr M, Donnenfeld E, Newton M, *et al.*: Excimer laser phototherapeutic keratectomy. *Cornea* 1996, 15:557–565.

31. Bialasiewicz AA, Schaudig U, Draeger J, *et al.*: Descemetocele after excimer laser phototherapeutic keratectomy in herpes simplex virus-induced keratitis: a clinicopathologic correlation. *Klin Monatsbl Augenheilkd* 1996, 208:120–123.

32. Zuckerman SJ, Aquavella JV, Park SB: Analysis of the efficacy and safety of excimer laser PTK in the treatment of corneal disease. *Cornea* 1996, 15:9–14.

33.• Moreira LB, Sanchez D, Trousdale MD, *et al.*: Aerosolization of infectious virus by excimer laser. *Am J Ophthalmol* 1997, 123:297–302.

These authors recovered HSV and adenovirus from adjacent culture plates after ablation through infected cell monolayers. They concluded that the potential for aerosolized infectious virus exists during excimer laser ablation.

34.• Hagen KB, Kettering JD, Aprecio RM, *et al.*: Lack of virus transmission by the excimer laser plume. *Am J Ophthalmol* 1997, 124:206–211.

In this study, an excimer laser was used to ablate a Pseudorabies virus-infected tissue culture plate while an uninfected tissue culture plate was in an inverted position over the infected plate. Pseudorabies virus is a porcine-enveloped herpes virus similar in structure and life cycle to HIV and HSV. The authors concluded that excimer laser ablation was unlikely to pose a health hazard to the surgeon.

35.• Taravella MJ, Weinberg A, Blackburn P, *et al.*: Do intact viral particles survive excimer laser ablation? *Arch Ophthalmol* 1997, 115:1028–1030.

In this study, excimer laser ablation of fibroblasts infected with attenuated VZV was performed. The laser plume was collected for polymerase chain reaction analysis and viral culture. While viral DNA was detected in the material trapped from the laser plume, live virus could not be demonstrated to have survived ablation. The authors concluded that attenuated VZV did not seem to survive excimer laser ablation, but felt that further study of other viruses was needed to fully assess the risk to the surgeon.

36. Liu C: Hyperopic shift and the use of masking agents in excimer laser superficial keratectomy [letter]. *Ophthalmol* 1992, 76:62–63.

37. Gartry D, Kerr Muir M, Marshall J: Hyperopic shift and the use of masking agents in excimer laser superficial keratectomy [letter]. *Br J Ophthalmol* 1992, 76:63.

38. Stark WJ, Chamon W, Kamp MT, *et al.*: Clinical follow-up of 193-nm ArF excimer laser photokeratectomy. *Ophthalmology* 1992, 99:805–812.

39. Sher NA, Bowers RA, Zabel RW, *et al.*: Clinical use of 193-nm excimer laser in the treatment of corneal scars. *Arch Ophthalmol* 1991, 109:491–498.

40. Meyer JC, Stulting RD, Thompson KP, *et al.*: Late onset of corneal scar after excimer laser photorefractive keratectomy. *Am J Ophthalmol* 1996, 121:529–539.

41.• Lipshitz I, Loewenstein A, Varssano D, *et al.*: Late onset corneal haze after photorefractive keratectomy for moderate and high myopia. *Ophthalmology* 1997, 104:369–373.

Decreased visual acuity and regression of refractive effect occurred in 18 of 1000 consecutive eyes secondary to late onset corneal haze. This haze appeared 4 to 12 months after PRK, and partially reversed with topical steroids or reoperation.

42. Tsubota K, Toda I, Itoh S: Reduction of subepithelial haze after photorefractive keratectomy by cooling the cornea. *Am J Ophthalmol* 1993, 115:820–821.

43.• Corbett MC, Verma S, O'Brart DP, *et al.*: Effect of ablation profile on wound healing and visual performance 1 year after excimer laser photorefractive keratectomy. *Br J Ophthalmol* 1996, 80:224–234.

This study randomized patients to 5- or 6-mm treatment zones during PRK for -3.00 or -6.00 D. The 6 mm group had a smaller hyperopic shift, a more predictable and stable refractive outcome, less haze, fewer halos, and fewer night vision problems when compared with the 5 mm group.

44. O'Brart DP, Corbett MC, Lohmann CP, *et al.*: The effects of ablation diameter on the outcome of excimer laser photorefractive keratectomy: a prospective, randomized, double-blind study. *Arch Ophthalmol* 1995, 113:438–443.

45. Rao SK, Mukesh BN, Bakshi H, *et al.*: Photorefractive keratectomy: the Sankara Nethralaya experience. *Ophthalmic Surg Lasers* 1996, 27:S444–S453.

46. Schipper I, Senn P, Niesen U: Are we measuring the right intraocular pressure after excimer laser photorefractive laser keratoplasty in myopia? *Klin Monatsbl Augenheilkd* 1995, 206:322–324.

47. Chatterjee A, Shah S, Bessant DA, *et al.*: Reduction in intraocular pressure after excimer laser photorefractive keratectomy: correlation with pretreatment myopia. *Ophthalmology* 1997, 104:355–359.

48. Mardelli PG, Piebenga LW, Whitacre MM, *et al.*: The effect of excimer laser photorefractive keratectomy on intraocular pressure measurements using the Goldmann applanation tonometer. *Ophthalmology* 1997, 104:945–948.

49.• Shahinian L, Jain S, Jager RD, *et al.*: Dilute topical proparacaine for pain relief after photorefractive keratectomy. *Ophthalmology* 1997, 104:1327–1332.

In total, 48 eyes of 34 patients were randomized to topical proparacaine 0.05% or placebo as needed for pain for 1 week after PRK. Patients reported significantly greater pain relief for a longer period in the treatment group. No difference in number of days to complete epithelial healing was present between groups.

50. Corbett MC, O'Brart DP, Marshall J: Do topical corticosteroids have a role following excimer laser photorefractive keratectomy for myopia. *J Refract Surg* 1995, 11:341–347.

51. Fagerholm P, Hamberg-Mystrom H, Tengroth B, *et al.*: Effect of postoperative steroids on the refractive outcome of photorefractive keratectomy for myopia with the Summit excimer laser. *J Cataract Refract Surg* 1994, 20:212–215.

52. Gartry DS, Kerr Muir MG, Lohmann CP, *et al.*: The effect of topical corticosteroids on refractive outcome and corneal haze after photorefractive keratectomy: a prospective, randomized, double-blind trial. *Arch Ophthalmol* 1992, 110:944–952.

53. Marques EF, Leite EB, Cunha-Vaz JG: Corticosteroids for reversal of myopic regression after photorefractive keratectomy. *J Refract Surg* 1995, 11:S302–S308.

54. O'Brart DP, Lohmann CP, Klonos G, *et al.*: The effects of topical corticosteroids and plasmin inhibitors on refractive outcome, haze, and visual performance after photorefractive keratectomy: a prospective, randomized, observer-masked study. *Ophthalmology* 1994, 101:1565–1574.

55. Barraquer JI: Queratoplastia refractiva. *Est e Inf. Oftal Inst Barraquer* 1949, 2:10.

56.• Salah T, Waring GO III, el-Maghraby A, *et al.*: Excimer laser in-situ keratomileusis (LASIK) under a corneal flap for myopia of 2 to 20 D. *Trans Am Ophthalmol Soc* 1995, 93:163–183.

Eighty-eight patients with refractive errors ranging from -2.00 to -20.00 D underwent LASIK with the Chiron Automated Corneal Shaper and the Summit Omnimed laser. Postoperative UCVA was 20/20 or better in 36% of eyes and 20/40 or better in 71% of eyes. Three eyes (3.6%) lost two lines or more of BSCVA.

57.•• Perez-Santonja JJ, Bellot J, Claramoante P, *et al.*: Laser in situ keratomileusis to correct high myopia. *J Cataract Refract Surg* 1997, 23:372–385.

The Chiron Automated Corneal Shaper and the VISX 20/20 laser with a multizone profile were used to treat 143 eyes with preoperative refractive error -8.00 to -20.00 D with LASIK. At 6 months, 46.4% of eyes saw 20/40 or better uncorrected. Refractive error within 1.00 D of emmetropia was achieved by 60% of all eyes, 72.4% of eyes with preoperative myopia of -8.00 to -11.92 D, 46% of eyes with preoperative myopia of -12.00 to -15.97 D, and 50% of eyes with preoperative myopia of -16.00 to -20.00 D.

58.• Pirzada WA, Kalaawry H: Laser in situ keratomileusis for myopia of -1 to -3.50 Diopters. *J Refract Surg* 1997, 13(Suppl 5):S425–S426.

Pirzada and Kalaawry reported their results of LASIK for low myopia (-1.00 to -3.50 D). Eighty-five eyes underwent LASIK using the Chiron microkeratome and the Nidek EC 5000, a "second generation" scanning laser. UCVA was 20/30 or better in 80% of eyes at 1 month and 93% of eyes at 6 months. One eye was complicated by corneal abscess formation with subsequent scarring and visual acuity of 20/100.

59. Perez-Santonja JJ, Sakla HF, Abad JL, *et al.*: Nocardial keratitis after laser in situ keratomileusis. *J Refract Surg* 1997, 13:314–317.

60. Mulhern MG, Condon PI, O'Keefe M: Endophthalmitis after astigmatic myopic laser in situ keratomileusis. *J Cataract Refract Surg* 1997, 23:948–950.

61. Watanabe H, Sato S, Maida N, *et al.*: Bilateral corneal infection as a complication of laser in situ keratomileusis. *Arch Ophthalmol* 1997, 115:1593–1594.

62. Pietila J, Makinen P, Pajari S, *et al.*: Excimer laser photorefractive keratectomy for hyperopia. *J Refract Surg* 1997, 13:504–510.

63. Dausch D, Smecka Z, Klein R, *et al.*: Excimer laser photorefractive keratectomy for hyperopia. *J Cataract Refract Surg* 1997, 23:169–176.

64.• Daya SM, Tappouni FR, Habid NE, *et al.*: Photorefractive keratectomy for hyperopia: six months results in 45 eyes. *Ophthalmology* 1997, 104:1952–1958.

Daya *et al.* treated 45 consecutive hyperopic eyes (with and without astigmatism) of up to +6.50 D spherical equivalent with the Chiron Keracor 116 excimer laser. At 6 months, 88% of PRK and 85% of PARK eyes were within 1.00 D of emmetropia. UCVA was 20/40 or better in 93% and 20/20 or better in 38% of all eyes. In 6.7% of eyes, loss of 2 lines of BSCVA occurred and no eye lost more than 2 lines of BSCVA. However, 13% of eyes gained two or more lines of BSCVA.

65. Jackson WB, Mintsioulis G, Apagpitos PJ, *et al.*: Excimer laser photorefractive keratectomy for low hyperopia: safety and efficacy. *J Cataract Refract Surg* 1997, 23:480–487.

66.• Suarez E, Torres F, Duplessie MD: LASIK for correction of hyperopia and hyperopia with astigmatism. *Int Ophthalmol Clin* 1996, 36:65–72.

Suarez *et al.* reported the results of LASIK on 326 eyes of 178 patients with or without astigmatism, using the Chiron Automated Corneal Shaper and the Coherent/Schwind Keratom II excimer laser. Preoperative hyperopia ranged from +1.00 to +8.50 D with astigmatism <0.75 D (group 1) or +1.00 to +6.50 D (group 2). At 3 months, UCVA of 20/40 or better was achieved in 72% of eyes in group 1, and 58% of eyes in group 2. Astigmatism in group 2 was <1.50 D in 71% postoperatively, compared with only 37% before surgery.

67.•• Koch DD, Kohnen T, McDonnell PJ, *et al.*: Hyperopia correction by noncontact holmium:YAG laser thermal keratoplasty. United States phase IIA clinical study with a 2-year follow-up. *Ophthalmology* 1997, 104:1938–1947.

Koch *et al.* reported the results of an FDA Phase IIA clinical study of noncontact Ho:YAG LTK. Twenty-eight eyes were treated to correct low to moderate (up to +3.88 D) of hyperopia and followed for 2 years. Treatments consisted of 1 (6-mm diameter) or 2 (6- and 7-mm diameter) symmetric octagonal rings of 8 spots per ring. At 2 years, the mean change in manifest refraction spherical equivalent was -0.53 D for the 1-ring group and -1.48 D for the 2-ring group. Unfortunately, a permanent refractive effect (liberally defined as >± 0.25 D) was not achieved in the 1-ring group in 41% of eyes at 1 year and 29% of eyes at 2 years. All eyes in the 2-ring group had some lasting effect, although the effect was generally small (-0.38 to -2.25 D). No eye lost two or more lines of BSCVA.

68. Goggin M, Lavery F. Holmium laser thermokeratoplasty for the reversal of hyperopia after myopic photorefractive keratectomy. *Br J Ophthalmol* 1997, 81:541–543.

69. Alio JL, Ismail MM, Artola A, *et al.*: Correction of hyperopia induced by photorefractive keratectomy using non-contact Ho:YAG laser thermal keratoplasty. *J Refract Surg* 1997, 13:13–16.

70. Habib MS, Speaker MG, Kaiser R, *et al.*: Myopic intrastromal photorefractive keratectomy with the neodymium-yttrium lithium fluoride picosecond laser in the cat cornea. *Arch Ophthalmol* 1995, 113:499–505.

71. Vogel A, Gunther T, Asiyo-Vogel M, *et al*: Studies of the development of refractive effects in intrastromal refractive corneal surgery with the picosecond laser. *Ophthalmologe* 1997, 94:467–474.

72. Marchi V, Gualano A, Zumbo G, *et al*: Intrastromal photorefractive keratectomy for myopia by Nd:YLF picosecond laser. *J Refract Surg* 1996,12:S284–S287.

73.• Ito M, Quantock AJ, Sameena M, *et al.*: Picosecond laser in situ keratomileusis with a 1053-nm Nd:YLF laser. *J Refract Surg* 1996,12:721–728.

The Nd:YLF laser was used on human donor eyes to fashion anterior corneal flaps and generate intrastromal lenticules, using 40 to 60 μJ pulses spaced 20 to 30 μm apart. The quality of the dissections, as evaluated by scanning electron microscopy, was enhanced when the smaller pulse separation of 20 μm was used.

74. Lipshitz I, Rephael B, Loewenstein A: Cutting the cornea with a waterjet keratome. *J Refract Surg* 1996, 12:184–186.

CHAPTER 3

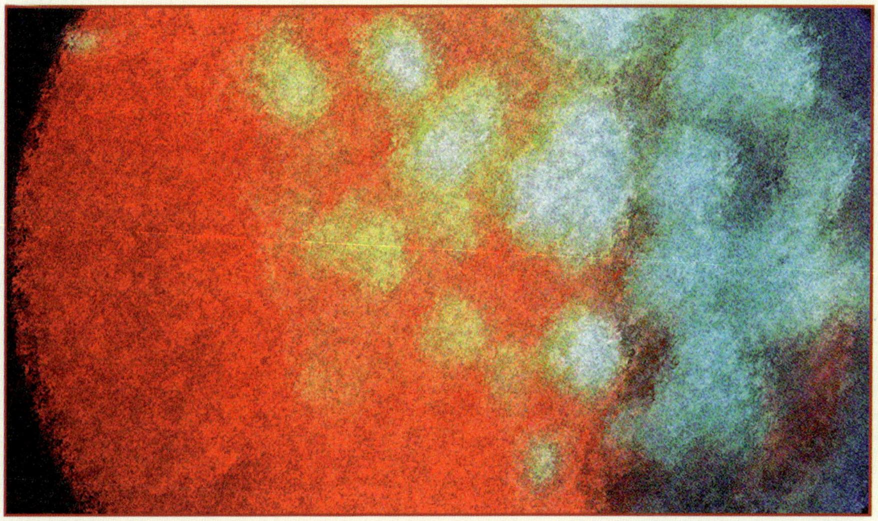

Lasers in Oculoplastic Surgery

Daniel A. Ebroon
Albert Hornblass

Lasers have assumed an integral role in the clinician's armamentarium for the treatment of many oculoplastic disorders. Whether for use on the lacrimal system, eyelids, or orbit, and whether for use in incising, excising, or remolding tissue, the laser is a necessary instrument for the modern oculoplastic surgeon. In contrast to many intraocular applications of the laser in which access of tissue is achieved without directly invading the globe, the laser as used in oculoplastic surgery offers a new way of affecting tissues that are relatively accessible. Therefore, application of this technology in many oculoplastic procedures offers disadvantages and advantages that differ from its use in many other ophthalmic settings. The astute surgeon applies techniques using the laser when the advantages offered are beneficial to the patient. This chapter provides an overview for the laser's use in oculoplastic surgery with emphasis placed on its relative merits compared with traditional surgical approaches.

CARBON DIOXIDE LASERS

The advent of the carbon dioxide (CO_2) laser and its increased use (Figs. 3-1 and 3-2) can largely be attributed to its hemostatic properties. The CO_2 laser operates at the invisible wavelength of 10,600 nm and its energy is absorbed by both intracellular and extracellular water. This energy raises the temperature to 100°C and flash boils the water. Soft tissue, composed of approximately 88% water, is vaporized within 0.1 mm of the application of the laser. Because the energy is absorbed by water and not by tissue, the color of the treated tissue has minimal relevance. With flash point boiling and tissue vaporization, blood vessels coagulate efficiently. In fact, vessels 0.5 mm in diameter or smaller are consistently sealed. Larger vessels can be sealed by applying a defocused laser beam to the end of a vessel for a few seconds. Hemostasis as achieved with this form of incision provides the surgeon with a clean surgical field and improved visibility.

Another major advantage of the CO_2 laser is the precision by which it can be applied. The collimated beam is coupled with a helium-neon laser that provides a red, coaxial guiding light beam. The laser, applied in a single pulse, penetrates 0.1 mm into soft tissues, thereby providing exceptional control over the depth of the incision. Unlike cutting with a blade, however, the depth of tissue penetration must be ascertained solely on visual clues. Alternatively, the use of a scalpel provides a sense of proprioception that helps the surgeon control the depth of the incision.

The laser can be applied in either a continuous wave or millisecond pulses. Millisecond bursts reduce the total energy delivered so that less thermal damage is produced, which may translate into better wound healing and less scar formation. Less thermal damage, however, may mean that larger-caliber vessels remain uncoagulated and, therefore, it is more difficult to achieve hemostasis. Of course, the amount of energy absorbed by the tissues, and consequently the amount of thermal damage produced, also depend on other factors. For example, slower movement of the laser beam while creating an incision translates into a greater amount of energy applied to a unit of tissue, with increased charring, increased coagulation, deeper ablation, and more thermal damage.

Disadvantages of the CO_2 laser include loss of proprioceptive feedback, greater expense, longer recovery

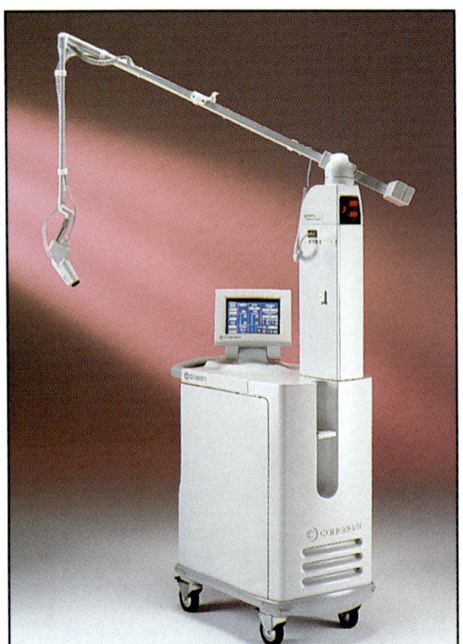

FIGURE 3-1. One example of a carbon dioxide laser is this Coherent Ultra-Pulse laser. (Coherent, Palo Alto, CA)

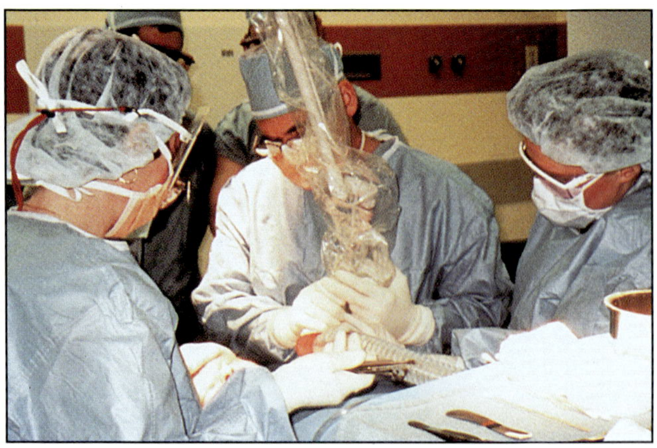

FIGURE 3-2. The carbon dioxide laser is pictured in use for facial resurfacing in the operating room. Note that all operating room personnel are wearing eye protection. The patient's eyes are protected with stainless steel contact lenses. The patient's oxygen is turned off to prevent it from igniting, and wet towels are placed around the surgical field.

for a wound to develop its tensile strength, and use of a bulky articulated arm for laser delivery. With regard to wound healing, incisions created with the CO_2 laser lag in tensile strength behind those created with a scalpel. This difference may be a consequence of the collateral thermal damage created by the laser. Furthermore, the laser's efficient ablation of blood vessels may retard early postoperative healing. At any rate, the cosmetic appearance and tensile strength of an incision created with a laser or scalpel are indistinguishable 3 weeks postoperatively.

Lymphangioma

The repertoire of disorders successfully treated with the CO_2 laser has grown as more surgeons have become assured of its utility. In the 1980s, it became clear that the CO_2 laser's hemostatic properties render it useful for excision of vascular lesions. For example, orbital lymphangiomas can be removed safely with a CO_2 laser [1,2]. These tumors are rarely encapsulated and can be infiltrative, friable, and quite close to orbital structures. The CO_2 laser can be used to debulk such tumors while minimizing risk to surrounding orbital structures because of the precision of the laser incision. The laser may be mounted on a surgical microscope to maximize the precision of laser delivery [1]. Power settings range from 500 mW to 15 W, with lower powers applied to intraconal lesions for safety.

Blepharoplasty

The CO_2 laser has many applications as an incisional instrument. Most procedures that require a skin incision can be transformed into laser procedures by cutting with the CO_2 laser. A prime example is blepharoplasty, a procedure in which the laser can be used for both incising skin and excising fat (Fig. 3-3).

A proposed incision line can be created with tiny spot burns placed about 5 mm apart in the upper lid crease. This is done with the laser set at 2 W in the single pulse mode. To make the incision, the power is turned to 6 W in the continuous wave mode. With a smooth motion, the skin and orbicularis are cut. Lower powers require more exposure time to create the incision; higher powers necessitate moving the handpiece faster at the expense of some loss of control for most surgeons. The surgeon must remember to maintain the handpiece perpendicular to the tissue plane being cut as well as to keep the laser beam in focus. This technique provides the cleanest incision both in terms of minimizing collateral thermal damage, as well as by maximally cauterizing vessels at the wound margin. It may also be that a finer incision heals with less scarring [3].

After the incision has been completed, the superior flap is grasped and tented superiorly, and the laser is used in a horizontal back-and-forth motion to create a plane between the orbicularis and the septum. Any small bleeding vessels can be coagulated by applying the laser directly to the open vessel. Defocusing the beam may help affect a larger area, with vessels still receiving enough energy to occlude. After the septum has been divided, redundant orbital fat is then grasped within a clamp and excised with the laser.

Because it takes a few weeks for the incision created with a laser to equal the tensile strength of an incision made with a scalpel, sutures may be removed around the eighth postoperative day. Some surgeons feel that the scar created with a laser is more prominent [3], but this varies with other surgeons' experience [4]. It is generally agreed that laser procedures have less ecchymosis, less edema, and, after the surgeon is comfortable with the equipment, faster intraoperative time.

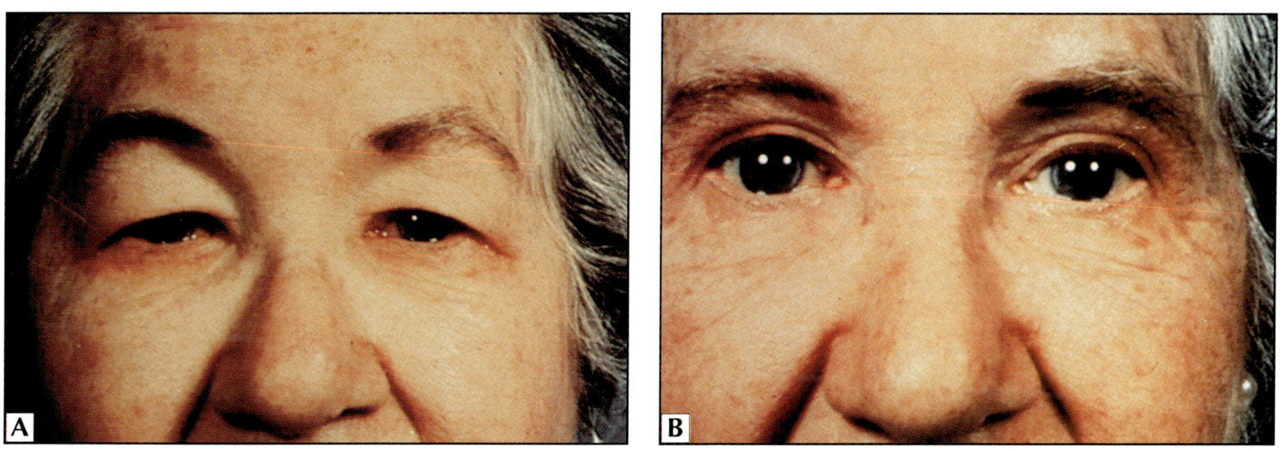

FIGURE 3-3. **A**, Preoperative photograph, **B**, postoperative photograph of a woman who underwent bilateral upper eyelid blepharoplasty using the Coherent (Palo Alto, CA) carbon dioxide laser as a cutting instrument. *See* text for details on the laser settings. (*Courtesy of* Stephen Bosniak, MD, Manhattan, NY.)

Ptosis and ectropion

The CO_2 laser as an incisional tool has been applied to ptosis surgery and ectropion repair with a lateral tarsal strip [5,6•]. As already described for blepharoplasty, the laser may be used to create clean, precise incisions with good hemostasis (*eg*, when creating a lateral canthotomy or cantholysis). Dissection through deeper tissues may be carried out as well, such as to expose the levator aponeurosis during ptosis repair [6•].

Xanthelasma

The CO_2 laser has been used for removal of xanthelasma palpebrarum. Deposits of fatty tissue in the superficial skin layer occur from heredity or from elevated systemic levels of cholesterol and triglycerides. Techniques to remove xanthelasma have traditionally consisted of excision with a scalpel or application of chemical treatment (*eg*, trichloroacetic acid or phenol) to remove the affected skin caustically. The CO_2 laser can be used to remove such lesions with excellent cosmetic results [7–9].

The laser may be prepared with a 1-mm spot size and a power setting at 6 W. Local anesthesia infiltrated into the subcutaneous plane helps isolate the treated area and protect the ciliary margin because water readily absorbs energy from CO_2 and shields underlying tissue. After the circumferential incision is made through the epidermis, a lower laser power can be used to undermine and remove the lesion. This can be performed either by decreasing the power to 4 W, or more quickly by defocusing the laser beam. Skin curettage may help remove affected tissue down to the dermis and, sometimes, the superficial fascial layer. The resulting defect can be left to heal by secondary intention with excellent cosmesis (Fig. 3-4).

Chalazions

Chalazions are extremely common focal accumulations of lipogranulomatous material within the eyelids that accumulate secondary to malsecretion of the meibomian glands. They are commonly treated with warm compresses, lid hygiene, corticosteroid injections, or incision and drainage. The CO_2 laser can be used to create a transconjunctival incision into the substance of a chalazion and then to vaporize the contents of the chalazion itself. Because no chalazion clamp is placed, no local anesthesia is necessary [10,11].

Capillary hemangioma

Capillary hemangiomas are the most common benign tumor in children. They are benign collections of vascular channels surrounded by proliferated endothelial cells and most often involve the upper lid. They usually

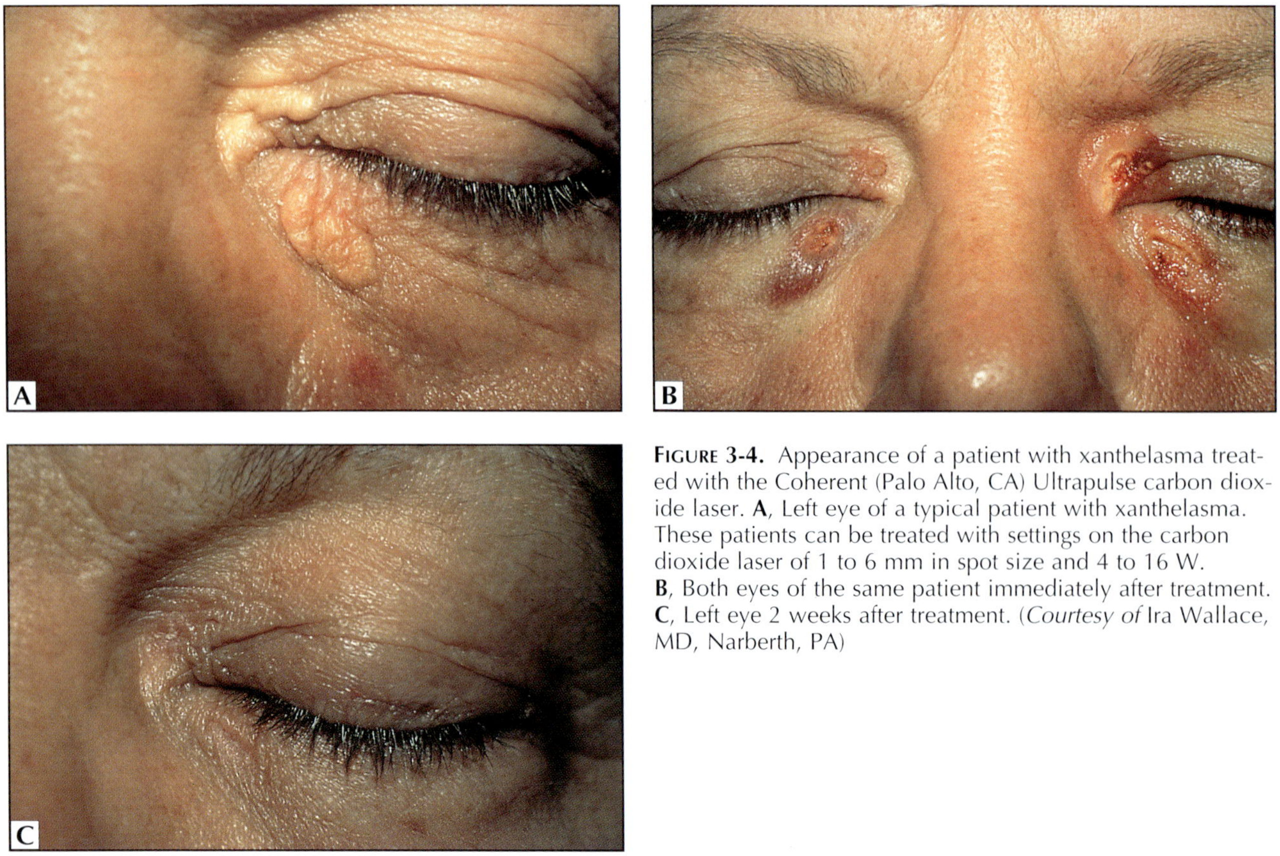

FIGURE 3-4. Appearance of a patient with xanthelasma treated with the Coherent (Palo Alto, CA) Ultrapulse carbon dioxide laser. **A**, Left eye of a typical patient with xanthelasma. These patients can be treated with settings on the carbon dioxide laser of 1 to 6 mm in spot size and 4 to 16 W. **B**, Both eyes of the same patient immediately after treatment. **C**, Left eye 2 weeks after treatment. (*Courtesy of* Ira Wallace, MD, Narberth, PA)

grow for the first 6 months of life, then slowly involute over the subsequent 4 or 5 years. Capillary hemangiomas must be treated if the visual axis is occluded, if a large amount of astigmatism exists, or if the lesion is cosmetically unacceptable. These lesions often regress with the use of injected steroids. Given the CO_2 laser's advantage in treating vascular lesions, it is a useful tool for this disorder.

A skin incision may be made within the lid crease overlying or near the capillary hemangioma. The incision may be made either with a scalpel or with the laser itself. With the skin retracted, the laser is used either freehand or mounted on an operating microscope to vaporize the hemangioma with minimal blood loss [10].

Meningiomas

Orbital meningiomas may arise from arachnoid villi surrounding the optic nerve or within the cranium, thus secondarily invading the orbit. These tumors are difficult to excise because they tend to adhere tightly to orbital structures. The advantage in using the CO_2 laser to remove such a tumor is the instrument's precision. A spot size of 1 mm or less may be used to meticulously dissect tumor away from structures such as the optic nerve or the globe [12].

Syringomas

Syringomas are smooth, flesh-colored, dome-shaped papules 1 to 3 mm in diameter that represent a collection of eccrine sweat glands and ducts. They most often appear periorbitally in women. They have been removed successfully by applying laser energy to the lesion in a pulsed or superpulsed mode [13,14]. First the skin is vaporized, revealing an underlying whitish cyst, which can be drained with a 25-gauge needle or ablated with the laser itself.

Exenteration

The CO_2 laser has been used to perform orbital exenterations. The laser's ability to seal off blood vessels and lymphatic channels offers the theoretical advantage of limiting both the hematogenous and lymphatic spread of orbital tumors. At powers of 4 to 14 W, bone is minimally affected by the laser. Therefore, the laser can be applied to bone adjacent to areas of tumor involvement, selectively destroying tumor cells and preserving bone [10]. At powers of 20 W, however, the laser can be used to pit the outer table of orbital bones in a grid pattern to stimulate granulation in areas of exposed bone.

Skin resurfacing

The use of the CO_2 laser for cosmetic skin resurfacing has increased dramatically over the last few years. The laser is applied to the skin around the eyes and the rest of the face, evenly ablating the epidermis and reticular dermis. When the dermis and epidermis reform, the skin appears smoother with fewer fine wrinkles. How the skin heals largely depends on its pigmentation, with fairer skinned people (*eg*, Fitzpatrick skin types I and II) healing more evenly and those with darker skin types healing with varying levels of pigmentation.

Patients designated for skin resurfacing must be chosen very carefully. In addition to assessing skin pigmentation, a thorough medical history must be taken to rule out certain entities that may recur or that may complicate the procedure. Laser skin resurfacing is contraindicated in patients with a history of herpes zoster ophthalmicus, connective tissue disorders, systemic lupus erythematosus, or severe facial burns. It is also vital to discuss thoroughly with the patient his or her expectations from the procedure, the anticipated postoperative course, and possible side effects.

Patients must be physically prepared for CO_2 laser resurfacing. They are pretreated with oral acyclovir and an antibiotic (*eg*, cephalexin) to help prevent infections. The skin is also treated with agents such as tretinoin and hydroquinone to promote smooth healing of the skin with even pigmentation. Use of a smoke evacuator deserves emphasis. Large skin surfaces ablated with the laser cause a plume that may contain vital viral particles. A smoke evacuator clears the vaporized tissue more quickly, which, in conjunction with a fine particle surgical mask, maximizes safety.

The laser is set on the superpulse mode, between 4 and 6 W. The size of the spot can be set as large as the surgeon chooses. Each pass with the laser ablates between 40 and 70 μm from the surface. Because eyelid skin is among the thinnest of the body, most surgeons feel one pass is enough to effect a desired result. Many surgeons apply a second pass to the shoulders of the deep rhytids temporal to the lateral canthal angle to achieve a greater effect on these wrinkles. The thicker skin of the rest of the face is treated with two passes.

Postoperative occlusive dressings may be placed; ice is used to minimize edema. The extent of postoperative erythema correlates well with the number of passes and with higher power setting. Erythema may take from several weeks to several months to dissipate, and in some cases longer. A green-based makeup may be used within a few days of treatment to camouflage redness. As already suggested, the major side effects of CO_2 laser resurfacing are persistent erythema, hyperpigmentation, hypopigmentation, hypertrophic scarring, herpes zoster reactivation, and bacterial infection.

Argon laser

The argon laser has been used successfully for the treatment of vascular skin lesions, pigmented skin lesions, and trichiasis. When stimulated by high voltage electricity, argon gas emits a blue-green light in the spectrum between 488 to 514 nm. This spectrum overlaps with the absorption spectrum of both hemoglobin and melanin, which absorb most of the argon laser energy applied to the skin. A small amount of energy is scattered throughout the skin and mucus membranes.

The argon laser is best used for ablating lesions in the skin and mucus membranes that contain melanin or hemoglobin. These molecules efficiently absorb argon laser energy and convert the energy to heat. This causes thermal damage to cells containing pigment and to the superficial cutaneous vasculature. The depth of thermal damage is directly proportional to the amount of vascularization or pigmentation in the treated area. A heavily pigmented tumor, for example, rapidly absorbs the laser energy and prevents its deeper penetration. Even in areas not heavily pigmented, the argon laser ablates to a depth of 1 to 2 mm. Consequently, the argon laser is more useful for superficial lesions, such as port wine stains, and less so for deep lesions, such as those found with the orbit.

Extreme caution should be used with the argon laser because it is readily absorbed by the retinal pigmented epithelium and can easily cause retinal damage if inadvertently directed into the eyes of the patient or operating room personnel. Therefore, the patient should wear protective contact lenses and all operating room personnel should wear protective glasses that absorb argon laser energy.

Trichiasis

The argon laser has been used successfully for the treatment of trichiasis. Epilation and electrolysis are also useful treatments, although each has its drawbacks. Epilation is usually temporizing because the lash follicle is unaffected and the lash grows back in 2 to 4 weeks [15]. Electrolysis, like the argon laser, is also a precise method for selectively ablating lashes, but its main drawback is a recurrence rate of nearly 50%. Cryotherapy has a success rate of 60% to 90% and is the treatment of choice for many patients; however, it is a grossly more destructive procedure that creates an inflammatory response. Cryotherapy has also been known to cause symblepharon formation and activation of herpes zoster [16]. It is best used in patients with extensive areas of trichiasis.

The argon laser has the advantage of allowing selective ablation of abnormal lashes while leaving adjacent normal lashes undisturbed [17]. This contrasts with cryotherapy, which is much less localized, involving larger areas of both normal and trichiatic lashes. The laser is also advantageous for patients in whom minimal inflammation is desired, such as those with Stevens–Johnson disease or ocular cicatricial pemphigoid.

The argon laser is set with a 50- to 100-µm spot size, 0.05 to 0.5 seconds, and powers that range from 300 mW to 1.5 W. Topical anesthesia with tetracaine drops may be used for most patients when the power setting is 1.0 W or less [18]. However, patients receiving close to 1.5 W per pulse may need infiltrative anesthesia to remain comfortable [19]. The globe is protected with a plastic shield and 15 to 60 laser pulses are applied to the base of each cilia. The eyelash shaft is destroyed first, forming a crater. The endpoint is reached when the ablation is at least 2 mm deep because this is where the lash follicle is located.

The success of initial therapy ranges from 59% to 93% and depends on the intensity of treatment [19–22, 23•,24]. A higher success rate may be achieved with higher powers of up to 1.5 W; however, this is attained at the dual expense of requiring infiltrating anesthesia and of risking a complication profile that includes eyelid dimpling and hypopigmentation of the lid margin. Furthermore, treating distichiasis is risky because laser applied to the marginal tarsus may cause severe eyelid notching [19]. Finally, a higher success rate is found when treating more focal trichiasis of less than 6 lashes. In sum, the argon laser is an excellent modality for treating focal trichiasis or trichiasis in any patient with a predisposition for an intense inflammatory response.

Port wine stain

The argon laser has been used by many surgeons for the treatment of port wine stains, a form of nevus flammeus. These are congenital vascular malformations that rarely regress. They may involve the periorbital skin as well as the skin of the rest of the face, forehead, occiput, and neck regions.

Skin involved in a port wine stain has varying amounts of abnormal vessels. In turn, the vessels themselves have varying amounts of circulating erythrocytes. Because the energy of the argon laser is largely absorbed by erythrocytes, the setting used on the laser varies greatly. Consequently, many surgeons first treat an inconspicuous area of a port wine stain with empiric test spots. The spot size is 0.5 to 1.0 mm and the power ranges from 1 to 5 W. Some patients require local anesthesia before treatment. Nonepinephrine-containing compounds should be used because epinephrine causes vasoconstriction, limiting the amount of hemoglobin target and preventing optimal treatment.

Skin blanches immediately after applying the laser. Some surgeons advocate chilling areas of skin before treatment as a way to improve results, theorizing that cooled dermal appendages resist collateral thermal damage. Over the next few days, extensive necrosis of the epidermis and dermis occurs. Within approximately 10 days, an eschar forms, loosens, and then falls off.

The congenitally abnormal vessels occlude over the 4 to 6 weeks after treatment.

Treated areas recanalize over subsequent months as the tissues undergo fibrosis in concert with the ingrowth of finer blood vessels. Treated skin can continue to lighten in appearance for 18 months after treatment with laser, although most of the effects are seen within the first 6 to 8 months [25]. The reported success rate for the argon laser is 60% to 75% [26]. Some clinical characteristics favor better clinical results; it seems that patients who are older and have darker purplish lesions tend to have better results than those who are younger and have pink lesions.

Capillary hemangioma

Capillary hemangiomas are difficult to excise surgically because of their tendency to bleed. The argon laser has been used successfully to remove such lesions on the upper lid [27,28]. The laser is set at a 1-mm spot size, 900 mW power, and a 1.0-second duration. A larger spot size seems to provide better hemostasis.

Punctal stenosis

The argon laser has been used near the punctum both for its recanalization and for its ablation. Punctal stenosis may be congenital or may be secondary to either traumatic or inflammatory insult. The argon laser has been used with settings of 200-μm spot size, 0.2-second exposure time, and up to 1500 mW of power to treat an occluded punctum [29]. The tissue overlying the punctum was treated repeatedly with the laser until it was vaporized, creating a crater that led to the medial wall of the canaliculus. The laser has also been used in patients with dry eyes to occlude puncta, but has been found to have only a small benefit because many more patients tend to recanalize compared with those treated with thermal occlusion [30,31].

Chloasma

Chloasma, or "the mask of pregnancy," is periorbital hyperpigmentation that occurs after pregnancy or with the use of oral contraceptives. Use of an argon laser may help blunt this hyperpigmentation. As with port wine stains, test shots are applied to choose a power setting and time of exposure empirically. A full treatment is given in 6 weeks if the patient has a good response to the test shots.

Phthiriasis pubis

Phthiriasis pubis, or crab louse, is a parasite that infects eyelashes. The louse is either in the form of a nit or an adult parasite. Traditional treatment consists of application with a petroleum ointment that smothers the adult parasite but is ineffective in killing the nit.

The argon laser has been used to kill phthiriasis pubis in one sitting by identifying the crab lice and killing them individually [32]. The laser can be set at a 200-μm spot size, 0.1-second exposure time, and 200 mW of power. Applying the laser to the junction of the louse's head and neck kills it. Application of the laser to the nit kills it as well, thereby minimizing the risk of recurrence.

Blepharopigmentation

Blepharopigmentation for cosmetic purposes involves implanting iron oxide pigment into eyelid skin near the lid margin. The argon laser can be used as a tool to remove pigment when it is no longer wanted [33]. The laser is set with a 50-μm spot size, 0.5-second exposure time, and between 300 to 800 mW of power. The purpose of the treatment is to create a 2- to 3-mm wide groove in the skin, ablating the pigmented area, and allowing the wound to heal by secondary intention. The true safety and efficacy of this treatment have not been determined.

YTTRIUM-ALUMINUM-GARNET LASERS

There are various forms of yttrium-aluminum-garnet (YAG) lasers including neodymium (Nd):YAG, holmium (Ho):YAG, and potassium-titanyl-phosphate (KTP):YAG. These lasers emit light near the infrared wavelengths (*eg*, Nd:YAG emits at 1060 nm). These wavelengths are absorbed mainly by protein; therefore, the YAG laser used on skin causes diffuse thermal damage as protein absorbs and scatters the laser energy. Consequently, the YAG laser is an imprecise instrument for tissues around the eye but is extremely effective in providing hemostasis [34].

The fiberoptic delivery system may be fitted with a sapphire tip that allows the surgeon to contact the delivery system to tissue. This tip provides a form of tactile sensation not offered by other lasers that is closer to the feel of a surgical scalpel [35]. An incision created with a YAG laser is not as strong in the first few weeks as one created with a scalpel. After 4 weeks, however, the tensile strength of the wound is nearly the same regardless of the modality used. Moreover, because the YAG laser does not shrink tissue, the wound can heal with minimal stress.

Dacryocystorhinostomy

Conventional dacryocystorhinostomy (DCR) with an external approach is a time honored, highly successful approach to nasolacrimal duct obstruction with a success rate of better than 90%. However, despite its popularity with many surgeons, it has drawbacks. It creates an external scar, may alter the medial canthal tendon structures, requires a certain recovery period for the resolution of postoperative edema and ecchymosis, and has significant intraoperative and postoperative risk for bleeding (sometimes sufficiently to necessitate a blood transfusion). For these reasons, some surgeons have turned to laser DCR.

Hornblass has used the surface contact YAG laser to make the skin incision, create a bony osteotomy, make nasal mucosal flaps, and make lacrimal sac flaps. Such an approach reduces the risk of intraoperative and postoperative bleeding. However, the cutaneous scar can be prominent, most probably as a consequence of the collateral thermal damage produced by the YAG laser.

Woog *et al.* [36] describe a technique of laser-assisted DCR with an endonasal approach. The patient is anesthetized with a nasal gauze soaked in 4% cocaine solution inserted into the nose. To minimize mucosal congestion, a solution of 1% lidocaine with epinephrine 1:100,000 is injected submucosally at the middle turbinate and in the lateral nasal wall anterior to the middle turbinate. After lacrimal punctal dilation, a 20-gauge fiberoptic light probe is threaded into the lacrimal sac. The lateral nasal wall is thereby transilluminated, helping to localize the lacrimal sac fossa.

The YAG laser is then inserted into the nose and guided to the area of transillumination along the lateral nasal wall. The laser is set between 0.5 to 1.0 J per pulse and delivered at a rate between 5 and 10 pulses per second. Each pulse has a duration of 250 ms and the power can range anywhere from 2.5 to 17 w. The laser energy is delivered through a quartz fiber tip 400 μm in diameter that is attached to the laser handpiece. Lower powers and pulse rates are used to remove nasal mucosa and higher settings are used to remove bone.

An intranasal burr or small rongeurs can facilitate removal of charred tissue and enlarge the osteotomy site, particularly in the area of the thicker anterior lacrimal crest. The osteotomy is enlarged to about 10 mm in diameter. Next, the medial wall of the lacrimal sac is identified, exposed, and removed either with the laser or with angled endoscopic forceps. This opening is enlarged to 10 mm as well. Both canaliculi are intubated with silicone tubes after the common internal punctum has been visualized with the endoscope. A C-Flex catheter may be placed at the common internal punctum as a sleeve to keep the silicone stents in place. The tubes are brought through the osteotomy and tied together with nylon sutures.

The success rate of endoscopic laser DCR is between 70% and 82%, which is lower than that of external DCR [37–39]. However, laser DCR offers the advantages of no external scar, faster recovery, and improved hemostasis.

Other authors have advocated using the YAG and other lasers to perform DCRs with a transcanalicular approach [40,41]. The main benefit to such an approach is that the laser energy is directed away from the globe and toward the nose, reducing the risk for injury to the globe. The main limitation of this technique is that, with laser tips small enough to thread into the canaliculus, it is very difficult to create bony osteotomies in adequate sizes.

Skin resurfacing

The erbium (Er):YAG laser has garnered attention for its use in skin resurfacing. This laser, at a wavelength of 2940 nm, resembles the CO_2 laser because it is readily absorbed by water [42]. However, the laser energy is also readily absorbed by collagen. Thus, as opposed to the CO_2 laser, the Er:YAG laser's energy is confined to a much smaller area of tissue [43,44]. Clinically, this may translate into a lower risk of side effects. Erythema or changes in pigmentation may be less likely with the Er:YAG laser if it affects tissue with less collateral thermal damage, making it an attractive instrument for laser skin resurfacing [45,46]. Further clinical studies are needed to assess this laser's efficacy in removing rhytids.

OTHER LASERS

The pulsed dye laser is a tunable laser that can be set at 580 nm to allow selective absorption by blood vessels. This wavelength maximizes absorption by oxyhemoglobin and minimizes absorption by melanin so that skin can be efficiently penetrated, helping to lower the risk of postoperative pigment changes or scarring. At the same time, blood vessels selectively absorb the laser energy and are coagulated.

This laser has been used successfully for treating periorbital port wine stains [47–49] and facial telangiectasis [50]. For port wine stains, the laser is set at 585-nm wavelength, a 450-ms duration, and a 5-mm spot size. An improvement of about 50% is seen with the first treatment, and 10% with each successive treatment. The settings for treating telangiectasis are 577-nm wavelength, 300-ms duration, and a 5-mm spot size. With such settings, more than 90% of patients need only a single treatment.

In direct contrast to the pulsed dye laser, the Q-switched ruby laser at 694 nm is selectively absorbed by pigment. A 20- to 40- nanosecond pulse duration matches the thermal relaxation time for melanosomes so that the energy is confined to the pigmented target. The ruby laser has been shown to be very useful in treating pigmented lesions such as the nevus of Ota [51], café-au-lait macules, and tattoos [52].

REFERENCES AND RECOMMENDED READING

Recently published papers of particular interest have been highlighted as:

- • Of interest
- •• Of outstanding interest

1. Kennerdell JS, Maroon JC, Garrity JA, *et al.*: Surgical management of orbital lymphangioma with the carbon dioxide laser. *Am J Ophthalmol* 1986, 102:308–314.
2. Jordan DR, Anderson RL: Carbon dioxide laser therapy for conjunctival lymphangioma. *Ophthalmic Surg* 1981, 18:728–730.
3. Baker SS, Muenzler WS, Small RG, *et al.*: Carbon dioxide laser blepharoplasty. *Ophthalmology* 1984, 91:238–244.
4. David LM, Sanders G: CO_2 laser blepharoplasty: a comparison to cold steel and electrocautery. *J Dermatol Surg Oncol* 1987, 13:110–114.
5. Baker SS, Pham RT: Lateral canthal suspension using the carbon dioxide laser. A modified technique. *Dermatol Surg* 1995, 21:107–113.
6. • Baker SS: Carbon dioxide laser ptosis surgery combined with blepharoplasty. *Dermatol Surg* 1995, 21:1065–1070.

The author describes a useful technique developed using the CO_2 laser on 82 patients with ptosis. He shows the efficacy of using the laser for ptosis correction combined with blepharoplasty.

7. Apfelberg DB, Maser MR, Lash II, *et al.*: Treatment of xanthelasma palpebrarum with the carbon dioxide laser. *J Dermatol Surg Oncol* 1987, 13:149–151.
8. Gladstone GJ, Beckman H, Elson LM, *et al.*: CO_2 laser excision of xanthelasma lesions. *Arch Ophthalmol* 1985, 103:440–442.
9. Ullmann Y, Har-Shai Y, Peled IJ: The use of CO_2 laser for the treatment of xanthelasma palpebrarum. *Ann Plast Surg* 1993, 31:504–507.
10. Wesley RE, Bond JB: Carbon dioxide laser in ophthalmic plastic and orbital surgery. *Ophthalmic Surg* 1985, 16:631–633.
11. Korn EL: Laser chalazion removal. *Ophthalmic Surg* 1988, 19:428–431.
12. Takizawa T, Yamazaki T, Miura N, *et al.*: Laser surgery of basal, orbital and ventricular meningiomas which are difficult to extirpate by conventional methods. *Neurol Med Chir* 1980, 20:729–737.
13. Wheeland RG, Bailin PL, Reynolds OD, *et al.*: Carbon dioxide (CO_2) laser vaporization of multiple facial syringomas. *J Dermatol Surg Oncol* 1986, 12:225–228.
14. Apfelberg DB, Maser MR, Lash H, *et al.*: Superpulse CO_2 laser treatment of facial syringomata. *Lasers Surg Med* 1987, 7:533–537.
15. Bartley GB, Bullock JD, Olsen TG, *et al.*: An experimental study to compare methods of eyelash ablation. *Ophthalmology* 1987, 94:1286–1289.
16. Wood JR, Anderson RL: Complications of cryosurgery. *Arch Ophthalmol* 1981, 99:460–463.
17. Berry J: Recurrent trichiasis: treatment with laser photocoagulation. *J Ophthalmic Surg* 1979, 10:36–38.
18. Arwan KJ: Argon laser treatment of trichiasis. *J Ophthalmic Surg* 1986, 17:658–660.
19. Gossman D, Yung R, Berlin J, *et al.*: Prospective evaluation of the argon laser in the treatment of trichiasis. *Ophthalmic Surg* 1992, 23:183–187.
20. Campbell DC: Thermoablation treatment for trichiasis using the argon laser. *Aust N Z J Ophthalmol* 1990, 18:427–430.
21. Huneke JW: Argon laser treatment for trichiasis. *Ophthalmic Plast Reconstr Surg* 1992, 8:50–55.
22. Bartley GB, Lowry JC: Argon laser treatment of trichiasis. *Am J Ophthalmol* 1992, 113:71–74.
23. • Elder MJ: The true rate of success in argon laser eyelash thermoablation. *Ophthalmic Surg Lasers* 1996, 27:888–890.

The author mathematically describes the true rate of recurrence per eyelash treated and gives support for the use of the argon laser in treating trichiasis. He bases his conclusion on the true rate of the laser's success, the minimal inflammation it generates, and the precision with which it can be applied.

24. Ladas ID, Karamaounas N, Vergados J, *et al.*: Use of argon laser photocoagulation in the treatment of recurrent trichiasis: long-term results. *Ophthalmologica* 1993, 207:90–93.
25. Wisnicki JL: Hemangiomas and vascular malformations. *Ann Plast Surg* 1984, 12:41–59.
26. Apfelberg DB: Argon laser treatment of port wine hemangiomas: summary of 10 years experience. In *Symposium on Vascular Malformations and Melanotic Lesions*. Edited by Williams HB. St. Louis: CV Mosby, 1983:95–100.
27. Gladstone GJ, Beckman H: Argon laser treatment of an eyelid margin capillary hemangioma. *Ophthalmic Surg* 1983, 14:944–946.
28. Hobby LW: Further evaluation of the potential of the argon laser in the treatment of strawberry hemangiomas. *Plast Reconstr Surg* 1983, 71:481–489.
29. Awan KJ: Laser punctoplasty for the treatment of punctal stenosis. *Am J Ophthalmol* 1985, 100:341–342.
30. Benson DR, Hemmady PB, Snyder RW: Efficacy of laser punctal occlusion. *Ophthalmology* 1992, 99:618–621.
31. Vrabec MP, Elsing SH, Aitken PA: A prospective randomized comparison of thermal cautery and argon laser for permanent punctal occlusion. *Am J Ophthalmol* 1993, 116:469–471.
32. Awan KJ: Argon laser phototherapy of phthiriasis palpebrarum. *Ophthalmic Surg* 1986, 17:813–814.
33. Tanenbaum M, Karas S, McCord CD: Laser ablation of blepharopigmentation. *Ophthalmic Plast Reconstr Surg* 1988, 4:49–56.

34. Peyman GA, Katoh N, Tawakol M, *et al*: Contact Nd:YAG laser for use in oculoplastic surgery. *Jpn J Ophthalmol* 1987, 31:635–645.

35. Diakuzono N, Joffe SN: Artificial sapphire probe for contact photocoagulation and tissue vaporization with the Nd:YAG laser. *Med Instrum* 1985, 19:173–178.

36. Woog JJ, Metson R, Puliafito CA: Holmium:YAG endonasal laser dacryocystorhinostomy. *Am J Ophthalmol* 1993, 116:1–10.

37. Kong YT, Kim TI, Kong BW: A report of 131 cases of endoscopic laser lacrimal surgery. *Ophthalmology* 1994, 101:1793–1800.

38. Boush GA Lemke BN, Dortzbach RK: Results of endonasal laser-assisted dacryocystorhinostomy. *Ophthalmology* 1994, 101:955–959.

39. Metson R, Woog JJ, Puliafito CA: Endoscopic laser dacryocystorhinostomy. *Laryngoscope* 1994, 104:269–274.

40. Levin PS, Stormo-Gipson J: Endocanalicular laser-assisted dacryocystorhinostomy. *Arch Ophthalmol* 1992, 110:1488–1490.

41. Silkiss RZ, Axelrod RN, Iwach AG, *et al.*: Transcanalicular THC:YAG dacryocystorhinostomy. *Ophthalmic Surg* 1992, 23:351–353.

42. Walsh JT, Deutsch TF: Er:YAG laser ablation: measurement of ablation rates. *Lasers Surg Med* 1989, 9:327–337.

43. Walsh JT, Flutte TJ, Deutsche TF: Er:YAG laser ablation of tissue: pulse duration and tissue type on thermal damage. *Lasers Surg Med* 1989, 314–326.

44. Hohenleuter HH: Fast and effective skin ablation: Er:YAG determination of ablation rates and thermal damage zones. *Lasers Surg Med* 1997, 20:242–247.

45. Khatri K: Comparison of erbium YAG and CO_2 lasers on wrinkle removal. *Lasers Surg Med Suppl* 1997, 9:1–66.

46. Ziering LL: Cutaneous laser resurfacing with the erbium YAG laser and the char-free carbon dioxide laser: a clinical comparison of 100 patients. *Int J Aesthet Restor Surg* 1997, 5:29–37.

47. Holy A, Geronemus RG: Treatment of periorbital port-wine stains with the flashlamp-pumped pulsed dye laser. *Arch Ophthalmol* 1992, 110:793–797.

48. Goldman MP, Fitzpatrick RE, Ruiz-Esparza J: Treatment of port-wine stains (capillary malformation) with the flashlamp-pumped pulsed dye laser. *J Pediatr* 1993, 122:71–77.

49. Alster TS, Wilson F: Treatment of port-wine stains with the flashlamp-pumped pulsed dye laser: extended clinical experience in children and adults. *Ann Plast Surg* 1994, 32:478–484.

50. Gonzalez E, Gange RW, Momtaz KT: Treatment of telangiectases and other benign vascular lesions with the 577 nm pulsed dye laser. *J Am Acad Dermatol* 1992, 27:220–226.

51. Chasy CJ, Nelson JS, Achauer BM: Q-switched ruby laser treatment of oculodermal melanosis (nevus Ota). *Plast Reconstr Surg* 1996, 98:784–790.

52. Tse Y, Levine VJ, McClain SA, *et al.*: The removal of cutaneous pigmented lesions with the Q-switched ruby laser and the Q-switched neodymium: yttrium-aluminum-garnet laser. A comparative study. *J Dermatol Surg Oncol* 1994, 20:795–800.

CHAPTER 4

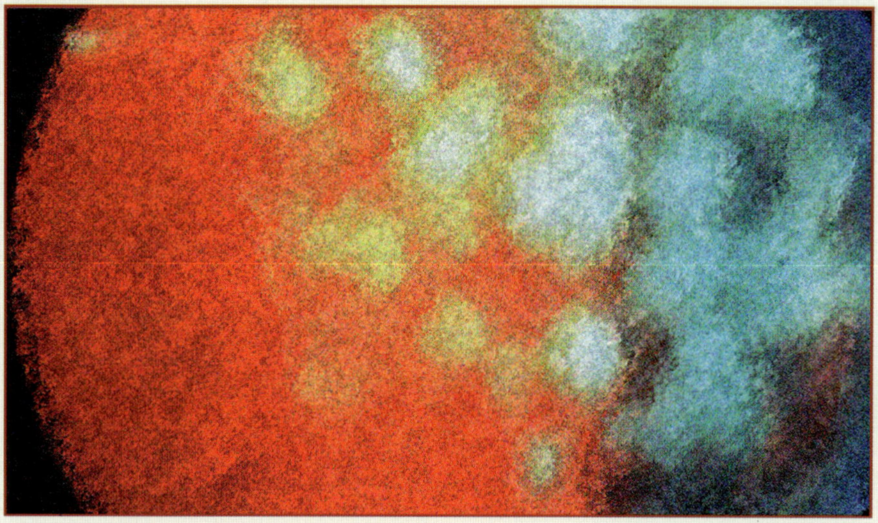

Lasers in the Treatment of Proliferative Retinopathies

SCOTT D. PENDERGAST
LAWRENCE J. SINGERMAN
HERNANDO ZEGARRA
JOHN H. NIFFENEGGER

Proliferative retinopathies represent a broad spectrum of retinal vascular diseases and are characterized by retinal ischemia and neovascularization of the posterior segment. Neovascularization can involve the optic disc or can emanate from retinal vessels, in particular, retinal veins. Although the pathophysiology of retinal neovascularization is not fully understood, retinal ischemia is a primary factor shared by an array of retinal disorders associated with the development of neovascularization. After neovascularization of the posterior segment has occurred, sight-threatening complications can ensue, *eg*, vitreous hemorrhage and tractional retinal detachment of the macula or peripheral retina. Before the development of laser photocoagulation, no effective treatment was available for proliferative retinopathies; today, laser therapy remains the safest and most effective form of treatment for this group of retinal disorders.

In the first section of this chapter we review characteristics of various lasers as well as the rationale for using laser photocoagulation in the treatment of the proliferative retinopathies. The second section highlights indications, treatment guidelines, and complications of photocoagulation in proliferative diabetic retinopathy (PDR) and other important retinal vascular diseases responsible for neovascularization. Previous studies that have expanded our knowledge of these disorders, particularly prospective randomized trials, are mentioned, but more recent studies, published between 1992 and the present, are emphasized.

LASERS AND WAVELENGTH SELECTION

Although photocoagulation has been employed for over 40 years to produce chorioretinal lesions for treatment of various retinal conditions, it was not until the late 1960s that Aiello *et al.* [1] reported scatter treatment with a ruby laser (694 nm) for management of PDR. In 1971, the argon laser (emitting at 488 and 514 nm) became commercially available and virtually replaced the ruby laser, owing to its more favorable wavelength and the fact that it emits blue-green light continuously. The Diabetic Retinopathy Study Research Group [2] clearly demonstrated the efficacy of scatter argon laser and xenon photocoagulation in reducing the risk of severe visual loss (defined as visual acuity of 5/200 or less) in patients with PDR. In this study, eyes treated with xenon photocoagulation had greater visual field loss and were more likely to lose two to four lines of visual acuity compared with eyes treated with argon laser. However, a subsequent study that used less extensive xenon photocoagulation did not show a higher incidence of complications in xenon-treated eyes [3]. Although xenon lasers have been superseded by argon and solid-state lasers in the United States, xenon arc devices are effective in the treatment of proliferative retinopathies and are still employed elsewhere.

As our understanding of the pathophysiology and treatment of proliferative retinopathies has evolved, and lasers that emit at various wavelengths have become available, interest has been increasing in the theoretical and practical advantages of specific wavelengths and laser systems for the treatment of proliferative retinopathies and macular disorders. The therapeutic effect of photocoagulation is achieved by converting light energy to thermal energy through absorption at a specific tissue site. In the case of retinal photocoagulation, the principal light absorbers are melanin, xanthophyll, and hemoglobin. Melanin best absorbs all wavelengths used for retinal photocoagulation. Because its extinction coefficient gradually decreases with increasing wavelength, deeper chorioretinal burns result from increasing wavelengths [4]. Xanthophyll is located in the inner and outer plexiform layers and concentrated in the macula. Macular xanthophyll absorbs blue light well and results in undesirable neurosensory retinal damage. Thus, argon blue-green laser (488 nm) has been superseded by higher wavelengths, such as argon green (514 nm), which absorbs xanthophyll poorly, and krypton laser (647 nm), which is not absorbed by xanthophyll. Hemoglobin absorbs blue, green, and yellow light well and absorbs red (647 nm) and infrared wavelengths (810 nm) poorly.

Based on the light-scattering properties of the ocular media (cornea and lens) as well as the absorption properties of pigmented structures in the retina, wavelengths between 510 and 600 nm are considered most favorable. For these wavelengths, melanin absorption is excellent, xanthophyll absorption in the inner retina is relatively low, and attenuation of radiation by the ocular media (cornea, lens, and vitreous hemorrhage, if present) is limited. Based on these considerations as well as laboratory investigations, several authors have concluded that a wavelength of 577 nm (yellow) is optimal. In our practice, we frequently use this wavelength to treat proliferative retinopathies when a tunable dye laser is available. However, histologic studies have shown similar tissue effects across a broad range of wavelengths and clinical studies have demonstrated similar clinical efficacy of xenon arc, argon, dye yellow, krypton, and diode lasers. Various authors have found the longer wavelengths (*eg*, yellow, krypton) to be advantageous in older patients with cataracts or if vitreous hemorrhage is present—situations in which treatment with argon green laser can be problematic [5,6•].

Argon, krypton, and tunable dye lasers

Early seminal studies established the efficacy of argon green laser for the treatment of proliferative retinopathies, including PDR and branch retinal vein occlusion. In addition, argon green laser has been shown to be effective in the management of choroidal neovascularization and diabetic macular edema. Owing to its versatility and proven efficacy for the treatment of retinal vascular disorders, argon green laser remains the most commonly used laser in the United States. In the mid 1970s, shortly after the introduction of argon green laser, the krypton laser was introduced as a red-light–emitting laser. More recently, variable wavelength (organic dye) lasers enabled the photocoagulator to rapidly tune the desired wavelength to facilitate the targeting of specific tissues (Fig. 4-1). Although krypton and tunable dye lasers have been shown to be as effective as argon green, no studies have demonstrated a significant difference in clinical efficacy among these modalities.

Diode laser

In the middle and late 1980s, advances in semiconductor technology led to the development of diode lasers emitting infrared wavelengths (790 to 950 nm). McHugh *et al.* [7] were the first to report results of diode laser in the treatment of retinal vascular disease. They successfully treated 33 eyes affected by PDR, diabetic macular edema, or retinal vein occlusion complicated by neovascularization using a diode laser emitting at 810 nm. More recent studies have established the efficacy of diode laser photocoagulation for the treatment of PDR [8] and retinopathy of prematurity (ROP) [9,10•]. A potential disadvantage of the diode laser is that higher power settings are needed to achieve uptake compared with those at 514 nm and 532 nm wavelengths [11]. This requirement, coupled with the deeper penetration of the near-infrared wavelength, can result in significant patient discomfort and may necessitate retrobulbar anesthesia.

Although a wavelength of 810 nm falls outside the optimal window of 510 to 600 nm, the diode laser offers some important ergonomic advantages. Argon, krypton, and tunable dye lasers rely on relatively bulky gas–ion tubes to generate a continuous laser wavelength. Given the low electrical–optical conversion efficiency, electrical energy consumption is high and forced cooling of the units by circulating water is necessary. As a result, these units tend to be large and require permanent installation. In contrast, laser energy for diode lasers is generated by gallium-aluminum-arsenide laser diodes. This solid-state laser has standard voltage requirements, weighs under 10 kg, has no external cooling requirements, and has power output of up to 3 W. Like argon laser, delivery systems include the slit lamp, indirect ophthalmoscope, and endolaser probes (Fig. 4-2). In addition, near-infrared wavelengths have the ability to penetrate the sclera and achieve uptake in the retinal pigment epithelium (RPE) and choroid. Transscleral probes are commercially available and have been used to perform transscleral retinopexy [12,13,14•]. Given its relatively low cost, durability, and compact size, use of the diode laser has increased dramatically over the past several years.

A very recent and promising application of semiconductor technology involves a diode-pumped solid-state laser (Fig. 4-3). This system uses a diode laser pump source to produce a near-infrared wavelength of 808 nm. A laser crystal converts this wavelength to 1064

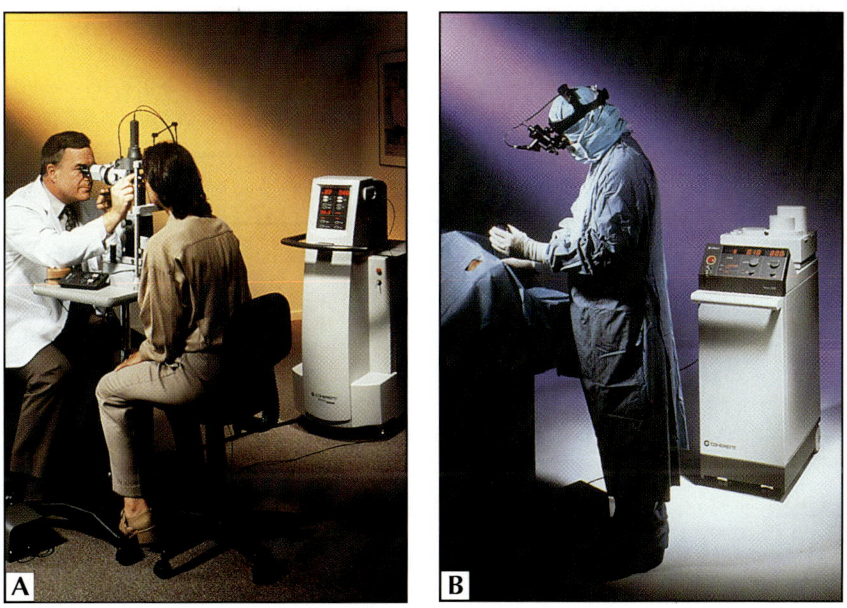

FIGURE 4-1. A, The Coherent Novus Omni laser mounted on a slit lamp allows instantaneous selection of green (521 nm), yellow (568 nm), and red (647 nm) wavelengths. **B**, The Coherent Novus 2000 laser (emitting blue-green or green wavelengths) is being used with a laser indirect ophthalmoscope in the operating room. (*Courtesy of* Coherent, Palo Alto, CA.)

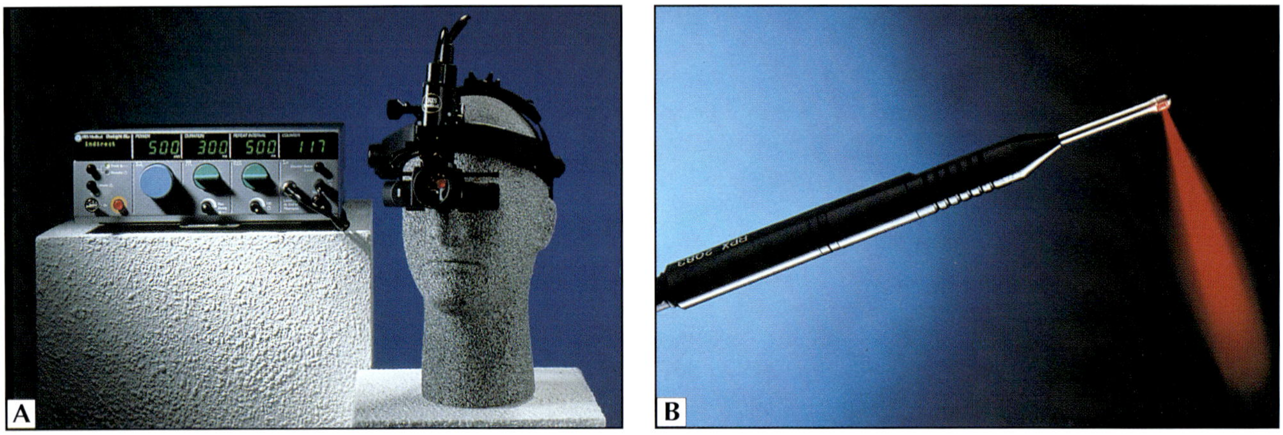

FIGURE 4-2. Ophthalmic diode lasers. **A**, Diode laser indirect ophthalmoscope. **B**, The Diopexy probe (Iris Medical, Mountain View, CA) for transscleral peripheral retinal photocoagulation.

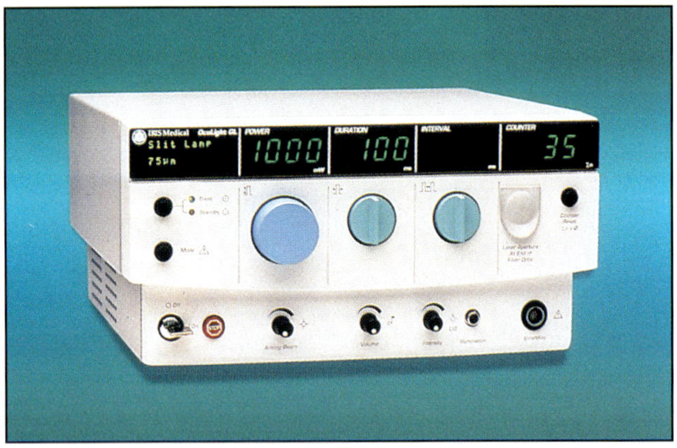

FIGURE 4-3. The Oculight GL solid-state laser delivers a 532-nm green wavelength. (Iris Medical, Mountain View, CA.)

nm and a doubling crystal produces a final wavelength of 532 nm. Thus, a green wavelength is now available that affords the ergonomic advantages inherent in a solid-state laser system.

Neodymium:yttrium-aluminum-garnet laser

The Q-switched neodymium:yttrium-aluminum-garnet (Nd:YAG) laser, emitting at 1064 nm, has been used extensively for approximately 15 years by surgeons operating in the anterior segment. Rather than emitting light that is absorbed by pigments and converted to thermal energy to destroy target tissues, the Nd:YAG laser produces high energy pulses of laser energy concentrated in time and space, resulting in tissue "photodisruption." This property has led investigators to use the Nd:YAG laser to perform successful membranotomies to treat subinternal limiting membrane hemorrhages [15,16] and to divide vitreous strands (vitreolysis) for recurrent vitreous hemorrhage and tractional retinal detachments involving or threatening the macula [17].

Continuous-wave Nd:YAG lasers enabled photocoagulators to produce thermal effects and have been used to treat PDR [18]. However, a recent controlled study found Nd:YAG (1064 nm) panretinal photocoagulation (PRP) to be ineffective for the treatment of PDR [19]. In 1988, Jalkh *et al.* [20] introduced the frequency-doubled Nd:YAG photocoagulation system. Using a potassium-titamyl-phosphate crystal, this solid-state laser produces a 532-nm monochromatic green wavelength by the doubling the frequency of a 1064-nm Nd:YAG wavelength. The efficacy and convenience of this laser have been documented in recent studies [21,22].

RATIONALE OF PHOTOCOAGULATION THERAPY FOR PROLIFERATIVE RETINOPATHIES

The pathophysiology of neovascularization is complex; a comprehensive discussion of the various mechanisms thought to play a role is beyond the scope of this chapter. Despite intensive research efforts, the exact pathogenesis of retinal neovascularization remains unclear. General agreement exists that retinal neovascularization is a nonspecific programmed response to chronic retinal hypoxia. A feature common to the proliferative retinopathies is capillary closure with resultant retinal ischemia and the release of a soluble angiogenic substance that induces neovascularization of the iris, retina, or optic nerve. Various hormones and growth factors have been implicated in the development of retinal neovascularization, including insulin-like growth factor [23], growth hormone [24], tumor necrosis factor-α [25], and basic fibroblast growth factor [26].

More recently, interest has been considerable in an endothelial cell-specific mitogen and angiogenic protein called vascular endothelial growth factor (VEGF). In 1994, Aiello *et al.* [27] observed elevated levels of VEGF in PDR and other ischemic retinal disorders. Subsequent studies showed that intraocular injection of VEGF could induce neovascularization of the iris [28] as well as retinal ischemia and microangiopathy in nonhuman primates [29•]. Furthermore, inhibition of VEGF in animal models suppresses neovascularization of the retina [30,31] and iris [32]. Finally, it has been shown that expression of VEGF is regulated by oxygen levels: VEGF mRNA expression is up-regulated under hypoxic conditions [33] and down-regulated by hyperoxia [34].

Panretinal photocoagulation, by modulating retinal blood flow and retinal oxygenation, may induce regression of neovascularization by one of several mechanisms. In diabetic retinopathy, for example, retinal blood flow alterations and loss of local autoregulation are well described in the literature [35]. Presumably, these circulatory abnormalities represent compensatory mechanisms responding to retinal hypoxia. Following PRP, retinal vasoconstriction with a significant reduction in retinal blood flow occurs [36,37]. Similarly, regional retinal blood flow has been shown to decrease following scatter photocoagulation [38]. In addition, previous studies have demonstrated local increases in preretinal oxygen tensions in regions overlying photocoagulated outer retina in animal models [39•,40] and in patients with PDR [41].

The mechanism for the regression of neovascularization following photocoagulation appears to be related to the restoration of inner retinal hypoxia and abnormal retinal blood flow, as well as its effect on retinal metabolism. Previous authors have theorized that destruction of the high-oxygen-consuming photoreceptor–RPE complex facilitates diffusion of oxygen from the choriocapillaris directly to the inner retina, thereby eliminating the hypoxic stimulus [42]. Retinal vasoconstriction following PRP correlates with regression of disc neovascularization and probably occurs in response to increased oxygenation [43]. Thus, responses in retinal blood flow [36] and retinal vasoconstriction are parameters that may be useful in assessing response to PRP.

An additional mechanism that may play an important role in the regression of neovascularization following photocoagulation involves release of an inhibitor of neovascularization by RPE cells. In 1985, Glaser *et al.* [44] identified a substance produced by RPE cells that prevents growth of new vessels and inhibits proliferation of vascular endothelial cells. More recent studies have shown that photocoagulation of cultured human RPE cells results in increased production of transforming growth factor-β_2, a growth factor that has been shown to inhibit vascular endothelial cell proliferation in vitro [45].

TREATMENT OF PROLIFERATIVE RETINOPATHIES

Diabetic retinopathy

It is estimated that of the 16 million people with diabetes in the United States, approximately half suffer from diabetic retinopathy. Each year 65,000 Americans progress to PDR and 24,000 new cases of blindness result due to complications of diabetic retinopathy, making it the leading cause of visual loss in working-age Americans [46]. Before development of laser photocoagulation, the vast majority of patients who developed PDR progressed to blindness because the only form of treatment available was pituitary ablation—a procedure associated with significant complications. The beneficial effect of laser photocoagulation has been quite dramatic, reducing the rate of blindness by over 90%. Although tight control of blood glucose levels has been proven to slow progression and reduce severity of PDR [47], laser photocoagulation is the safest and most effective form of treatment available to treat PDR after neovascularization has been established.

Indications for treatment

The Diabetic Retinopathy Study [2] was a multicenter randomized prospective clinical trial begun in 1971 to investigate whether laser photocoagulation could prevent severe visual loss (visual acuity less than 5/200 on two consecutive visits) in the eyes of 1758 patients with PDR. This study demonstrated a 60% reduction in severe visual loss in eyes treated with PRP versus untreated eyes. A later study identified a subgroup of eyes with "high risk" characteristics: 1) neovascularization of the disc of moderate to severe degree (measuring approximately one third of the disc areas in size or larger); 2) any neovascularization of the disc associated with preretinal or vitreous hemorrhage; and 3) neovascularization elsewhere of moderate to severe degree (occupying greater than half the disc area) if associated with preretinal or vitreous hemorrhage [48]. The Diabetic Retinopathy Study group [2] concluded that eyes with such characteristics should be treated promptly with full scatter photocoagulation.

Although treatment guidelines for high-risk retinopathy are well established, the optimal management of eyes with early PDR and severe nonproliferative diabetic retinopathy (NPDR) is somewhat equivocal. The Early Treatment Diabetic Retinopathy Study [49] evaluated the effect of early PRP in eyes with mild to severe NPDR and early PDR (*ie*, less than high-risk PDR). Early treatment of non–high-risk eyes was associated with a small reduction in the rate of severe visual loss (2.6% versus 3.7%) and lowered the risk of requiring vitrectomy and progression of retinopathy compared with untreated eyes after 5 years of follow-up. Because adverse effects were observed in treated eyes immediately after treatment (*eg*, decreased visual acuity and visual field loss), the study did not recommend early scatter photocoagulation for eyes with mild or moderate NPDR provided careful follow-up could be maintained. For eyes with more severe retinopathy, the study recommended consideration of scatter photocoagulation.

In clinical practice, the timing of PRP in patients with non–high-risk PDR must be individualized. Eyes with rubeosis are generally treated promptly to prevent neovascular glaucoma. Many photocoagulators will treat patients demonstrating early PDR or severe NPDR, particularly under the following circumstances: 1) patients with a history of noncompliance or poor follow-up; 2) PDR developing during pregnancy; 3) moderate to severe NPDR in one eye and a history of severe PDR with visual loss in the fellow eye; 4) juvenile patients with diabetes; and 5) rapid progression of retinopathy. Most eyes with early PDR and severe NPDR will require treatment within 3 to 5 years and early treatment, even if limited, will often prevent progression of disease.

Initial treatment guidelines

We generally perform PRP using dye yellow or argon green wavelengths as discussed earlier. A wide-angle lens, such as the Rodenstock Panfunduscopic (G. Rodenstock Instrument GmBH, Munich, Germany) or the Volk Quadraspheric (Mentor, OH), provides an inverted and reversed view of the entire posterior pole and midperipheral retina. A Goldmann three-mirror lens can also be used, particularly for treating the peripheral retina, but care must taken to orient the lens appropriately to avoid inadvertent treatment of the macula. The Diabetic Retinopathy Study [2] protocol used 500-μm spots spaced one half to one burn width apart, and recommended approximately 1200 burns. However, most ophthalmologists today apply more extensive treatment, generally 1600 to 2000 burns in two or more sessions (Fig. 4-4). In patients with severe PDR, 2000 to 3000 applications are often necessary (Fig. 4-5). In the first session, we generally treat the inferior retina first in case the patient develops a vitreous hemorrhage before the next session—a complication that could prevent adequate treatment. The pulse duration is generally set at 0.05 to 0.2 seconds with a spot size of 400 to 500 μm spaced about one burn width apart. If a Rodenstock or Quadraspheric lens is used, the spot size selector on the rotating cylinder should be set on 300 to 350 μm to account for magnification effect. An initial power setting of 200 mW is used and increased incrementally until a burn of moderate intensity is achieved. Burns of excessive intensity can result in patient discomfort and increase the risk of adverse effects, such as rupture of Bruch's membrane, choroidal hemorrhage, choroidal effusions, and visual field loss [50]. The laser applications are placed at least one disc diameter nasal to the optic disc and at least two disc diameters temporal to the center of the fovea. However, it may advisable to treat more peripherally (*ie*, at least three disc diameters temporal to the center of the fovea) to prevent diminished retinal sensitivity in the 15° and 30° central visual field, particularly in eyes with less severe disease [50]. It is useful to demarcate the temporal border of the macu-

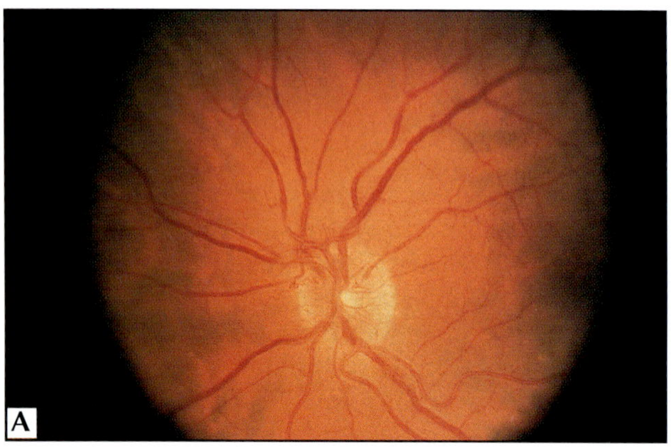

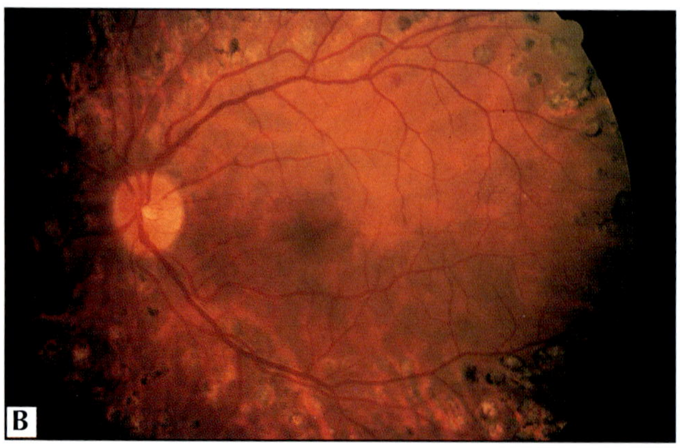

FIGURE 4-4. A, Left eye of a patient with proliferative diabetic retinopathy with neovascularization of the disk before treatment. **B**, Following moderate panretinal photocoagulation consisting of approximately 1500 burns, the neovascularization shows nearly complete regression.

la by placing several arcuate rows of burns to facilitate identification and prevent inadvertent treatment within the macula. After 800 to 1000 burns have been applied, the patient returns in 1 to 3 weeks for a second session, at which time the superior retina is treated. Because studies have linked capillary nonperfusion and ischemia in the midperipheral retina to retinal neovascularization [51], it is important to treat this region fully.

Indications and guidelines for supplemental treatment

No consensus exists regarding the optimal number of burns to achieve the desired goal of regression of neovascularization while minimizing adverse sequelae. Although PRP will ideally induce complete regression of neovascularization, frequently only a partial response is achieved (Fig. 4-4). For example, in the Diabetic Retinopathy Study [2], only 21% of treated eyes with moderate or severe neovascularization of the disc had complete regression of new vessels after 1 year. Various authors have evaluated the time course of regression of neovascularization following full PRP and have developed protocols concerning augmentation of laser treatment [52,53]. Doft and Blankenship [52] demonstrated that within 3 weeks of treatment, 72% of high-risk eyes showed regression to less than three risk factors. Furthermore, of the eyes that failed to show this early favorable response, 64% continued to have high-risk characteristics after 6 months of follow-up. Similar results have been shown in a later study, with regression or disappearance of neovascularization of the disc occurring in approximately 45% to 71% of eyes (response rate varies with severity of the disc neovascularization) 8 weeks after initial treatment and 36% to 60% of eyes after 2 years of follow-up [54].

In eyes with severe PDR that fail to respond to conventional PRP, some authors have suggested incremental, extensive PRP [53,55]. Vine [53] reported a series of 23 eyes with severe PDR that failed to respond to PRP of approximately 3000 burns. After incremental augmentation of about 1000 to 2000 burns per session every 6 to 8 weeks, almost half of the eyes eventually responded favorably after a mean of 7550 burns. Eyes that failed to respond tended to have a poor prognosis. Aylward *et al.* [55] reported similar results involving 28 eyes that required a mean of 7225 burns (and up to 11,513 burns) to achieve a favorable response. In a prospective randomized trial, 35 eyes that failed to respond to initial PRP were randomized to augmentation of PRP versus no supplemental treatment. Although faster regression was initially observed in the former group, no difference in retinopathy risk factors was observed after 1 year of follow-up [56]. Therefore, eyes with high-risk PDR should be treated with full PRP and monitored closely at 6 to 8 week intervals. If the disease stabilizes or improves, further observation is usually indicated. If existing neovascularization worsens, new neovascularization develops, or new vitreous hemorrhage occurs, supplemental or "fill-in" PRP should be considered.

The treatment technique for supplemental PRP is essentially the same as for initial treatment. A spot size of 400 to 500 µm is used and 700 to 1000 burns are placed between existing burns. Again, areas of elevated neovascularization, hemorrhage, and photocoagulation scars should be avoided. If necessary, the peripheral retina anterior to the equator can be treated using a laser-indirect ophthalmoscope with scleral depression, cryotherapy, or the recently developed transscleral diode laser probe [13,14]. In severe, resistant cases, one to two rows of 200-µm burns can be placed just

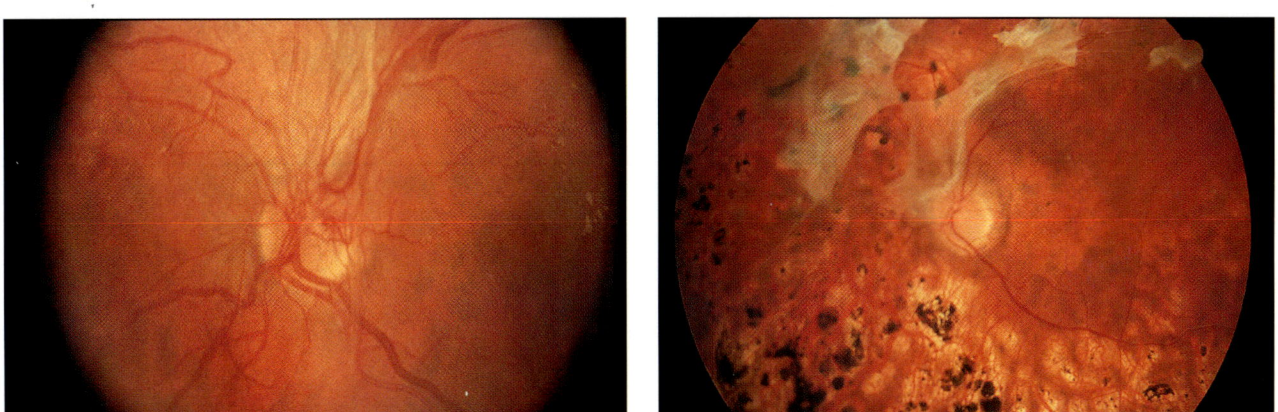

FIGURE 4-5. A, A patient with proliferative diabetic retinopathy with florid neovascularization of the disk and fibrovascular proliferation resulting in retinal traction superior to the disc. **B**, Following panretinal photocoagulation consisting of approximately 3000 burns, the neovascularization has regressed, leaving remnant fibroglial tissue superiorly.

inside the vascular arcades and treatment can be extended to within two disc diameters of the center of the fovea. Although 50% to 70% of resistant nonresponsive eyes improve following aggressive supplemental PRP with or without added cryoablation, some eyes ultimately require vitrectomy.

Complications

Decreased central visual acuity and visual field loss are the most common and significant complications following PRP. The Diabetic Retinopathy Study group [2] observed decreased visual acuity of two or more lines in 10% of eyes undergoing PRP and found it was much more common in the xenon-treated group compared with the group of eyes treated with the argon laser [2,57,58]. Similarly, visual field constriction occurred in 5% of eyes treated with argon laser and 50% of eyes in the xenon-treated group [58]. In addition, subjective complaints of nyctalopia were also described in these early studies and have been confirmed in dark adaptation studies [59].

More recent studies have documented decreased visual acuity following PRP due to the development or exacerbation of macular edema. In a series involving 175 consecutive eyes treated with PRP, McDonald and Shatz [60] reported increased macular edema in 43% of treated eyes 6 to 10 weeks following treatment. Persistent macular edema was observed in 27% of treated eyes, of which 33% had lost two or more lines of visual acuity. However, other authors report improvement in macular edema and visual acuity after PRP alone when peripheral PRP is performed in multiple sessions over several months in eyes with adequate macular perfusion [61]. In patients with PDR and macular edema, we frequently perform grid or focal macular photocoagulation before or at the time of PRP to prevent worsening of macular edema. In addition, burns should be applied more peripherally and intense treatment should be avoided, particularly in patients over age 50 who may be more likely to suffer worsening of macular edema following PRP.

Two less common causes of decreased visual acuity following PRP include inadvertent foveal burns and macular detachment. The former is a rare but potentially devastating complication and usually results from sudden eye movement during treatment. Occasionally, patients may require retrobulbar anesthesia to prevent excessive ocular movements during treatment. In addition, the photocoagulator must always be cognizant of the retinal landmarks and anatomy, particularly when using a three-mirror lens. Decreased visual acuity due to tractional detachment of the macula was reported by the Diabetic Retinopathy Study group [2] and was more frequently observed in eyes treated with xenon arc photocoagulation. Elliott and Flanagan [62] described macular detachment in 13 eyes after argon laser treatment for PDR. In most cases, these eyes were initially undertreated and subsequently underwent extensive treatment after progression of neovascular proliferation. Thus, early aggressive treatment may help prevent this complication.

Visual field loss is a common, predictable complication of PRP. Early reports documented some visual field dysfunction in most patients undergoing argon or xenon arc photocoagulation, with severe visual field loss occurring in patients treated with xenon arc [2]. In addition, studies have correlated the severity of visual field loss with the extent or distribution of laser photocoagulation [49,50,58,63]. Visual field impairment is sufficiently severe that 50% to 89% of patients fail to meet requirements of driving license tests, particularly patients treated with xenon laser [63]. Hulbert and Vernon [63] suggested that treating early PDR using 200-μm burns appears less likely to jeopardize driving license requirements. Interestingly, a more recent study documented the presence of decreased visual field sensitivity in patients with pre-PDR and early PDR prior to PRP [64]. Following standard PRP, significant impairment of visual fields occurred but subjective complaints were few and functional impairment was minimal.

Finally, several rare but potentially serious complications of scatter photocoagulation exist. In most cases, these complications are related to excessive burn intensity and can be prevented by employing appropriate parameters and avoiding direct treatment of pigmented areas or hemorrhage. Ciliary body and choroidal detachment have been reported following extensive photocoagulation applied in a single session [65]. In severe cases, massive choroidal effusions may occasionally result in angle-closure glaucoma [66]. In a recent study, Gentile *et al.* [67] identified low-lying ciliochoroidal effusions in 59% of eyes after PRP for PDR using ultrasound biomicroscopy. Risk factors associated with the development of choroidal effusion included number of laser applications, shorter axial length, and percentage of retinal surface area treated. Interestingly, low-lying ciliochoroidal detachment has been detected in 90% of diabetic eyes 3 days following sector PRP applied in a single quadrant (208 to 331 burns) [68]. In both studies the effusions spontaneously disappeared within 3 to 14 days in all cases.

Chorioretinal and choriovitreal neovascularization are rare complications of photocoagulation for proliferative retinopathies [69,70]. Histologic studies have demonstrated choroidal neovascularization passing through discontinuities in Bruch's membrane into the retina [71]. Disruption of Bruch's membrane was associated with areas of intense focal treatment. Treatment of chorioretinal neovascularization is frequently accompanied by increased growth of the vessels into the vitreous cavity with resulting vitreous hemorrhage [69,71,72]. Due to the futility and risk of re-treatment, laser photocoagulation of choroidal neovascularization in this setting should generally be avoided.

Retinal vein occlusions

Branch and central retinal vein occlusions represent a common cause of visual loss in older patients. Retinal vein occlusions frequently result in extensive capillary dropout and retinal ischemia, which stimulates neovascularization of the iris, retina, or optic disc. The clinical features and treatment strategies of complications related to retinal vein occlusions are discussed in Chapter 6.

Retinopathy of prematurity

Retinopathy of prematurity is a retinal vascular disorder affecting infants of low birth weight and short gestational age [73]. Other factors, most notably oxygen exposure, have also been implicated [74]. Very recently, missense mutations in the Norrie's disease gene have also been implicated in the pathogenesis of advanced ROP [75]. Incidence of ROP is increasing because survival rates for infants at the highest risk are increasing. In the multicenter Cryotherapy for ROP study [76], 65.8% of infants weighing less than 1251 g at birth showed evidence of some form of ROP, 16.5% had stage 3 disease, and 2.1% of infants developed unfavorable outcomes as defined later in this chapter. Despite advances in our understanding and management of ROP, it remains a leading cause of blindness in children in the United States.

The Cryotherapy for ROP study [76] was a multicenter prospective randomized trial that clearly demonstrated the benefit of peripheral cryoablation in eyes with threshold disease, defined as five or more contiguous or eight cumulative clock hours of stage 3 ROP in zone 1 or 2 in the presence of posterior retinal vascular dilation and tortuosity (plus disease). Cryotherapy reduced the incidence of adverse outcomes (*eg*, retinal fold involving the macula, retinal detachment involving the posterior pole, or retrolental mass) by approximately 50% [77]. The beneficial effect of cryotherapy for both structural and functional outcomes has been confirmed on long-term follow-up [78•].

Advantages of laser photocoagulation over cryotherapy

Although the benefits of cryoablation clearly outweigh the risks of treatment in eyes with threshold ROP, this form of therapy carries significant morbidity and is associated with significant ocular and systemic complications. Ocular complications include conjunctival laceration and subconjunctival and vitreous hemorrhage. In addition, cryotherapy typically causes severe lid edema and conjunctival chemosis that often last for several days. Bilateral massive proliferation of conjunctival tissue affecting visual development has also been reported following cryotherapy for ROP [79]. Due to the manipulation of the globe required to perform cryoablation, particularly in eyes with posterior disease, significant pain and exhaustion can result. Systemic complications, such as bradycardia, cyanosis, hypoxemia, and apnea are not uncommon during cryotherapy and occurred in approximately 10% of patients in the Cryotherapy for ROP study [80]. More severe complications, including respiratory and cardiopulmonary arrest, have also been reported. Recently, investigators have suggested that general anesthesia may reduce the risk of systemic complications during cryotherapy [81].

When an adequate indirect laser delivery system became available in the late 1980s, interest was immediate in applying this modality for the treatment of threshold ROP. The practical and theoretical advantages of laser photocoagulation include 1) decreased risk of ocular and systemic complications because less manipulation of the globe is required; 2) technical ease of laser therapy compared with cryotherapy, particularly in eyes with posterior disease; 3) less inflammation and vitreous contraction stimulated by cryoablation; and 4) less damage to adjacent structures. Finally, long-term studies have shown that eyes treated with cryotherapy have a significantly higher incidence of myopia and high myopia compared with eyes treated with laser [82•,83], and visual acuities tend to be reduced in eyes treated with cryotherapy compared with untreated fellow eyes that spontaneously regressed [78•]. In a small pilot study involving six patients undergoing cryotherapy in one eye and laser therapy in the fellow eye, mean visual acuities were 20/150 and 20/40, respectively [84].

Early studies demonstrated that peripheral argon laser photocoagulation was effective in treating threshold ROP and appeared to be as effective as cryotherapy [85,86]. Two independent prospective randomized studies showed that diode laser photocoagulation was at least as effective as cryotherapy in treating threshold ROP [9,10]. The Laser ROP Study Group [87] performed meta-analysis on 293 eyes treated with argon or diode laser photocoagulation for threshold ROP and reported a favorable result in 91.6% of eyes compared with 80.8% for eyes treated with cryotherapy.

Because of the significant ergonomic advantages of solid-state laser discussed earlier, use of diode laser photocoagulation for ROP has greatly expanded over the last several years. This modality allows treatment to be performed in the neonatal intensive care unit (NICU) in the presence of neonatologists and NICU support staff who deal with critically ill infants on a regular basis. In addition, diode lasers can be easily transported to multiple hospitals, thereby avoiding the risks and expense associated with transferring neonates to treatment centers.

Published studies have documented the advantages of laser therapy for posterior ROP [88,89]. Posterior ROP is generally defined as the presence of at least one clock hour (a 30° sector) of extraretinal fibrovascular proliferation within zone 1, defined as a circle centered on the optic disc with a radius of twice the distance from the disc to the fovea. In the Cryotherapy for ROP study [80], eyes with zone-1 disease responded poorly to cryotherapy—treatment only reduced the rate of unfavorable outcomes in eyes with posterior threshold ROP from 92% to 75% at 3 months of follow-up. In contrast, Capone *et al.* [89] reported favorable outcomes in 83% of eyes with zone 1 threshold ROP treated with diode laser. Diode laser has also been advocated for the early treatment of posterior ROP in an effort to prevent progression to more advanced stages. Fleming *et al.* [88] treated 18 eyes of nine infants with prethreshold posterior ROP, and none of the eyes developed unfavorable outcomes. A recent prospective multicenter randomized trial evaluated the role of indirect laser photocoagulation (argon or diode) for the treatment of prethreshold posterior ROP [90•]. Of the 19 eyes undergoing early treatment, 16% developed unfavorable outcomes compared with 18% in eyes treated after reaching threshold disease. Because the vast majority of untreated eyes progress to threshold disease within 1 week, early treatment should be considered. However, in situations in which an infant is too unstable to undergo early laser, no disadvantage seems to exist in delaying treatment until threshold ROP is reached.

Treatment guidelines

Laser photocoagulation for threshold ROP is performed on one or both eyes using either argon or diode laser through an indirect delivery system. The procedure can be performed in the NICU or the operating room under either general anesthesia or intravenous sedation. In either case, adequate analgesia must be achieved and vital signs and oxygenation status must be closely monitored during treatment. An infant lid speculum is inserted, and a cotton-tipped applicator or Flynn scleral depressor (Starz Instrument Co., St. Louis, MO) is useful for manipulating the eye and performing scleral depression to facilitate treatment of the anterior avascular retina. Although a 28-diopter (D) lens has been traditionally used, a 40-D lens offers certain advantages. Ferrone and Trese [91] calculated that a 40-D, hand-held lens would create a spot size of 565 μm compared with 365 μm for a 28-D hand-held lens. The larger spot size afforded by the former lens reduces the risk of excessively hot burns and requires fewer applications, thereby reducing the time of the procedure. In addition, the larger field of view (64° versus 55°) facilitates examination and treatment of the infant's retina [91].

The entire peripheral avascular retina is treated with scatter photocoagulation from just anterior to the ridge to the ora serrata for 360° (Fig. 4-6). Burns are placed one half to one burn width apart and should be of no more than moderate intensity (*ie*, a dull gray to creamy white lesion). The fibrovascular ridge and any areas of preretinal hemorrhage should be avoided. The average number of burns applied generally varies from 500 to 1400, delivered in a single session whenever possible. However, the number of spots required varies greatly depending on the location of the fibrovascular ridge, the hand-held lens used (*ie*, spot size), and the intensity of treatment deemed necessary. Some investigators have advocated more intense treatment, with spots placed one quarter of a burn width apart, in eyes judged to have severe disease [92]. However, in our experience, spots placed one half of a burn width apart generally become confluent over time due to delayed lateral spread, particularly when a diode laser is used. Finally, transscleral diode laser has been shown to be as effective as transpupillary diode laser for the treatment of threshold ROP [12]. Although this modality is usually unnecessary, it could prove useful in cases in which the view is limited by vitreous hemorrhage or poor pupil dilation.

Complications

Various potential complications of indirect laser photocoagulation for ROP exist, including corneal burns, iris burns, lens burn with cataract formation, preretinal or vitreous hemorrhage, choroidal hemorrhage, choroidal neovascularization, and inadvertent photocoagulation of the fovea [86]. In terms of diabetic retinopathy, many or all of these complications can be prevented if excessively hot burns are avoided. Preretinal and vitreous hemorrhage is relatively common following indirect laser therapy, occurring in up to 10% to 20% of cases [9,86]. Hemorrhage is associated with treatment near the ridge and typically clears spontaneously within 2 weeks.

A less common but more problematic complication involves transient lenticular opacities and cataract formation following both argon [93,94] and diode [95] laser photocoagulation. In the case of argon laser therapy, high absorption of energy within the persisting tunica vasculosa lentis appears to increase the risk of cataract formation. Cataract formation is less common following diode laser and has been safely performed in eyes with persistent tunica vasculosa lentis [92]. Although the wavelength generated by a diode laser system (810 nm) is poorly absorbed by hemoglobin, cataracts have been reported following treatment. Fankhauser [96] has attributed this phenomenon to high-power density within the anterior segment that is generated by compression of the laser beam by the indirect imaging system. Finally, visual field loss has been reported following cryotherapy and laser photocoagulation, but it is typically mild, with treated eyes showing a loss of 6° to 10° compared with untreated fellow eyes [97].

Proliferative sickle cell retinopathy

Sickle cell disease is caused by point mutations in the hemoglobin gene and affects approximately 10% of the black population in the United States. Under anoxic or acidotic conditions, abnormal hemoglobin subunits polymerize within erythrocytes, resulting in increased rigidity of blood cells and the characteristic sickle shape. Increased blood viscosity can lead to sluggish flow, erythrocyte aggregation, and eventual vaso-occlusion of vessels in all susceptible tissues. Classic ocular findings include conjunctival vessel abnormalities, iris atrophy, and retinal abnormalities. Proliferative sickle cell retinopathy (PSCR) is the most serious ocular complication and develops in up to 11% of patients with sickle cell disease and 70% of patients with sickle cell hemoglobin C disease [98]. Although macular ischemia has been documented in patients with sickle cell disease, retinal ischemia and neovascularization are nearly always peripheral. Peripheral arteriolar occlusions lead to the formation of arteriolar-venular anastomoses and neovascular proliferation that is classically fan-shaped

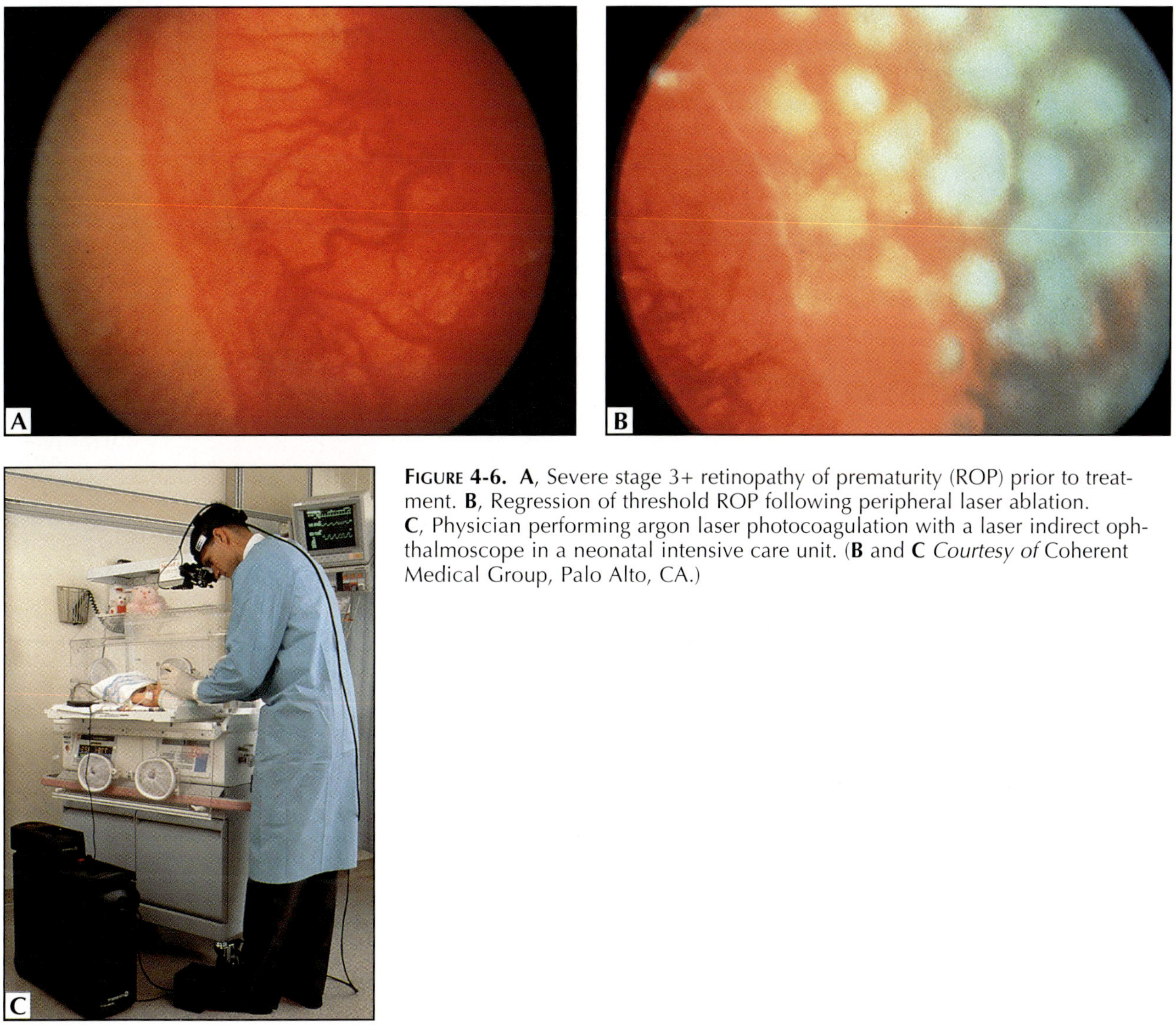

FIGURE 4-6. **A**, Severe stage 3+ retinopathy of prematurity (ROP) prior to treatment. **B**, Regression of threshold ROP following peripheral laser ablation. **C**, Physician performing argon laser photocoagulation with a laser indirect ophthalmoscope in a neonatal intensive care unit. (**B** and **C** *Courtesy of* Coherent Medical Group, Palo Alto, CA.)

and thus often termed "sea-fan" neovascularization. Although neovascularization frequently autoinfarcts and has a more benign natural history compared with other proliferative retinopathies, recurrent vitreous hemorrhage and tractional retinal detachment can result in severe visual loss.

Treatment guidelines and complications

Laser photocoagulation is the most commonly used treatment modality for peripheral neovascularization associated with PSCR. Two general techniques have been advocated to induce regression of neovascularization: feeder vessel photocoagulation and scatter photocoagulation. Several prospective randomized clinical trials have demonstrated that feeder vessel photocoagulation using either argon blue-green or xenon arc laser reduces the incidence of vitreous hemorrhage and visual loss in patients with PSCR [99–101]. The technique used in these studies involved intense treatment of the feeder arteriole followed by treatment of the draining venule after segmentation of the arteriole had been achieved. Repeat photocoagulation was performed several weeks later if the arteriole could not be segmented. Generally, a spot size of 500 µm and a duration of 0.2 seconds were the settings used. Although this technique was shown to be effective, the intense burns necessary to segment retinal vessels commonly resulted in complications, including preretinal and vitreous hemorrhages, vitreoretinal traction, retinal tears, and retinal detachment [99–102]. However, choroidal neovascularization is the most common complication encountered following this technique, particularly in eyes treated with xenon arc photocoagulation. Jampol *et al.* [99] reported an incidence of 80% for this complication following xenon treatment and, in a follow-up study involving eyes treated with argon blue-green laser, 11% of eyes developed choroidal neovascularization. Although flat chorioretinal neovascularization is typically benign, choriovitreal neovascularization can result in recurrent vitreous hemorrhage or retinal detachment with significant visual loss [103,104]. Because laser photocoagulation of choroidal neovascularization is problematic and can stimulate further growth into the vitreous, this treatment is not recommended.

Scatter laser photocoagulation has also been advocated for the treatment of PSCR (Fig. 4-7). Given that

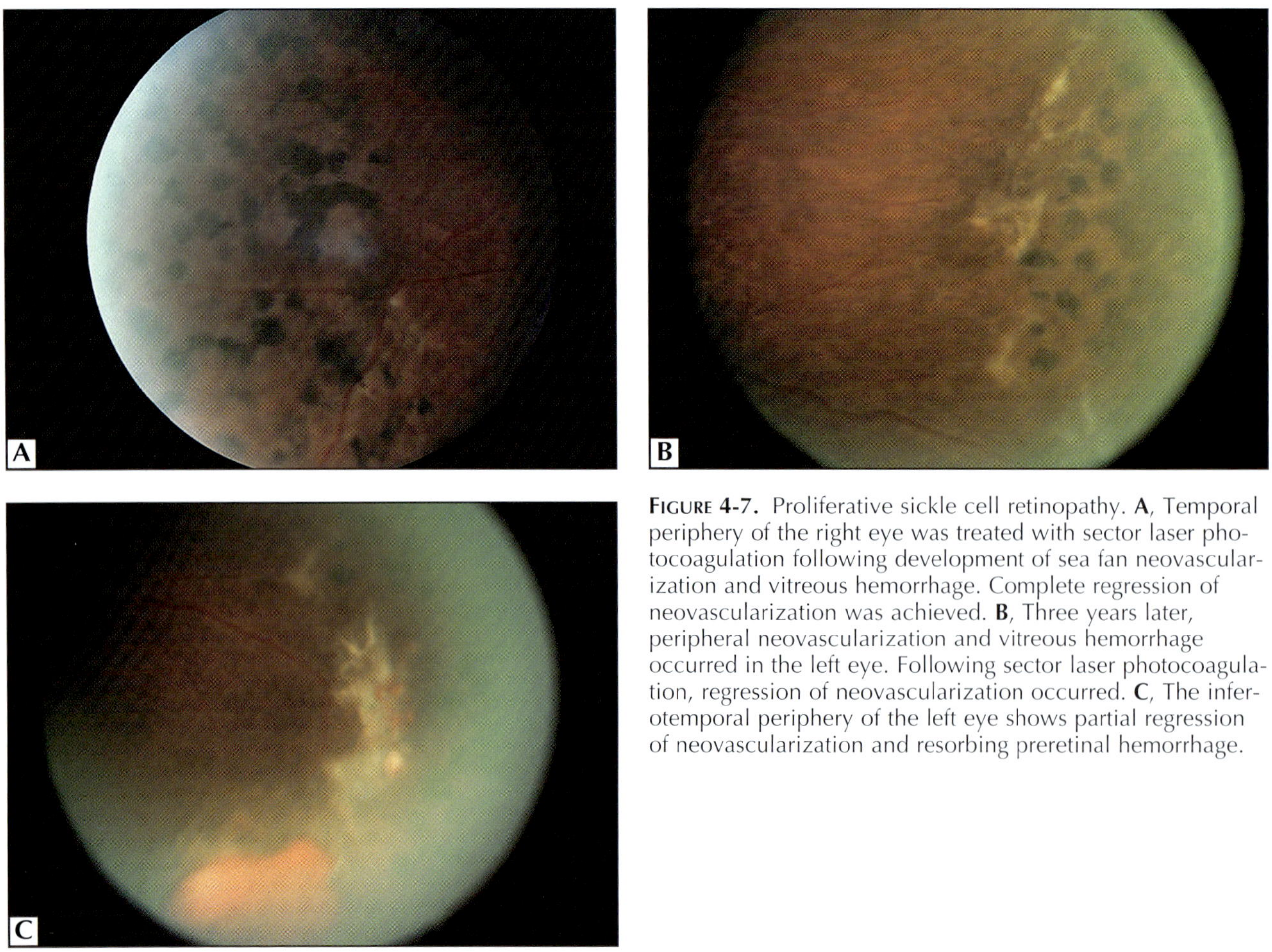

FIGURE 4-7. Proliferative sickle cell retinopathy. **A**, Temporal periphery of the right eye was treated with sector laser photocoagulation following development of sea fan neovascularization and vitreous hemorrhage. Complete regression of neovascularization was achieved. **B**, Three years later, peripheral neovascularization and vitreous hemorrhage occurred in the left eye. Following sector laser photocoagulation, regression of neovascularization occurred. **C**, The inferotemporal periphery of the left eye shows partial regression of neovascularization and resorbing preretinal hemorrhage.

scatter laser photocoagulation is easier to perform and is not associated with severe complications associated with feeder vessel photocoagulation, the former technique has gained widespread acceptance in recent years. Rednam *et al.* [105] treated 45 sea fans in 21 eyes with PSCR using localized scatter laser photocoagulation and achieved partial or complete regression in 78% of sea fans. In a more recent randomized prospective trial, 174 eyes were treated with localized scatter photocoagulation using argon blue-green laser [106]. Partial or complete regression occurred in 81% of eyes and the incidence of vitreous hemorrhage and prolonged loss of visual acuity was significantly reduced in treated eyes compared with untreated control eyes. In both studies, 500-μm burns of moderate intensity were spaced one burn width apart and were placed around all sea fans without treating the neovascularization or feeder vessel itself. Treatment extended from one disc diameter posterior to one disc diameter anterior to the sea fan and one clock hour to each side.

Circumferential scatter laser photocoagulation also appears to be effective in the treatment of PSCR. Cruess *et al.* [107] performed scatter laser photocoagulation in the zone of capillary nonperfusion and extended treatment to the ora serrata for 360°. Following treatment of 40 eyes, complete or partial regression occurred in 83% of sea fans and only one de novo sea fan developed during the follow-up period of 1.4 years. In a follow-up study, these favorable results persisted after a mean follow-up of 3.3 years [108]. Although these studies suggest that peripheral circumferential laser photocoagulation is effective in inducing regression of neovascularization and may prevent the development of de novo lesions, prospective randomized trials are lacking. Because circumferential treatment theoretically increases the risk of complications (*eg*, macular pucker and vitreous traction), localized scatter laser photocoagulation is generally favored. However, in cases in which a patient's reliability or ability to return for follow-up is in question, Jampol *et al.* [109] recommend consideration of circumferential treatment.

Less common proliferative retinopathies

Although ocular disorders discussed thus far encompass the overwhelming majority of proliferative retinopathies, a multitude of vascular, hereditary, and ocular inflammatory diseases exist that predispose to the development of neovascularization. Because many of these conditions are uncommon, controlled studies documenting the efficacy of various treatment modalities are often lacking and therefore clinicians must frequently extrapolate from published data based on the treatment of more ordinary ocular disorders, such as diabetic retinopathy and retinal vein occlusions. Although a detailed discussion of these less familiar ocular diseases is beyond the scope of this chapter, a few of them warrant brief mention.

Central retinal artery occlusion

Patients with central retinal artery occlusion (CRAO) typically present in the seventh decade of life with sudden, unilateral, painless visual loss. Ophthalmoscopy reveals retinal arteriolar narrowing and segmentation ("boxcarring") associated with retinal whitening and edema. A "cherry-red spot" in the macula is another classic finding. Although neovascularization of the optic disc and iris following CRAO was thought to be uncommon, more recent evidence suggests that incidence of iris neovascularization is approximately 16% to 18% [110]. Duker and Brown [111] treated three eyes with neovascularization of the disc using PRP, and regression of the vessels occurred in all three eyes. In a retrospective study, the same authors evaluated the role of PRP for iris neovascularization after CRAO [112]. Eleven of 17 eyes (65%) showed regression of new vessels. However, eyes treated before neovascular glaucoma developed showed better results, with complete regression of vessels in 89% of eyes. Despite the lack of a control group, these results suggest that PRP is effective for the treatment of iris neovascularization following CRAO because most eyes developing this complication progress to neovascular glaucoma without treatment. Furthermore, it has been shown that additional PRP is effective in cases of neovascularization of the iris when it follows CRAO occurring in eyes with regressed PDR that have been previously treated with scatter laser photocoagulation [113].

Familial exudative vitreoretinopathy

Familial exudative vitreoretinopathy (FEVR) is a vitreoretinal dystrophy characterized by premature arrest of vascularization of the peripheral retina. It is inherited as an autosomal dominant or X-linked recessive trait with high penetrance and variable expressivity. Mild forms of the disease are often asymptomatic and show only peripheral vascular abnormalities such as a peripheral avascular zone, vitreoretinal adhesions, arteriovenous anastomoses, supernumerous vascular branching, and a V-shaped area of retinochoroidal degeneration. More severe manifestations include neovascularization, subretinal and intraretinal hemorrhage and exudates, and vascularized preretinal membranes that can lead to retinal folds, macula ectopia, and retinal detachment. FEVR tends to be a variably progressive disorder and, despite the lack of adequate natural history studies, appears to stabilize after adulthood has been reached. Although FEVR is an uncommon entity, it represents a significant cause of retinal detachment in patients under 30 years of age.

There is a paucity of studies evaluating the results of surgical intervention in eyes with subretinal exudate or retinal detachment related to FEVR. Early studies involving a small number of eyes advocated peripheral cryotherapy to ablate hyperpermeable vessels associated with the peripheral fibrovascular tissue to prevent progression of FEVR [114]. The largest series to date has been recently reported by Pendergast and Trese [115•]. The study consisted of 40 eyes of 26 patients with FEVR that were treated with laser photocoagulation with or without vitreoretinal surgery. Peripheral laser ablation was performed using either diode or argon laser through an indirect delivery system. Laser burns of moderate intensity with a spot size of approximately 500 µm spaced one half to one burn width apart were applied to the peripheral avascular retina, sparing the vascular ridge. In eight of 15 eyes undergoing laser as initial treatment for FEVR, the subretinal exudate resolved and no additional therapy was required. Six of these eight eyes responding to laser alone were stage 2B (avascular retinal periphery with extraretinal vascularization and exudate) and two eyes were stage 4B (subtotal exudative retinal detachment involving the fovea). The authors concluded that, in a subset of eyes with FEVR, peripheral laser ablation is beneficial and may prevent progression to more advanced stages of disease.

Incontinentia pigmenti

Incontinentia pigmenti, or Bloch-Sulzberger syndrome, is a rare X-linked dominant condition characterized by congenital cutaneous anomalies occurring in successive stages. Ocular manifestations occur in approximately 35% of cases and frequently result in severe visual loss. A characteristic feature is premature arrest of the peripheral retinal vasculature and the development of peripheral neovascularization and, in many cases, tractional retinal detachment. Previous authors have reported regression of neovascularization following cryotherapy or laser photocoagulation [116–118]. Owing to the paucity of cases reported, no standard treatment guidelines have been established. Some authors have advocated treatment of the neovascular or hemorrhagic mass directly [116], whereas others have reported success following treatment of the peripheral avascular retina alone [118]. Although peripheral laser or cryotherapy appears to be beneficial in many cases, the response to treatment is variable and delayed total retinal detachments have been observed following initially successful treatment [117]. Thus, early diagnosis and intervention are important and patients must observed for an indefinite period for signs of progression of the vascular abnormalities.

Ocular ischemic syndrome

Ocular ischemic syndrome (OIS) is a potentially blinding condition that primarily affects older men. The condition is usually unilateral and results from obstruction or stenosis of the ipsilateral carotid artery. Color Doppler imaging studies have documented markedly reduced central retinal and posterior ciliary artery peak systolic velocities as well as reversal of ophthalmic artery blood flow associated with internal carotid artery stenosis [119]. Visual acuity is variably affected, ranging from 20/20 to no light perception. OIS is characterized by a constellation of signs, including corneal edema, anterior chamber cell and flare, rubeosis, cataract, retinal arteriolar attenuation or pulsation, retinal venous dilation without tortuosity, midperipheral dot blot hemorrhages, and optic disc neovascularization. In most cases, fluorescein angiography reveals increased artiovenous circulation times and delayed choroidal filling.

Treatment of OIS is difficult and remains controversial. Iris neovascularization has been observed in up to 87% of patients with OIS on initial presentation [120•] and is associated with a poor visual prognosis [121]. Treatment modalities, including panretinal photocoagulation and carotid artery surgery, have aimed at reducing the ischemic drive for iris neovascularization and preventing development of neovascular glaucoma. Unfortunately, few studies have evaluated the efficacy of PRP for OIS and therefore the role of PRP remains uncertain. Johnson *et al.* [122] reported four cases of OIS that responded favorably to PRP, with regression of proliferative retinopathy, iris neovascularization, and stabilization of visual acuity. Sivalingam *et al.* [121] advocate PRP in eyes with iris neovascularization and an open angle. However, Mizener *et al.* [120•] assert that, based on animal studies, uveal ischemia alone can produce iris neovascularization and therefore no scientific rationale exists for retinal photocoagulation in these cases. These authors therefore reserve PRP for eyes with neovascularization associated with retinal capillary dropout and nonperfusion documented on fluorescein angiography. Although optimal treatment for OIS has not yet been established, most retinologists routinely perform PRP in eyes with OIS and neovascularization of the iris or disc.

CONCLUSIONS

Laser photocoagulation remains the treatment of choice for the spectrum of ocular disorders characterized by retinal ischemia and neovascularization. Timely and appropriate treatment of PDR, ROP, retinal vein occlusions, and other proliferative retinopathies has dramatically reduced incidence of severe visual loss due to complications associated with the development of neovascularization of the iris, disc, or retina. Although the clinical efficacy of wavelengths ranging from 514 nm (argon blue-green) to 810 nm (diode) is similar, longer wavelengths are often advantageous in eyes with media opacity. Diverse delivery systems have become available, including slit lamp, laser-direct ophthalmoscope, endolaser, and transscleral probes, thus facilitating treatment in a variety of clinical settings. Finally, the recent availability of portable solid-state laser systems in both green and infrared wavelengths has further expanded the role of laser photocoagulation in outpatient clinics and NICUs.

Effective treatment of the proliferative retinopathies depends on early identification and adequate photocoagulation, regardless of the laser system used. Following treatment, patients must be carefully monitored to assess clinical response and to determine whether supplemental laser photocoagulation is necessary.

REFERENCES AND RECOMMENDED READING

Recently published papers of particular interest have been highlighted as:

- • Of interest
- •• Of outstanding interest

1. Aiello LM, Beetham WP, Balodimos MC, *et al.*: Ruby laser photocoagulation in treatment of diabetic proliferating retinopathy: preliminary report. In *Symposium on the Treatment of Diabetic Retinopathy* [Bulletin 1890]. Edited by Goldberg MF, Fine SL. Washington, DC: Public Health Service; 1969:437–463.

2. The Diabetic Retinopathy Study Research Group: Photocoagulation treatment of proliferative diabetic retinopathy: the second report of diabetic retinopathy study findings. *Ophthalmology* 1978, 85:82–106.

3. Okun E, Johnston GP, Boniuk I, *et al.*: Xenon arc photocoagulation of proliferative diabetic retinopathy (a review of 2688 consecutive eyes in the format of the diabetic retinopathy study—DRS). *Trans Am Ophthalmol Soc* 1983, 81:229–245.

4. Mainster MA: Wavelength selection in macular photocoagulation: tissue optics, thermal effects, and laser systems. *Ophthalmology* 1986, 93:952–958.

5. The Krypton Argon Regression Neovascularization Study Research Group: Randomized comparison of krypton versus argon scatter photocoagulation for diabetic disc neovascularization. The Krypton Argon Regression Neovascularization Study report number 1. *Ophthalmology* 1993, 100:1655–1664.

6.• Atmaca LS, Idil A, Gunduz K: Dye laser treatment in proliferative diabetic retinopathy and maculopathy. *Acta Ophthalmol Scand* 1995, 73:303–307.

This study compared the efficacy of various dye laser wavelengths in the treatment of PDR and diabetic macular edema. Regression of neovascularization and visual acuity results were equivalent among eyes treated with dye yellow, dye red, or a combination of the two wavelengths.

7. McHugh JD, Marshall J, Ffytche TJ, *et al.*: Initial clinical experience using a diode laser in the treatment of retinal vascular disease. *Eye* 1989, 3:516–527.

8. Bandello F, Brancato R, Trabucchi G, *et al.*: Diode versus argon-green laser panretinal photocoagulation in proliferative diabetic retinopathy: a randomized study in 44 eyes with a long follow-up time. *Graefes Arch Clin Exp Ophthalmol* 1993, 231:491–494.

9. McNamara JA, Tasman W, Vander JF, Brown GC: Diode laser photocoagulation for retinopathy of prematurity. Preliminary results. *Arch Ophthalmol* 1992, 110:1714–1716.

10.• White JE, Repka MX: Randomized comparison of diode laser photocoagulation versus cryotherapy for threshold retinopathy of prematurity: 3-year outcome. *J Pediatr Ophthalmol Strabismus* 1997, 34:83–87.

In this prospective randomized trial, laser photocoagulation appeared to have an outcome at least comparable with that of cryotherapy when the patients were examined 3 years following therapy. Visual acuity and refractive error data suggested a small but significant advantage of laser photocoagulation over cryotherapy.

11. Ludwig K, Lasser T, Sakowski H, *et al.*: Continuous wave laser photocoagulation at different wavelengths: equivalent power settings in edematous and nonedematous retina. *Lasers Light Ophthalmol* 1994, 6:159–167.

12. Obana A, Lorenz B, Birngruber R: Transscleral and indirect ophthalmoscope diode laser retinal photocoagulation: experimental quantification of the therapeutic range for their application in the treatment of retinopathy of prematurity. *Graefes Arch Clin Exp Ophthalmol* 1993, 231:378–383.

13. McHugh D, Schwartz S, Dowler J, *et al.*: Diode laser contact transscleral retinal photocoagulation: a clinical study. *Br J Ophthalmol* 1995, 79:1083–1087.

14.• Dowler J, Hamilton AMP: Contact transscleral diode laser panretinal photocoagulation in the management of proliferative diabetic retinopathy in eyes with cataract. *Laser Light Ophthalmol* 1996, 7:216.

The transscleral diode laser is useful for applying peripheral laser photocoagulation, particularly in patients with significant media opacity.

15. Raymond LA: Neodymium:YAG laser treatment for hemorrhages under the internal limiting membrane and posterior hyaloid face in the macula. *Ophthalmology* 1995, 102:406–411.

16. Ezra E, Dowler JG, Burgess F, *et al.*: Identifying maculopathy after neodymium: YAG membranotomy for dense diabetic premacular hemorrhage. *Ophthalmology* 1996, 103:1568–1574.

17. Jagger JD, Hamilton AMP, Polkinghorne P: Q-switched neodymium YAG laser vitreolysis in the therapy of posterior segment disease. *Graefes Arch Clin Exp Ophthalmol* 1990, 228:222–225.

18. Okisaka S, Kashima K, Kimura T, *et al.*: Retinal photocoagulation using the Nd YAG laser. In *Documents of Ophthalmic Procedures*, Series 36. Edited by Birngruber R, Gabel P. The Hague: Dr. W. Junk Publishers; 1984:71–80.

19. Menchini U, Lanzetta P, Soldano F, *et al.*: Continuous wave Nd:YAG laser photocoagulation in proliferative diabetic retinopathy. *Br J Ophthalmol* 1995, 79:642–645.

20. Jalkh AE, Pfibsen K, Pomerantzeff O, *et al.*: A new solid-state, frequency doubled neodymium-YAG photocoagulation system. *Arch Ophthalmol* 1988, 106:847–849.

21. McMullen WW, Garcia CA: Comparison of retinal photocoagulation using pulsed frequency-doubled neodymium-YAG and argon green laser. *Retina* 1992, 12:265–269.

22. Roider J, Schiller M, el Hifnawi ES, Birngruber R: Retinal photocoagulation with a pulsed, frequency-doubled Nd:YAG laser (532 nm). *Ophthalmologe* 1994, 91:777–782.

23. Danis RP, Bingaman DP: Insulin-like growth factor-1: retinal microangiopathy in the pig eye. *Ophthalmology* 1997, 104:1661–1669.

24. Smith LE, Kopchick JJ, Chen W, *et al.*: Essential role of growth hormone in ischemia-induced retinal neovascularization. *Science* 1997, 276:1706–1709.

25. Spranger J, Meyer-Schwickerath R, Klein M, *et al.*: TNF-alpha level in the vitreous body. Increase in neovascular eye diseases and proliferative diabetic retinopathy. *Med Klin* 1995, 90:134–137.

26. Frank RN, Amin RH, Eliott D, *et al.*: Basic fibroblast growth factor and vascular endothelial growth factor are present in epiretinal and choroidal neovascular membranes. *Am J Ophthalmol* 1996, 122:393–403.

27. Aiello LP, Avery RL, Ariggs PG, *et al.*: Vascular endothelial growth factor in ocular fluids of patients with diabetic retinopathy and other retinal disorders. *N Engl J Med* 1994, 331:1480–1487.

28. Tolentino MJ, Miller JW, Gragoudas ES, *et al.*: Vascular endothelial growth factor is sufficient to produce iris neovascularization and neovascular glaucoma in a nonhuman primate. *Arch Ophthalmol* 1996, 114:964–970.

29.• Tolentino MJ, Miller JW, Gragoudas ES, *et al.*: Intravitreous injections of vascular endothelial growth factor produce retinal ischemia and microangiopathy in an adult primate. *Ophthalmology* 1996, 103:1820–1828.

This paper discusses multiple intraocular injections of VEGF–produced vascular abnormalities typical of diabetic retinopathy and other ischemic retinopathies, including venous beading, hemorrhage, capillary occlusion with ischemia, and intraretinal vascular proliferation.

30. Aiello LP, Pierce EA, Foley ED, *et al.*: Suppression of retinal neovascularization in vivo by inhibition of vascular endothelial growth factor (VEGF) using soluble VEGF-receptor chimeric proteins. *Proc Natl Acad Sci USA* 1995, 92:10457–10461.

31. Frank RN, Amin R, Kennedy A, Hohman TC: An aldose reductase inhibitor and aminoguanidine prevent vascular endothelial growth factor expression in rats with long-term galactosemia. *Arch Ophthalmol* 1997, 115:1036–1047.

32. Adamis AP, Shima DT, Tolentino MJ, *et al.*: Inhibition of vascular endothelial growth factor prevents retinal ischemia-associated iris neovascularization in a nonhuman primate. *Arch Ophthalmol* 1996, 114:66–71.

33. Aiello LP, Nothrup JM, Keyt BA, *et al.*: Hypoxic regulation of vascular endothelial growth factor in retinal cells. *Arch Ophthalmol* 1995, 113:1538–1544.

34. Pierce EA, Foley ED, Smith LE: Regulation of vascular endothelial growth factor by oxygen in a model of retinopathy of prematurity. *Arch Ophthalmol* 1996, 114:1219–1228.

35. Feke GT, Buzney SM, Ogaswara H, *et al.*: Retinal circulatory abnormalities in type 1 diabetes. *Invest Ophthalmol Vis Sci* 1994, 35:2968–2975.

36. Grunwald JE, Brucker AJ, Petrig BL, Riva CE: Retinal blood flow regulation and the clinical response to panretinal photocoagulation in proliferative diabetic retinopathy. *Ophthalmology* 1989, 96:1518–1522.

37. Mendivil A, Cuartero V: Ocular blood flow velocities in patients with proliferative diabetic retinopathy after scatter photocoagulation. Two years of follow-up. *Retina* 1996, 16:222–227.

38. Fujio N, Feke GT, Goger DG, McMeel JW: Regional blood flow reduction following half fundus photocoagulation treatment. *Br J Ophthalmol* 1994, 78:335–338.

39.• Pournaras CJ: Retinal oxygen distribution. Its role in the physiopathology of vasoproliferative microangiopathies. *Retina* 1995, 15:332–347.

Reduced oxygen partial pressure measurements of the ischemic retina in experimental branch retinal vein occlusion confirmed the hypothesis that tissue hypoxia triggers neovascularization. Laser photocoagulation over the ischemic retinal area restored oxygen partial pressures to baseline values.

40. Funatsu H, Wilson CA, Berkowitz BA, Sonkin PL: A comparative study of the effects of argon and diode laser photocoagulation on retinal oxygenation. *Graefes Arch Clin Exp Ophthalmol* 1997, 235:168–175.

41. Stefansson E, Machemer R, de Juan E Jr., *et al.*: Retinal oxygenation and laser treatment in patients with diabetic retinopathy. *Am J Ophthalmol* 1992, 113:36–38.

42. Weiter JJ, Zuckerman R: The influence of the photoreceptor-RPE complex on the outer retina. *Ophthalmology* 1980, 87:1133–1139.

43. Wilson CA, Stefansson E, Klombers L, *et al.*: Optic disc neovascularization and retinal vessel diameter in diabetic retinopathy. *Am J Ophthalmol* 1988, 106:131–134.

44. Glaser BM, Campochiaro PA, Davis JL, Sato M: Retinal pigment epithelial cells release an inhibitor of neovascularization. *Arch Ophthalmol* 1985, 103:1870–1875.

45. Yoshimura N, Matsumoto M, Shimizu H, *et al.*: Photocoagulated human retinal pigment epithelial cells produce an inhibitor of vascular endothelial cell proliferation. *Invest Ophthalmol Vis Sci* 1995, 36:1686–1691.

46. Who is at greatest risk for diabetic retinopathy? *Ocular Surg News* 1997, 1:21.

47. The Diabetes Control and Complications Trial: The effect of intensive diabetes treatment on the progression of diabetic retinopathy in insulin-dependent diabetes mellitus. *Arch Ophthalmol* 1995, 113:36–51.

48. Diabetic Retinopathy Study Research Group: Four risk factors for severe visual loss in diabetic retinopathy. The third report from the Diabetic Retinopathy Study. *Arch Ophthalmol* 1979, 97:654–655.

49. Early Treatment Diabetic Retinopathy Study Research Group: Early photocoagulation for diabetic retinopathy. ETDRS report number 9. *Ophthalmology* 1991, 98:766–785.

50. Theodossiadis GP, Boudouri A, Georgopoulos G, Koutsandrea C: Central visual field changes after panretinal photocoagulation in proliferative diabetic retinopathy. *Ophthalmologica* 1990, 201:71–78.

51. Shimizu K, Kobayaski Y, Muraoka K: Midperipheral fundus involvement in diabetic retinopathy. *Ophthalmology* 1981, 88:601–612.

52. Doft BH, Blankenship G: Retinopathy risk factor regression after laser panretinal photocoagulation for proliferative diabetic retinopathy. *Ophthalmology* 1984, 91:1453–1457.

53. Vine AK: The efficacy of additional argon laser photocoagulation for persistent, severe proliferative diabetic retinopathy. *Ophthalmology* 1985, 92:1532–1537.

54. Theodossiadis GP, Ismiridis KJ: Time span of regression or disappearance of optic disc neovascularisation in proliferative diabetic retinopathy after panretinal argon laser photocoagulation and results over a two-year follow-up. *Fortschr Ophthalmol* 1987, 84:465–467.

55. Aylward GW, Pearson RV, Jagger JD, Hamilton AM: Extensive argon laser photocoagulation in the treatment of proliferative diabetic retinopathy. *Br J Ophthalmol* 1989, 73:197–201.

56. Doft BH, Metz DJ, Kelsey SF: Augmentation laser for proliferative diabetic retinopathy that fails to respond to initial panretinal photocoagulation. *Ophthalmology* 1992, 99:1728–1734.

57. The Diabetic Retinopathy Study Research Group: Preliminary report on effects of photocoagulation therapy. *Am J Ophthalmol* 1976, 81:383–396.

58. The Diabetic Retinopathy Study Research Group: Photocoagulation treatment of proliferative diabetic retinopathy. Clinical application of Diabetic Retinopathy Study (DRS) findings. DRS report number 8. *Ophthalmology* 1981, 88:583–600.

59. Pender PM, Benson WE, Compton H, Cox GB: The effects of panretinal photocoagulation on dark adaptation in diabetics with proliferative retinopathy. *Ophthalmology* 1981, 88:635–638.

60. McDonald HR, Shatz H: Macular edema following panretinal photocoagulation. *Retina* 1985, 5:5–10.

61. Gardner TW, Eller AW, Friberg TR: Reduction of severe macular edema in eyes with poor vision after panretinal photocoagulation for proliferative diabetic retinopathy. *Graefes Arch Clin Exp Ophthalmol* 1991, 229:323–328.

62. Elliott A, Flanagan D: Macular detachment following laser treatment for proliferative diabetic retinopathy. *Graefes Arch Clin Exp Ophthalmol* 1990, 228:438–441.

63. Hulbert MFG, Vernon SA: Passing the DVLC field regulations following bilateral panretinal photocoagulation in diabetics. *Eye* 1992, 6:456–460.

64. Henricsson M, Heijl A: The effect of panretinal laser photocoagulation on visual acuity, visual fields and on subjective visual impairment in preproliferative and early proliferative diabetic retinopathy. *Acta Ophthalmol (Copenh)* 1994, 72:570–575.

65. Doft BH, Blankenship GW: Single versus multiple treatment sessions of argon laser panretinal photocoagulation for proliferative diabetic retinopathy. *Ophthalmology* 1982, 89:772–779.

66. Blondeau P, Pavan PR, Phelps CD: Acute pressure elevation following panretinal photocoagulation. *Arch Ophthalmol* 1981, 99:1239–1241.

67. Gentile RC, Stegman Z, Liebmann JM, *et al.*: Risk factors for ciliochoroidal effusion after panretinal photocoagulation. *Ophthalmology* 1996, 103:827–832.

68. Yuki T, Kimura Y, Nanbu S, *et al.*: Ciliary body and choroidal detachment after laser photocoagulation for diabetic retinopathy. A high-frequency ultrasound study. *Ophthalmology* 1997, 104:1259–1264.

69. Galinos SO, Asdourian GK, Woolf MB, *et al.*: Choroido-vitreal neovascularization after argon laser photocoagulation. *Arch Ophthalmol* 1975, 93:524–530.

70. Chandra SR, Bresnick GH, Davis MD: Choriovitreal neovascular ingrowth after photocoagulation for proliferative diabetic retinopathy. *Arch Ophthalmol* 1980, 98:1593–1599.

71. Wallow I, Johns K, Barry P, *et al.*: Chorioretinal and choriovitreal neovascularization after photocoagulation for proliferative diabetic retinopathy. A clinicopathologic correlation. *Ophthalmology* 1985, 92:523–532.

72. Benson WE, Townsend RE, Pheasant TR: Choriovitreal and subretinal proliferations: complications of photocoagulation. *Ophthalmology* 1979, 86:283–289.

73. Palmer EA, Flynn JT, Hardy RJ, *et al.*: Incidence and early course of retinopathy of prematurity. The Cryotherapy for Retinopathy of Prematurity Cooperative Group. *Ophthalmology* 1991, 98:1628–1640.

74. Hammer ME, Mullen PW, Fergusen JG, *et al.*: Logistic analysis of risk factors in acute retinopathy of prematurity. *Am J Opthalmol* 1986, 102:1–6.

75. Shastry BS, Pendergast SD, Hartzer MK, *et al.*: Identification of missense mutations in the Norrie disease gene associated with advanced retinopathy of prematurity. *Arch Ophthalmol* 1997, 115:651–655.

76. Cryotherapy for Retinopathy of Prematurity Cooperative Group: The natural ocular outcome of premature birth and retinopathy. Status at 1 year. *Arch Ophthalmol* 1994, 112:903–912.

77. Cryotherapy for Retinopathy of Prematurity Cooperative Group: Multicenter trial of cryotherapy for retinopathy of prematurity. Preliminary results. *Arch Ophthalmol* 1988, 106:471–479.

78.• Cryotherapy for Retinopathy of Prematurity Cooperative Group: Multicenter trial of cryotherapy for retinopathy of prematurity. Snellen visual acuity and structural outcome at 5-1/2 years after randomization. *Arch Ophthalmol* 1996, 114:417–424.

Results of this study supported the long-term efficacy of cryotherapy for threshold ROP. However, preliminary data suggested an adverse effect of treatment on visual acuity, with fewer treated eyes having visual acuity of 20/40 or better (13%) compared with control eyes (17%).

79. Watanabe H, Tsukamoto Y, Saito Y, *et al.*: Massive proliferation of conjunctival tissue after cryotherapy for retinopathy of prematurity [letter]. *Arch Ophthalmol* 1997, 115:278–279.

80. Cryotherapy for Retinopathy of Prematurity Cooperative Group: Multicenter trial of cryotherapy for retinopathy of prematurity. Three-month outcome. *Arch Ophthalmol* 1990, 108:195–204.

81. Haigh PM, Chiswick ML, O'Donoghue EP: Retinopathy of prematurity: systemic complications associated with different anaesthetic techniques at treatment. *Br J Ophthalmol* 1997, 81:283–287.

82.• Knight-Nanan DM, O'Keefe M: Refractive outcome in eyes with retinopathy of prematurity treated with cryotherapy or diode laser: 3 year follow up. *Br J Ophthalmol* 1996, 80:998–1001.

After 3 years of follow-up, 94.1% of patients had myopia following cryotherapy and 45.5% of patients had myopia following diode laser treatment. In the cryotherapy group, 55% of patients were highly myopic (more than -6.00 D), whereas in the laser group no high myopes appeared. Although efficacy of these two treatment modalities was similar, diode laser had the added benefit of reducing myopia in the treatment of ROP.

83. Laws F, Laws D, Clark D: Cryotherapy and laser treatment for acute retinopathy of prematurity: refractive outcomes, a longitudinal study. *Br J Ophthalmol* 1997, 81:12–15.

84. Ross RD, Page TP, Trese MT: Visual outcome of bilateral threshold stage 3 retinopathy of prematurity (ROP) randomized to laser or cryotherapy [poster presentation]. American Academy of Ophthalmology Meeting, Chicago, IL. *Ophthalmology* 1996, 103(Suppl):186.

85. Landers MBD, Semple HC, Ruben JB, Serdahl C: Argon laser photocoagulation for advanced retinopathy of prematurity. *Am J Ophthalmol* 1990, 110:429–431.

86. McNamara JA, Tasman W, Brown GC, Federman JL: Laser photocoagulation for stage 3+ retinopathy of prematurity. *Ophthalmology* 1991, 98:576–580.

87. Laser ROP Study Group: Laser therapy for retinopathy of prematurity [letter]. *Arch Ophthalmol* 1994, 112:154–156.

88. Fleming TN, Runge PE, Charles ST: Diode laser photocoagulation for prethreshold, posterior retinopathy of prematurity. *Am J Ophthalmol* 1992, 114:589–592.

89. Capone A Jr, Diaz-Rohena R, Sternberg P Jr, *et al.*: Diode-laser photocoagulation for zone 1 threshold retinopathy of prematurity. *Am J Ophthalmol* 1993, 116:444–450.

90.• Vander JF, Handa J, McNamara JA, *et al.*: Early treatment of posterior retinopathy of prematurity. A controlled trial. *Ophthalmology* 1997, 104:1731–1736.

This prospective, multicenter, randomized trial evaluated the potential benefits of early laser treatment for prethreshold posterior ROP. An unfavorable structural outcome occurred in 16% of early treatment eyes and 18% of eyes treated when threshold ROP developed. Because all eyes with posterior ROP and any neovascularization progressed to threshold disease, usually within 1 week, little advantage appears to derive from delaying treatment.

91. Ferrone PJ, Trese MT: Examination and treatment of patients with pediatric retinal disease [letter]. *Retina* 1997, 17:168–169.

92. Seiberth V, Linderkamp O, Vardarli I, *et al.*: Diode laser photocoagulation for threshold retinopathy of prematurity in eyes with tunica vasculosa lentis. *Am J Ophthalmol* 1995, 119:748–751.

93. Campolattaro BN, Lueder GT: Cataract in infants treated with argon laser photocoagulation for threshold retinopathy of prematurity [letter; comment]. *Am J Ophthalmol* 1995, 120:264–266.

94. Christiansen SP, Bradford JD: Cataract in infants treated with argon laser photocoagulation for threshold retinopathy of prematurity. *Am J Ophthalmol* 1995, 119:175–180.

95. Christiansen SP, Bradford JD: Cataract following diode laser photoablation for retinopathy of prematurity [letter]. *Arch Ophthalmol* 1997, 115:275–276.

96. Fankhauser F: Laser therapy for retinopathy of prematurity [letter]. *Arch Ophthalmol* 1997, 115:1344.

97. Quinn GE, Miller DL, Evans JA, *et al.*: Measurement of Goldmann visual fields in older children who received cryotherapy as infants for threshold retinopathy of prematurity. *Arch Ophthalmol* 1996, 114:425–428.

98. Fox PD, Dunn DT, Morris JS, Serjeant GR: Risk factors for proliferative sickle retinopathy. *Br J Ophthalmol* 1990, 74:172–176.

99. Jampol LM, Condon P, Farber M, *et al.*: A randomized clinical trial of feeder vessel photocoagulation of proliferative sickle cell retinopathy. I. Preliminary results. *Ophthalmology* 1983, 90:540–545.

100. Condon P, Jampol LM, Farber MD, *et al.*: A randomized clinical trial of feeder vessel photocoagulation of proliferative sickle cell retinopathy. II. Update and analysis of risk factors. *Ophthalmology* 1984, 91:1496–1498.

101. Jacobson MS, Gagliano DA, Cohen SB, *et al.*: A randomized clinical trial of feeder vessel photocoagulation of sickle cell retinopathy. A long-term follow-up. *Ophthalmology* 1991, 98:581–585.

102. Jampol LM, Goldberg MF: Retinal breaks after photocoagulation of proliferative sickle cell retinopathy. *Arch Ophthalmol* 1980, 98:676–679.

103. Dizon-Moore RV, Jampol LM, Goldberg MF: Chorioretinal and choriovitreal neovascularization. Their presence after photocoagulation of proliferative sickle cell retinopathy. *Arch Ophthalmol* 1981, 99:842–849.

104. Fox PD, Acheson RW, Serjeant GR: Outcome of iatrogenic choroidal neovascularisation in sickle cell disease. *Br J Ophthalmol* 1990, 74:417–420.

105. Rednam KR, Jampol LM, Goldberg MF: Scatter retinal photocoagulation for proliferative sickle cell retinopathy. *Am J Ophthalmol* 1982, 93:594–599.

106. Farber MD, Jampol LM, Fox P, *et al.*: A randomized clinical trial of scatter photocoagulation of proliferative sickle cell retinopathy. *Arch Ophthalmol* 1991, 109:363–367.

107. Cruess AF, Stephens RF, Magargal LE, Brown GC: Peripheral circumferential retinal scatter photocoagulation for treatment of proliferative sickle retinopathy. *Ophthalmology* 1983, 90:272–278.

108. Kimmel AS, Magargal LE, Stephens RF, Cruess AF: Peripheral circumferential retinal scatter photocoagulation for the treatment of proliferative sickle retinopathy. An update. *Ophthalmology* 1986, 93:1429–1434.

109. Jampol LM, Farber M, Rabb MF, Serjeant G: An update on techniques of photocoagulation treatment of proliferative sickle cell retinopathy. *Eye* 1991, 5:260–263.

110. Duker JS, Sivalingam A, Brown GC, Reber R: A prospective study of acute central retinal artery obstruction. The incidence of secondary ocular neovascularization. *Arch Ophthalmol* 1991, 109:339–342.

111. Duker JS, Brown GC: Neovascularization of the optic disc associated with obstruction of the central retinal artery. *Ophthalmology* 1989, 96:87–91.

112. Duker JS, Brown GC: The efficacy of panretinal photocoagulation for neovascularization of the iris after central retinal artery obstruction. *Ophthalmology* 1989, 96:92–95.

113. Vander JF, Brown GC, Benson WE: Iris neovascularization after central retinal artery obstruction despite previous panretinal photocoagulation for diabetic retinopathy. *Am J Ophthalmol* 1990, 109:464–468.

114. Gow J, Oliver GL: Familial exudative vitreoretinopathy. An expanded view. *Arch Ophthalmol* 1971, 86:150–155.

115.• Pendergast SD, Trese MT: Familial exudative retinopathy: Results of surgical management. *Ophthalmology* 1998; *in press.*

This is the largest study to date reporting results of laser and vitreoretinal surgery for FEVR.

116. Nix RR, Apple DJ: Proliferative retinopathy associated with incontinentia pigmenti. *Retina* 1981, 1:156–161.

117. Catalano RA, Lopatynsky M, Tasman WS: Treatment of proliferative retinopathy associated with incontinentia pigmenti [letter]. *Am J Ophthalmol* 1990, 110:701–702.

118. Rahi J, Hungerford J: Early diagnosis of the retinopathy of incontinentia pigmenti: successful treatment by cryotherapy. *Br J Ophthalmol* 1990, 74:377–379.

119. Ho AC, Lieb WE, Flaharty PM, *et al.*: Color Doppler imaging of the ocular ischemic syndrome. *Ophthalmology* 1992, 99:1453–1462.

120.• Mizener JB, Podhajsky P, Hayreh SS: Ocular ischemic syndrome. *Ophthalmology* 1997, 104:859–864.

This recent study provides an excellent discussion of the clinical features and management of OIS and the factors influencing its development.

121. Sivalingam A, Brown GC, Magargal LE: The ocular ischemic syndrome. III. Visual prognosis and the effect of treatment. *Int Ophthalmol* 1991, 15:15–20.

122. Johnston ME, Gonder JR, Canny CL: Successful treatment of the ocular ischemic syndrome with panretinal photocoagulation and cerebrovascular surgery. *Can J Ophthalmol* 1988, 23:114–119.

CHAPTER 5

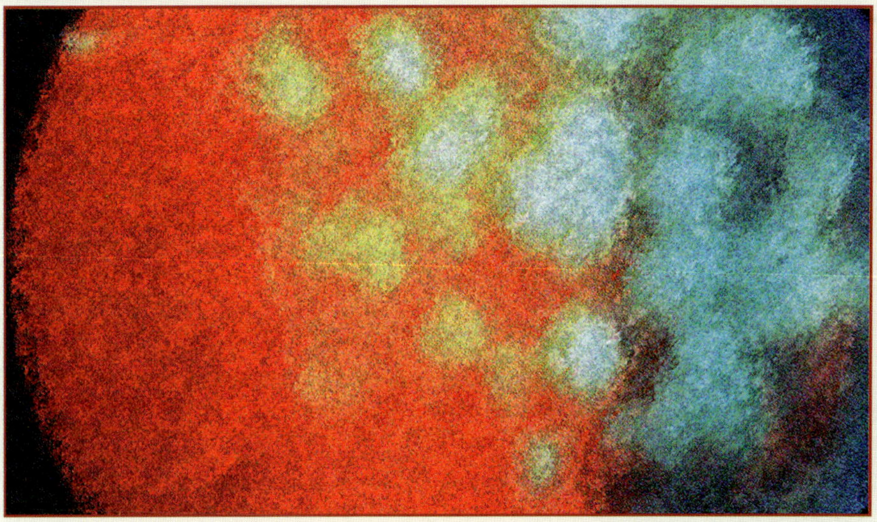

Laser Treatment of Diabetic Macular Edema

ROBERT P. MURPHY

Laser surgery has been used in the practice of ophthalmology with increasing success over the past three decades. Since the first publication of the Diabetic Retinopathy Study (DRS) Research Group in 1976 detailed the beneficial effects of scatter photocoagulation for proliferative diabetic retinopathy, great progress has been made in reducing visual loss resulting from diabetic retinopathy through improved laser treatment. Additional reports from the DRS Group and subsequent randomized controlled clinical trials have established the use and expanded and refined the indications and techniques of laser photocoagulation for various stages of diabetic retinopathy, including diabetic macular edema. The Early Treatment Diabetic Retinopathy Study (ETDRS) [1–5] was a multicenter prospective randomized clinical trial that began shortly after the DRS was completed. The ETDRS has provided a wealth of information that allows the treating ophthalmologist to accurately diagnose the severity of retinopathy through clinical examination and to assess risk factors of retinopathy progression and risk of visual loss based on the level of retinopathy. Moreover, the ETDRS tested multiple strategies and types of laser treatment that documented marked reductions in vision loss. For example, we now know that eyes with clinically significant macular edema have a better visual prognosis in general if focal laser treatment is applied before scatter laser treatment. The DRS and the ETDRS groups developed many of the data presented in this chapter. By applying the results of these remarkable clinical trials, it is now possible to reduce even further the rates of visual loss caused by diabetes. This chapter addresses the current indications, methods, and results of laser therapy for diabetic macular edema.

PATHOPHYSIOLOGY OF DIABETIC MACULAR EDEMA

Blood–retinal barriers normally restrict the passage of molecules and fluid from the vasculature into the retina. These blood–retinal barriers are found in two locations: the tight junctions between retinal vascular endothelial cells (inner blood–retinal barrier) and the tight junctions between adjacent retinal pigment epithelial (RPE) cells (outer blood–retinal barrier). In addition, active transport mechanisms move fluid from the eye across the RPE into the bloodstream.

Disruption of the blood–retinal barriers results in the accumulation of plasma components within the extracellular space of the retina. Histologically, macular edema is defined as an abnormal collection of fluid in the extracellular compartment of the retina in the macular region. The exact mechanism of leakage as it relates to histologic changes remains poorly understood. Accumulation of fluid within the macular area may be related to leakage of perifoveal capillaries or to more distant retinal vascular leakage. Distinct retinal microaneurysms or larger areas of abnormal telangiectatic retinal capillaries may leak and produce macular edema. The leakage also may be secondary to abnormalities in the RPE barrier, but mechanisms at this level are understood even less. Breakdown of the inner and outer blood–retinal barriers permits extravasation of ions, along with both small and larger molecular weight molecules. The presence of these osmotically powerful substances in the retina creates an oncotic gradient, which permits further extravasation of fluid into the retina.

Macular edema is evaluated clinically by slit lamp biomicroscopy, which demonstrates retinal thickening. In chronic cases, one may see cyst-like spaces within the retina. Distribution of retinal thickening may be described as focal or diffuse depending on its extent. Examining the macula with stereoscopic technique is essential to definitive diagnosis of macular edema. It is important to determine whether the center of the macula is thickened, because prognosis and management vary with central involvement. Most observers agree the best way to determine macular thickening is with the stereoscopic view provided by a macular contact lens at the biomicroscope. Indirect lenses such as a 78- or 90-diopter lens at the biomicroscope are helpful in screening diabetic patients for diabetic macular edema. If macular thickening is detected using these lenses, it is undoubtedly present; more subtle thickening, however, can be missed. Examination with the indirect ophthalmoscope is not effective to detect thickening.

Fluorescein angiography for diabetic macular edema should be obtained immediately after the clinical diagnosis of macular edema has been made and while treatment is being planned. Fluorescein angiography can be helpful in identifying areas of leakage. When the inner blood–retinal barrier is intact, fluorescein dye remains within the retinal vasculature. Disruption of endothelial cell tight junctions, however, permits extravasation of dye into the retina. Angiographically, this pattern of dye leakage around the macula assumes a characteristic petaloid pattern produced by the obliquely arranged middle retinal layers, that is, the outer plexiform layer of Henle. Although this characteristic fluorescein pattern is most often seen after cataract surgery, more diffuse, irregular patterns of dye leakage are seen in other forms of retinal vascular disease, such as diabetic retinopathy.

LASERS

Photocoagulation exerts its therapeutic effect on the macula by heating the retina and the underlying choroid to produce coagulation necrosis, which, in turn, produces a scar. An inner retinal effect is found at the level of retinal capillaries and microaneurysms with focal treatment using a shorter wavelength, such as green or yellow. Invariably, an outer retinal effect occurs at the same time because of the burn created at the level of the RPE. The exact biochemical and pathophysiologic processes that determine therapeutic response are poorly understood. The conversion of light to heat energy at a particular tissue site is a function of effective light absorption at that site [6]. The pigments involved with light absorption during macular photocoagulation are xanthophyll (inner/outer plexiform layers of the retina), melanin (RPE and choroidal melanocytes), and hemoglobin (in retinal and choroidal blood vessels).

Wavelength selection helps determine where light will be absorbed to produce its desired effect. Blue wavelengths are absorbed by xanthophyll in the inner retinal layers, whereas other visible wavelengths—red, yellow, and green—are absorbed by RPE (mostly by melanin) [6]. Although melanin may absorb light most effectively, its ability to do so varies little with change in wavelength [6]. Because xanthophyll, located primarily around the macula, absorbs blue light better than it does green or yellow, the latter wavelengths are preferred for macular laser treatments to avoid damage to the inner retinal layers. Hemoglobin has poor red light absorption, whereas blue, yellow, and green wavelengths are more easily absorbed. With vitreous, intraretinal, or subretinal hemorrhages, krypton red may provide a selective advantage because, theoretically, it can penetrate hemorrhagic tissues with less damage.

Argon green (514-nm), krypton yellow (568-nm), and krypton red (647-nm) wavelength lasers are currently the most commonly used lasers in the treatment of retinal disorders. Most collaborative randomized retinal studies used the argon laser, but the advantages of the krypton yellow and red laser wavelengths in penetrating cataracts and hemorrhages while sparing the inner retinal layers have established the utility of these wavelengths in the management of retinal diseases. The krypton yellow wavelength is particularly useful in treating diabetic macular edema because it penetrates cataracts well without lens uptake or beam divergence from the cataract. With the yellow wavelengths, beam divergence from edematous retina is lessened, permitting better control of the laser spot on the retina. Various longer wavelength lasers are available, including diode lasers. Recent publications suggest that these may also be effective in treating macular edema [7]. The treatment benefit demonstrated in most of the collaborative studies resulted from treatment with blue-green or green wavelength lasers.

DIABETIC MACULAR EDEMA

Diabetic macular edema is the leading cause of visual impairment in individuals with diabetic retinopathy [8–10]. It is estimated that 10% of people with diabetes have macular edema [11]. Although uncommon in the first 7 years of diabetes, it becomes increasingly frequent after 10 years. For individuals with disease duration of 15 years, the prevalence of edema (defined as thickening within one disc diameter of the center of the macula) rises to approximately 30%. Patients with later diabetes onset who are not taking insulin are less likely to have macular edema [11]. The risk of having macular edema increases with time and with increasing severity of retinopathy [11].

The usefulness of laser treatment for diabetic macular edema began to be apparent when three prospective randomized clinical trials demonstrated a treatment benefit [12–15]. Studies by Patz [12], Blankenship [13], and the Multicentered Controlled Study [14] all demonstrated reduction of visual loss with photocoagulation for diabetic macular edema compared with patients who did not receive treatment. All studies were relatively small, but the conclusions were similar. The study authors agreed that a larger, more rigorous study was warranted, and all supported a prospective randomized clinical trial with longer follow-up. One such study was the ETDRS [1–5]. With 3711 persons observed for over 7 years, the ETDRS was designed to evaluate multiple laser treatment strategies for diabetic macular edema. Information from ETDRS reports on macular edema remains the best source of natural history data for this condition and offers the clearest guidelines for the management and laser treatment of macular edema.

Clinically, diabetic macular edema is defined as abnormal thickening of the macula with fluid. Diagnosis is based on stereoscopic evaluation of the macula at the biomicroscope. Fluorescein angiography is not required to make the diagnosis; in some cases angiographic leakage in the macula is not associated with clinical edema. Thickening of the macula must be determined from clinical experience. Hard exudates are often (but not always) associated with macular edema and can frequently be a useful clinical clue. Chronic edema can cause microcystic changes in the retina, especially in the central macula.

Fluorescein angiography is usually needed to determine patterns of leakage. Discrete leakage from individual microaneurysms or localized microvascular abnormalities is called "focal" leakage. Less well-localized leakage from larger areas of abnormal retinal capillaries is termed "diffuse" leakage. Diffuse leakage can come from localized areas of the macula or, in severe cases, from the entire macular area. Macular edema can also be observed as associated with distinct microaneurysms or larger areas of abnormal capillaries.

Macular edema ranges widely in severity. To identify the more severe and visually threatening forms of macular edema, the ETDRS [1–5] developed the term "clinically significant macular edema" (CSME) to define retinal thickening that involves or threatens the center of the macula. Visual acuity is not part of the definition. Macular edema is assessed by stereo contact-lens biomicroscopy or stereo photography. The ETDRS definition of "clinically significant" macular edema includes one or more of the following three criteria (Table 5-1):

1. Thickening of the retina at or within 500 μm of the center of the macula
2. Hard exudates at or within 500 μm of the center of the macula, if associated with thickening of adjacent retina (but not residual hard exudates remaining after disappearance of retinal thickening)
3. A zone or zones of retinal thickening one disc area or larger in size, any part of which is within one disc diameter of the center of the macula

However, in more recent analyses of ETDRS data, eyes with macular edema that involves the center of the macula have been evaluated separately. Such eyes may be designated as having "central macular involvement" with edema and appear to be at highest risk of visual loss without treatment [10]. Investigators in the ETDRS used argon blue-green and argon green wavelengths for macular treatment. Tunable dye lasers have been developed, allowing for a selection of a variety of wavelengths. Some investigators prefer yellow for treating individual microaneurysms. In general, the longer wavelength lasers appear to be less suitable for treatment of diabetic macular edema unless opacities in the optical media prevent adequate treatment with the shorter laser wavelengths.

Natural history

Slow progression of the edema with attendant progressive loss of central vision is the usual course. In rare cases, regression can be spontaneous. Hard exudates can disappear without treatment but more commonly tend to aggregate in the center of the macula. Chronic hard exudates in the macula can lead to hyperplasia of the RPE and, in some cases, vascularized fibrous proliferation in the center of the macula. Focal laser treatment can reduce the rate of moderate visual loss.

Early Treatment Diabetic Retinopathy Study and diabetic macular edema

Study design

The ETDRS [1–5] was designed to answer three clinical questions regarding diabetic retinopathy:

1. When in the course of diabetic retinopathy is it most effective to initiate photocoagulation therapy?
2. Is photocoagulation effective in the treatment of macular edema?
3. Is aspirin effective in altering the course of diabetic retinopathy?

Information regarding the first two questions relate to macular edema. Between April 1980 and July 1984, the ETDRS enrolled 3711 patients with diabetes mellitus and bilateral diabetic retinopathy. This review concentrated on those patients who entered the ETDRS with macular edema who had visual acuity of 20/200 or better and mild to severe nonproliferative diabetic retinopathy or early proliferative diabetic retinopathy. One eye was randomly assigned to early photocoagulation in one of three possi-

TABLE 5-1 EARLY TREATMENT DIABETIC RETINOPATHY STUDY DEFINITIONS

Macular edema	Thickening of retina within 1 disc diameter of the center of the macula; or hard exudates ≥ standard photograph 3 in standard 30° photographic field centered on the macula (field 2), with some hard exudates within 1 disc diameter of the center of the macula
Clinically significant macular edema	Retinal thickening at or within 500 μm of the center of the macula; or hard exudates within 500 μm of the center of the macula, if associated with thickening of the adjacent retina; or a zone or zones of retinal thickening 1 disc area in size, at least part of which was within 1 disc diameter of the center
Severe visual loss	Visual acuity < 5/200 at two consecutive follow-up visits (scheduled at 4-month intervals)
Moderate visual loss	Loss of 15 or more letters between baseline and follow-up visit, equivalent to doubling the initial visual angle (*ie*, 20/20 to 20/40 or 20/50 to 20/100)

***Data from* Early Treatment Diabetic Retinpathy Study Research Group [1–5].**

ble treatments: (1) initial mild scatter, (2) initial full scatter, or (3) initial focal laser treatment. The initial type of laser treatment could subsequently be followed by another type of laser treatment. For example, eyes treated initially with focal treatment could have full scatter treatment later, or eyes initially treated with scatter treatment could have focal treatment later. The other eye was assigned to deferral of photocoagulation.

The primary endpoint for comparing the effects of laser treatment on macular edema was the development of "moderate visual loss," defined as a loss of 15 or more letters on the ETDRS chart (Fig. 5-1, Table 5-1) between baseline and follow-up visit, equivalent to a doubling of the visual angle [1,4]. Scatter laser treatment used in the ETDRS could be "mild" or "full," depending on the number of burns placed. Mild scatter treatment consisted of 400 to 650 burns spaced more than one burn width apart, whereas full scatter consisted of 1200 to 1600 burns spaced one-half the width of a burn apart. The spot-size diameter used was 500 μm, creating burns of moderate intensity. The treatment technique described by the ETDRS for macular edema specified argon blue-green or argon green laser applications (Table 5-2). Treatable lesions consisted of 1) microaneurysms, 2) focal leaks, or 3) diffuse leakage, all causing thickening of the retina and identified using slit lamp biomicroscopy or fluorescein angiography. Focal leakage and microaneurysms were treated directly using 50- to 100-μm burns of 0.1-second duration or less. The goal of treatment was to achieve whitening around larger microaneurysms. Achieving a color change in smaller microaneurysms was not required. Milder rather than more intense laser burns were recom-

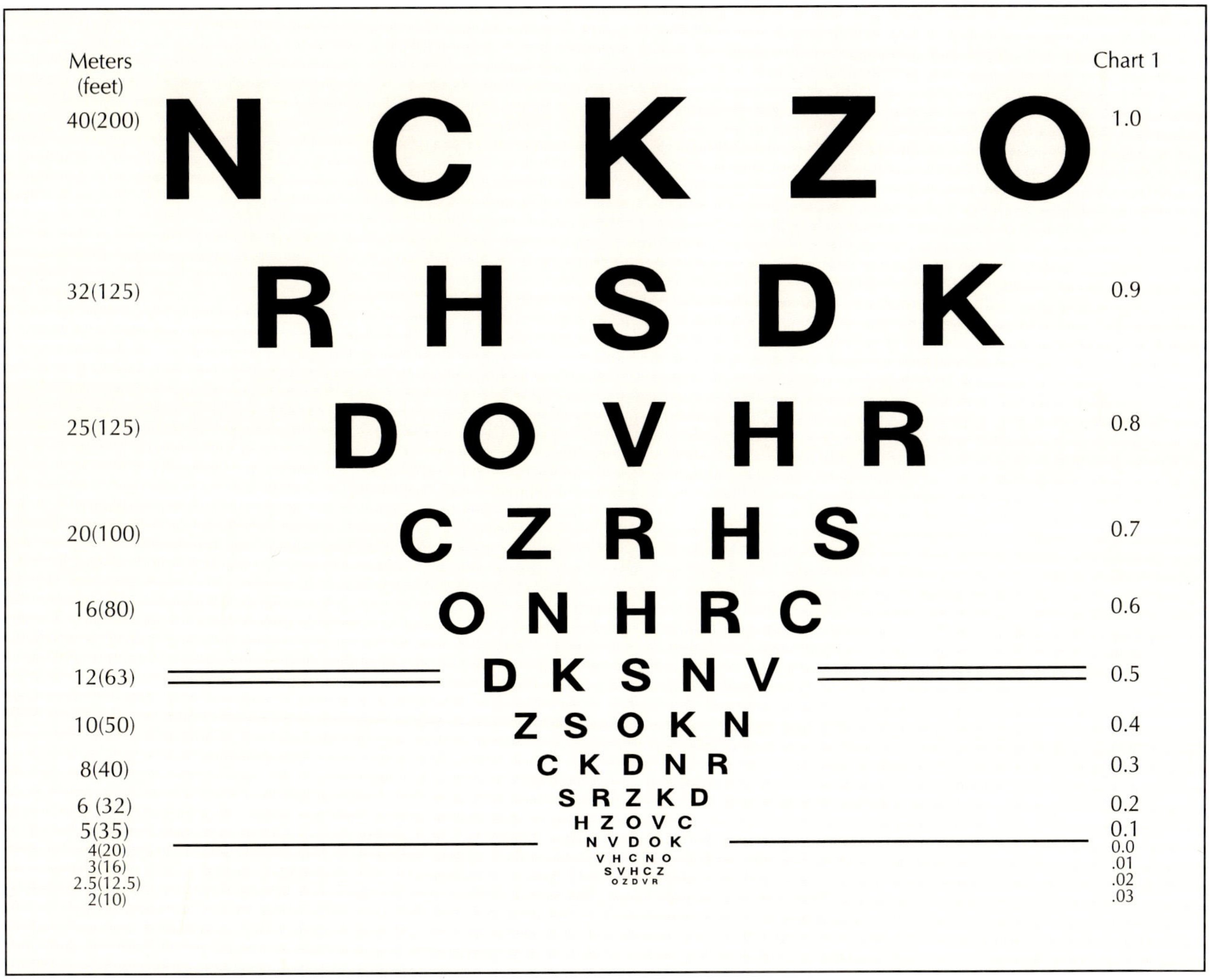

FIGURE 5-1. Early Treatment Diabetic Retinopathy Study (ETDRS) [1–5]. One of three ETDRS visual acuity charts used in the ETDRS study. Moderate visual loss, defined as a loss of 15 or more letters (three lines) on the ETDRS chart, is equivalent to a doubling of the visual angle. Moderate visual gain, defined as a gain of 15 or more letters (three lines) is equivalent to halving the visual angle.

TABLE 5-2 EARLY TREATMENT DIABETIC RETINOPATHY STUDY TECHNIQUES: BURN CHARACTERISTICS

Focal	Direct	Grid
Size, *μm*	50–100	< 200 (at retina)
Exposure, *s*	0.05–0.1	0.05–0.1
Intensity	Sufficient to whiten or darken large microaneurysms	Mild
Number	Sufficient to satisfactorily treat all focal leaks	Sufficient to cover areas of diffuse leakage and nonperfusion
Placement	500–3000 μm from center of fovea	Spaced greater than one burn width apart 500–3000 μm from center of fovea
Episodes, *n*	1	1
Indications for follow-up treatment	Presence of CSME and treatable lesions at ≥ 4 months	Presence of CSME and treatable lesions at ≥ 4 months

CSME—clinically significant macular edema.
***Data from* Early Treatment Diabetic Retinopathy Research Group [1–5].**

mended. Initial laser treatment avoided areas within 500 μm of the center of the macula, but treatment could be extended to within 300 μm of the center of the fovea at later treatment sessions if edema persisted. Areas of diffuse leakage received a grid pattern, using 50- to 200-μm spot size and spacing them at least one burn width apart. Grid treatments were not placed within 500 μm of the center of the macula or within 500 μm of the disc margin but could be placed in the papillomacular bundle.

In summary, the ETDRS treatment recommendations for macular edema followed these guidelines:

1. Treat leaking microaneurysms with focal photocoagulation using small, mild burns. More diffuse areas of leakage are treated with scatter or grid patterns of photocoagulation.
2. Reevaluate each patient every 2 to 4 months.
3. Re-treat at intervals of 3 to 4 months if CSME persists. The need to re-treat is common; additional treatment follows the same protocol.

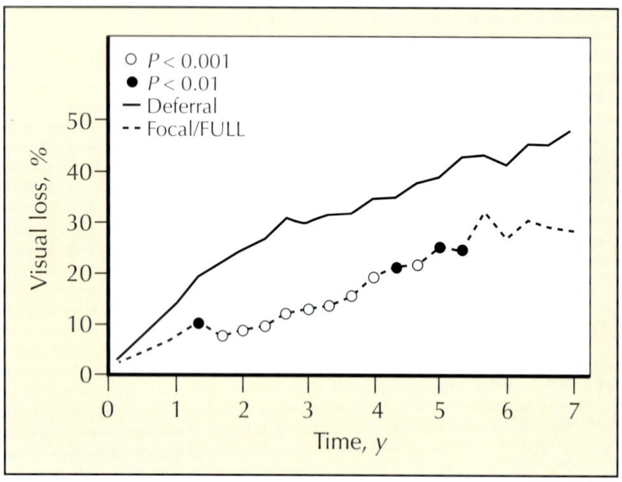

FIGURE 5-2. Occurrence of moderate visual loss in eyes with less severe retinopathy and central macular edema, immediate focal photocoagulation and delayed full scatter treatment (*dotted line*) versus deferral of photocoagulation (*solid line*). The beneficial effect of focal photocoagulation as the initial laser treatment strategy is clearly demonstrated; this treatment strategy is associated with the best visual outcome. Focal treatment decreases the risk of moderate visual loss by over 50%. The beneficial treatment effect is sustained for the 7-year study period.

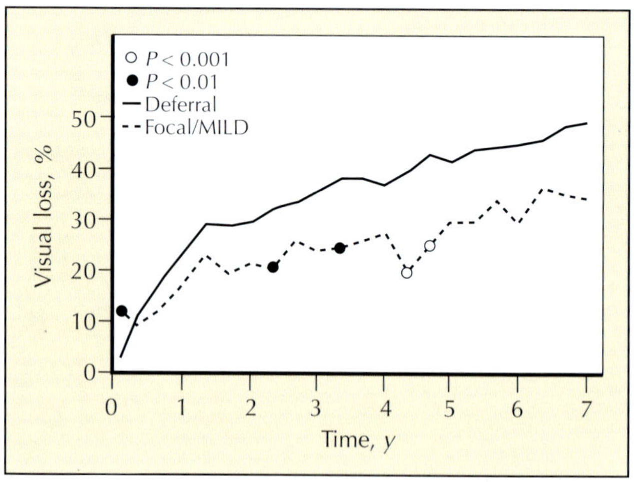

FIGURE 5-3. Occurrence of moderate visual loss in eyes with more severe retinopathy and central macular edema, immediate focal photocoagulation and delayed mild scatter treatment (*dotted line*) versus deferral of photocoagulation (*solid line*). The beneficial effect of focal photocoagulation becomes evident only after the first year following treatment, but treated eyes develop less visual loss than untreated eyes.

Study results

The ETDRS [1–5] showed that focal photocoagulation of clinically significant diabetic macular edema substantially reduces the risk of visual loss. At 3 years of follow-up, 29% of eyes with less severe retinopathy and macular edema with central thickening developed moderate visual loss (equal to or greater than a doubling of the visual angle) (Fig. 5-2). In contrast, only 13% of similar eyes treated with focal laser treatment as the initial treatment strategy developed such a degree of visual loss. This difference was evident from the first year of follow-up and continued throughout the 7-year follow-up period. The benefit of treatment was statistically significant at each follow-up visit. Focal treatment also increases the chance of visual improvement, decreases the frequency of persistent macular edema, lessens loss of color vision, and causes only minor visual field losses.

For eyes with macular edema that was *not* clinically significant, little difference between treated and untreated eyes was found in development of moderate visual loss in the first 2 years of follow-up. After 2 years, treated eyes developed moderate visual loss at approximately half the rate of untreated eyes. Any difference between the two groups after 2 years is probably due to the development of central macular edema. It seems reasonable, therefore, to defer laser treatment in eyes that do not have CSME, but to observe them carefully at intervals of 4 months. Eyes that subsequently develop CSME should be considered for laser treatment [1]. A similar but somewhat less pronounced treatment effect was found in eyes with macular edema and more severe retinopathy (Fig. 5-3).

Full scatter photocoagulation as an initial treatment for eyes with macular edema and less severe retinopathy was a poorer treatment strategy. For these eyes, an initial adverse effect on the risk of moderate visual loss appeared in the first 2 years when full scatter photocoagulation was initiated before focal treatment (Fig. 5-4). Visual outcome in these eyes was never better than the outcome for the deferred treatment group. In eyes with less severe retinopathy and macular edema with central involvement who received mild scatter treatment initially followed by focal treatment, a beneficial effect on the risk of moderate visual loss was seen, but only after about 4 years following treatment (Fig. 5-5).

Eyes receiving focal laser treatment were also more likely to have improved vision. Only 5% of untreated eyes gained three or more lines of vision, whereas 17% of treated eyes experienced this degree of improvement. These data suggest that the main benefit of focal laser treatment for diabetic edema is prevention of further visual loss, with only a small chance of visual

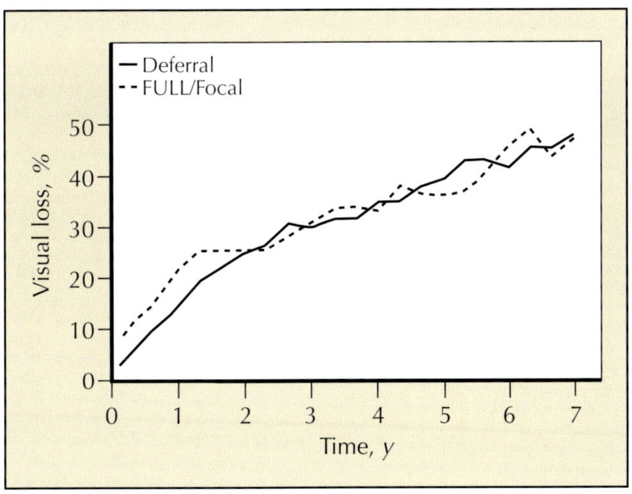

FIGURE 5-4. Occurrence of moderate visual loss in eyes with less severe retinopathy and central macular edema, immediate full scatter treatment followed by focal photocoagulation (*dotted line*) versus deferral of photocoagulation (*solid line*). The adverse effect of full scatter photocoagulation as an initial treatment strategy on moderate visual loss is seen. Eyes with central macular edema treated with full scatter treatment develop more moderate visual loss initially than deferral eyes; after the first year, the rates of moderate visual loss are similar in treated and untreated eyes. Visual acuity in eyes treated with this strategy is considerably worse that similar eyes receiving focal treatment as the initial strategy (*see* Fig. 5-2.)

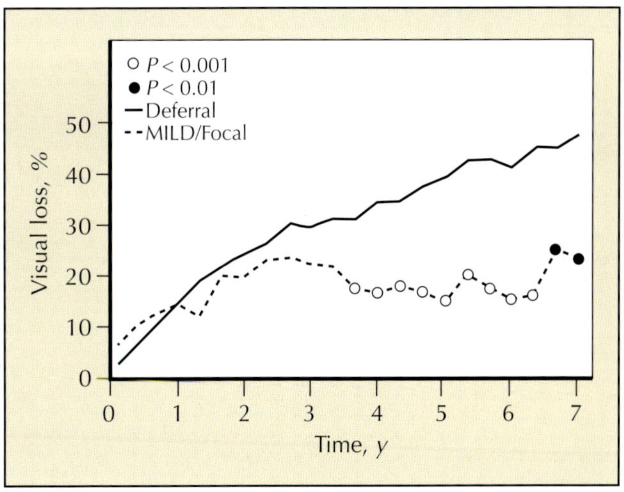

FIGURE 5-5. Occurrence of moderate visual loss in eyes with less severe retinopathy and central macular edema, immediate mild scatter treatment followed by focal photocoagulation (*dotted line*) versus deferral of photocoagulation (*solid line*). Here, the beneficial effect of photocoagulation can also be seen, but not until 4 years following initial treatment (*see* Fig. 5-2).

improvement. For this reason, treatment is recommended for eyes that have developed CSME or macular edema with central involvement before there has been a decrease in visual acuity.

The beneficial effects of treatment demonstrated in the ETDRS report support the following:

1. Focal photocoagulation treatment as an initial treatment strategy should be considered for all eyes with CSME and mild or moderate nonproliferative diabetic retinopathy.
2. Scatter treatment, or panretinal photocoagulation, was not shown to be effective for macular edema in the ETDRS. It may, in fact, worsen the visual acuity in untreated eyes. Some patients also had side effects such as mild decreases in central and peripheral vision following scatter treatment.
3. In cases of macular edema with more severe nonproliferative or proliferative retinopathy requiring immediate scatter treatment, the strategy associated with the least visual loss was a combination of mild scatter and focal treatment at the same sitting.

The ETDRS has shown the beneficial effects of focal laser treatment with delayed scatter photocoagulation in the management of diabetic macular edema (Fig. 5-6). Focal

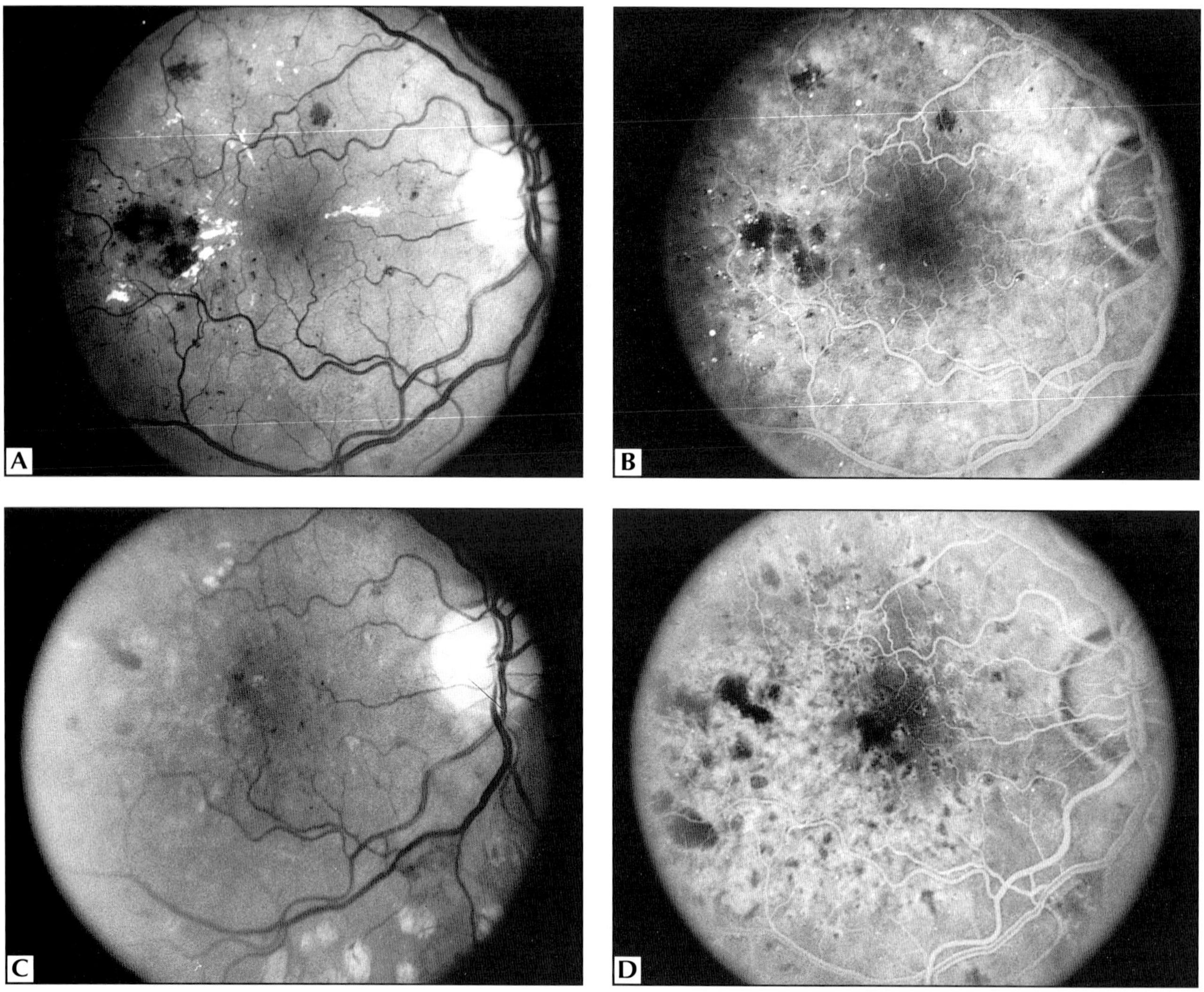

FIGURE 5-6. A, Pretreatment red-free photograph of an eye with multiple retinal hemorrhages, microaneurysms, and lipid exudates in the posterior pole. Stereo photography is required to recognize retinal thickening. **B,** Pretreatment fluorescein angiogram of the same eye shows blockage of fluorescence in the areas of retinal hemorrhage. Multiple microaneurysms can be seen temporal to the fovea. **C,** Red-free photograph of the same eye 3 years after focal laser photocoagulation to areas of leakage. Note reabsorption of intraretinal hemorrhages and reabsorption of lipid exudates temporal to fovea. Only small residual foci of intraretinal hemorrhage remain around the fovea. **D,** Posttreatment fluorescein angiogram clearly shows areas of laser treatment. Focal laser burns corresponding to treated microaneurysms are seen temporally and superiorlyt to the fovea. A grid pattern of laser burns has also been applied inferiorly. In comparison with *panel B,* disappearance of microaneurysms temporal to the fovea may be seen. A small focus of intraretinal hemorrhage remains temporal to fovea.

laser photocoagulation should be considered for all eyes with CSME and mild or moderate nonproliferative diabetic retinopathy or with more severe nonproliferative or proliferative retinopathy. In clinical practice, patients sometimes present with both proliferative retinopathy and diabetic macular edema. The ETDRS results suggest that, in general, focal laser treatment should be placed first for the diabetic macular edema. If the severity of retinopathy requires scatter laser treatment, it should be placed in sessions, divided as conservatively as possible. An eye that presents with macular edema and florid proliferative retinopathy must be treated with both focal initial treatment and aggressive scatter photocoagulation as indicated. Delay of treatment is not usually advisable in these cases. However, if an eye presents with central macular edema and early proliferative retinopathy without vitreous hemorrhage, the clinician could consider placing focal laser treatment and then gradually applying scatter treatment in divided sessions spaced as far apart as the treating ophthalmologist deems safe. Most ophthalmic laser surgeons believe that scatter laser treatment placed nasal to the optic nerve has less effect on macular edema. In cases requiring both focal and scatter treatment, one could consider treating the nasal quadrants with scatter photocoagulation first, carefully monitoring both visual acuity and status of macular edema. Additional scatter treatment is then placed gradually in the remaining quadrants.

Macular edema in more ischemic eyes

Severe and very severe nonproliferative diabetic retinopathy (NPDR) are specific terms used in the ETDRS to define eyes with more extensive levels of retinal ischemia. These eyes have a higher risk of progression to proliferative retinopathy and a higher risk of further visual loss. These ischemic eyes can be diagnosed by clinical examination alone; fundus photography and fluorescein angiography are not required for the diagnosis. A good clinical approximation of severe NPDR can be defined using the "4-2-1" rule. If any one of the following features is present, the eye has severe NPDR (Fig. 5-7):

1. Severe intraretinal hemorrhages (equal to or worse than to ETDRS standard photograph IIA) present in all four quadrants (midperipheral retinal areas), or
2. Venous beading in two or more quadrants, or
3. Moderately severe intraretinal microvascular abnormalities (equal to or worse than ETDRS standard photograph 8A) in one or more quadrant(s)

Eyes have very severe NPDR if two or three of the above features are present. Eyes with severe NPDR, very severe NPDR, and early proliferative retinopathy comprise the group with "more advanced retinopathy." Eyes with high-risk proliferative retinopathy and macular edema were not considered in this ETDRS analysis.

Eyes with macular edema and less severe retinopathy had a lower rate of moderate visual loss (a three-line decrease on the ETDRS chart comparable with a doubling of the visual angle) than did similar eyes with more severe retinopathy. Without treatment, the 3-year rates of moderate visual loss were 21.1% for eyes with less severe retinopathy and 27.1% for eyes with more severe retinopathy. Initial focal treatment reduced the rates of moderate visual loss in both groups. With treatment, the 3-year rate of moderate visual loss was approximately 12% for eyes with less

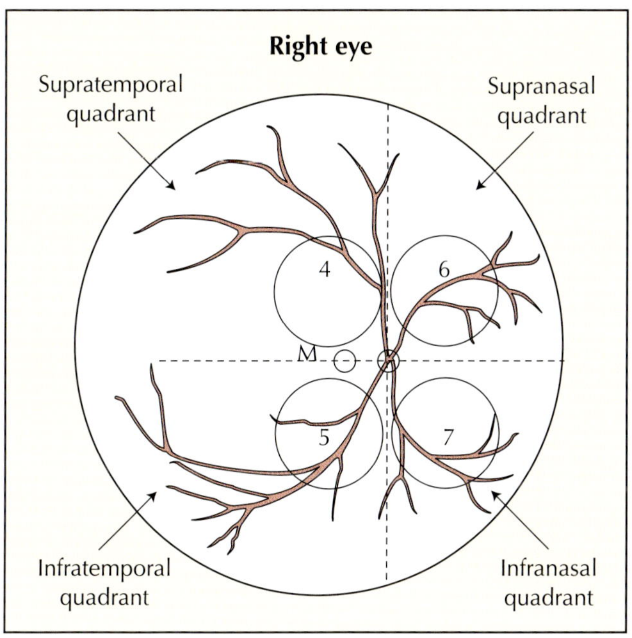

FIGURE 5-7. Circles labeled 4 through 7 indicate the location of the four midperipheral photographic fields used to grade presence, extent, and severity of intraretinal hemorrhages, venous beading, and intraretinal microvascular abnormalities to determine the level of nonproliferative diabetic retinopathy. Moderate intraretinal hemorrhages in all four fields, venous beading in two fields, or intraretinal microvascular abnormalities in just one of the fields qualify the eye for the severe nonproliferative retinopathy group using the 4:2:1 rule. M—macula.

severe retinopathy, compared with 22% for eyes with more severe retinopathy. The 5-year rates of moderate visual loss for eyes with macular edema treated with initial focal treatment were approximately 21% (less severe retinopathy) and 25% (more severe retinopathy).

For both the less severe and more severe retinopathy groups, initial focal laser treatment appeared to reduce the overall risk of moderate visual loss compared with deferral of photocoagulation. This beneficial effect of early photocoagulation was statistically significant, beginning with the first year of follow-up in eyes with macular edema and less severe retinopathy assigned to immediate focal photocoagulation with delayed scatter, and occurring later for eyes with macular edema and more severe retinopathy. However, the latter group received focal treatment and scatter treatment at the initial treatment. Eyes with less severe retinopathy initially received only focal treatment; they received scatter treatment later if they progressed to more severe retinopathy. The results presented are limited to eyes with retinal thickening that involved the center of the macula at the baseline visit (the group of eyes for which focal photocoagulation is generally recommended based on previous ETDRS reports). At all time points, eyes with less severe retinopathy and macular edema treated with immediate focal treatment fared better than those in which therapy was deferred. At 2 and 3 years' follow-up, the differences between treated and untreated eyes were statistically significant; treated eyes had half the rate of moderate visual loss.

In the first few months following focal laser treatment and scatter treatment, eyes with more severe retinopathy did not fare as well as eyes with less severe retinopathy. At 6 weeks and 4 months following treatment, treated eyes demonstrated an excessive degree of moderate visual loss compared with eyes with the same degree of retinopathy that had treatment deferred. At 6 weeks after initial focal treatment, over 8% of treated eyes developed moderate visual loss, compared with less than 2% in the deferral group, a difference that was considered statistically significant. At 4 months after initial focal treatment, over 12% of treated eyes had moderate visual loss, compared with 6% in the deferral group, a difference that also was considered statistically significant. At follow-up 1 year after treatment, treated eyes were slightly less likely to have moderate visual loss compared with deferral eyes, and by 4 years had a significantly lower rate of moderate visual loss than eyes assigned to deferred treatment.

The treating surgeon should know before treatment whether the eye being considered for treatment of diabetic macular edema has less severe or more severe retinopathy. Using the ETDRS retinopathy classification, the retinopathy level can quickly and accurately be determined. Treating ophthalmologists should be aware that between 10% and 15% of eyes with more severe retinopathy may develop moderate visual loss immediately after initial focal laser treatment if scatter treatment is performed at the same time. The initial adverse effect was less in eyes receiving mild scatter treatment than in eyes receiving full scatter treatment, suggesting the adverse effect of scatter with focal treatment is dose related. With longer follow-up, these eyes fare better with treatment than without treatment, but the risk of moderate initial visual loss should be discussed with the patient prior to treatment. Immediate scatter treatment should be avoided whenever possible in eyes with macular edema and more severe retinopathy, even if the eyes also receive focal treatment at that time. Other possible strategies to lower the risk of immediate moderate visual loss include reducing the number of focal treatment spots at each treatment session and providing more treatment sessions while carefully monitoring the visual acuity. Sectored macular treatment may also reduce the risk of driving the macular edema and intraretinal lipid (hard exudates) into the center and may be helpful in reducing this initial visual loss. More investigation is needed to develop and test treatment strategies to reduce the risk of moderate visual loss in eyes with more severe retinopathy and diabetic macular edema.

COMPLICATIONS OF LASER TREATMENT

Complications of the treatment of diabetic macular edema were evaluated in the ETDRS but were, in general, few and difficult to measure. However, in individual cases this treatment is not without complications. Development of scotomas after focal laser therapy close to the center of the macula is a well-recognized problem. Recently, other complications have been reported. Fortunately, these are uncommon and, for the most part, avoidable. Choroidal neovascularization has been reported following treatment of diabetic macular edema by Varley *et al.* [16]. Lewis *et al.* [17] presented a series of eight patients with choroidal neovascularization that developed from previous laser scars. The choroidal neovascularization was diagnosed 2 weeks to 5 months after treatment, and despite further laser treatment, visual acuity remained poor. Schatz *et al.* [18] described enlargement of laser scars following grid laser treatments for diffuse diabetic macular edema. They reported eleven patients with progressive enlargement of focal photocoagulation scars and decreased visual acuity months to years after treatment. Enlargement of the scars into the central macula as well as hyperplastic changes in the RPE were seen in these eyes. This type of scar can be formed only by relatively intense laser applications. Excessively intense laser burns are to be avoided in the macula to avoid this potential complication. Both complications—choroidal neovascularization and enlargement of laser scars—can be prevented with avoidance of intense laser applications in the macula.

Another potentially vision-limiting complication following laser photocoagulation of diabetic macular edema is the development of submacular fibrosis. Han *et al.* [19] reported on ten eyes and Guyer *et al.* [20] reported on seven eyes with subretinal fibrous strands emanating from the treated areas. In some eyes, these strands extended from laser scars, suggesting a role of the laser treatment in this process. This complication is associated with a decline in visual acuity. Again, avoidance of excessively intense laser applications will avoid this complication. However, Fong *et al.* [21] found that retinal hard exudates of a severe degree were much more likely than laser treatment to be associated with the development of subretinal fibrosis. They evaluated 109 eyes in 96 persons in the ETDRS [21] who developed subretinal fibrosis during the course of the study. In this study, the largest of its kind, the development of subretinal fibrosis was directly related to photocoagulation in only nine of the 109 eyes. Development of subretinal fibrosis was strongly related to the presence of extensive, severe degrees of hard exudates in the macula before fibrosis developed. Of the eyes in which fibrosis developed, 7% had very severe degrees of hard exudates in the macula before development of fibrosis, compared with 2.5% of the eyes with clinically significant macular edema in which fibrosis did not develop ($P<0.001$). Subretinal fibrosis developed in 31% of the eyes with this severe degree of hard exudates, but in only 0.05% of eyes without severe hard exudates.

SYSTEMIC CONSIDERATIONS

New data from the ETDRS [22,23] demonstrate a very strong relationship between elevated serum lipid levels and retinal hard exudate in diabetic retinopathy. Of 3711 patients enrolled in the ETDRS, the first 2709 persons enrolled had serum lipid levels measured at the time of the baseline examination. Measurements included baseline fasting serum lipid levels, best-corrected visual acuity, and assessment of retinal thickening and hard exudate from stereoscopic macular photographs. Patients with elevated total serum cholesterol levels or serum low-density lipoprotein cholesterol levels at baseline were twice as likely to have retinal hard exudates as were patients with normal levels. These patients were also at higher risk of developing hard exudates during the course of the study. Severity of hard exudates was found to be a separate, additive risk factor for visual loss. The risk of losing visual acuity was associated with the extent and severity of hard exudate even after adjusting for the extent of macular edema.

For persons with diabetes, elevated serum lipid levels are associated with an increased risk of retinal hard exudates. Retinal hard exudates are frequently a feature of diabetic macular edema, which is well known to place eyes at risk for visual loss. This ETDRS analysis [22,23] clearly demonstrates that increasing levels of retinal hard exudates act as an independent, additive risk factor for visual loss. These data also suggest that lowering serum lipids may decrease the risk of hard exudate formation and thereby lower the risk of visual loss in patients with diabetic retinopathy. In addition, reducing the risk of further visual loss from lipemic macular edema is another motivating factor to lower serum lipid levels in persons with diabetic retinopathy and elevated serum lipid levels. Because lowering blood glucose levels is known to lower the risk of retinopathy progression, the ophthalmologist should communicate with and coordinate the care of persons with diabetes with their endocrinologist or primary care provider [24]. Using this "team" approach to achieve ideal levels of blood glucose and lower abnormally elevated blood lipids can significantly reduce the risk of retinopathy progression and further reduce the risk of visual loss.

REFERENCES AND RECOMMENDED READING

Recently published papers of particular interest have been highlighted as:
- • Of interest
- •• Of outstanding interest

1. Early Treatment Diabetic Retinopathy Study Research Group: Photocoagulation for diabetic macular edema. Early Treatment Diabetic Retinopathy Study Report Number 1. *Arch Ophthalmol* 1985, 103:1796–1806.
2. Early Treatment Diabetic Retinopathy Study Research Group: Treatment techniques and clinical guidelines for photocoagulation of diabetic macular edema. Early Treatment Diabetic Retinopathy Study Report Number 2. *Ophthalmology* 1987, 94:761–774.
3. Early Treatment Diabetic Retinopathy Study Research Group: Photocoagulation for diabetic macular edema. Early Treatment Diabetic Retinopathy Report Number 4. *Int Ophthalmol Clin* 1987, 27:265–272.
4. Early Treatment Diabetic Retinopathy Study Research Group: Early treatment diabetic retinopathy study design and baseline patient characteristics. Early Treatment Diabetic Retinopathy Study Report Number 7. *Ophthalmology* 1991, 98(Suppl):741–756.
5. Early Treatment Diabetic Retinopathy Study Research Group: Early photocoagulation for diabetic retinopathy. Early Treatment Diabetic Retinopathy Report Number 9. *Ophthalmology* 1991, 98(Suppl):766–785.
6. Mainster MA: Wavelength selection in macular photocoagulation: tissue optics, thermal effects, and laser systems. *Ophthalmology* 1986, 93:952–958.
7. Akduman L, Olk RJ: Diode laser (810 nm) versus argon green (514 nm) modified grid photocoagulation for diffuse diabetic macular edema. *Ophthalmology* 1997, 104:1433–1441.
8. Ferris FL III, Patz A: Macular edema: a complication of diabetic retinopathy. *Surv Ophthalmol* 1984, 28:452–461.
9. Bresnick GH: Diabetic maculopathy: a critical review highlighting diffuse macular edema. *Ophthalmology* 1983, 90:1301–1317.
10. Bresnick GH: Diabetic macular edema: a review. *Ophthalmology* 1986, 93:989–997.
11. Klein R, Klein BEK, Moss SE, *et al.*: The Wisconsin epidemiologic study of diabetic retinopathy, IV. Diabetic macular edema. *Ophthalmology* 1984, 91:1464–1474.
12. Patz A, Schatz H, Berkow JW, *et al.*: Macular edema: an overlooked complication of diabetic retinopathy. *Trans Am Acad Ophthalmol Otolaryngol* 1973, 77:34–42.
13. Blankenship GW: Diabetic macular edema and argon laser photocoagulation: a prospective randomized study. *Ophthalmology* 1979, 86:69–78.
14. Multicentered Controlled Study: Photocoagulation in treatment of diabetic maculopathy. *Lancet* 1975, 2:1110–1113.
15. Townsend C, Bailey J, Kohner E: Xenon arc photocoagulation for the treatment of diabetic maculopathy: interim report of a multicentre controlled clinical study. *Br J Ophthalmol* 1980, 64:385–291.
16. Varley MP, Frank E, Purnell EW: Subretinal neovascularization after focal argon laser for diabetic macular edema. *Ophthalmology* 1988, 95:567–573.
17. Lewis H, Schachat AP, Haimann MH, *et al.*: Choroidal neovascularization after laser photocoagulation for diabetic macular edema. *Ophthalmology* 1990, 97:503–511.
18. Schatz H, Madeira D, McDonald R, Johnson RN: Progressive enlargement of laser scars following grid laser photocoagulation for diffuse diabetic macular edema. *Arch Ophthalmol* 1991, 109:1549–1551.
19. Han DP, Mieler WF, Burton TC: Submacular fibrosis after photocoagulation for diabetic macular edema. *Am J Ophthalmol* 1992, 113:513–521.
20. Guyer DR, D'Amico DJ, Smith CW: Subretinal fibrosis after laser photocoagulation for diabetic macular edema. *Am J Ophthalmol* 1992, 113:652–656.
21. Fong DS, Segal PP, Myers FM, *et al.*, for the Early Treatment Diabetic Retinopathy Study Research Group: Subretinal fibrosis in diabetic macular edema. ETDRS report 23. *Arch Ophthalmol* 1997, 115:873–877.
22. Chew EY, Klein ML, Ferris FL, *et al.*, for the Early Treatment Diabetic Retinopathy Study Research Group: Association of elevated serum lipid levels with retinal hard exudate in diabetic retinopathy. *Arch Ophthalmol* 1996, 114:1079–1084.
23. Ferris FL, Chew EY, Hoogwerf BJ; for the Early Treatment Diabetic Retinopathy Study Research Group: Serum lipids and diabetic retinopathy. *Diabetes Care* 1996, 19:1291–1293.
24. Diabetes Control and Complications Trial Research Group: The effect of intensive treatment of diabetes on the development and progression of long-term complications in insulin-dependent diabetes mellitus. *N Engl J Med* 1993, 329:977–986.

CHAPTER 6

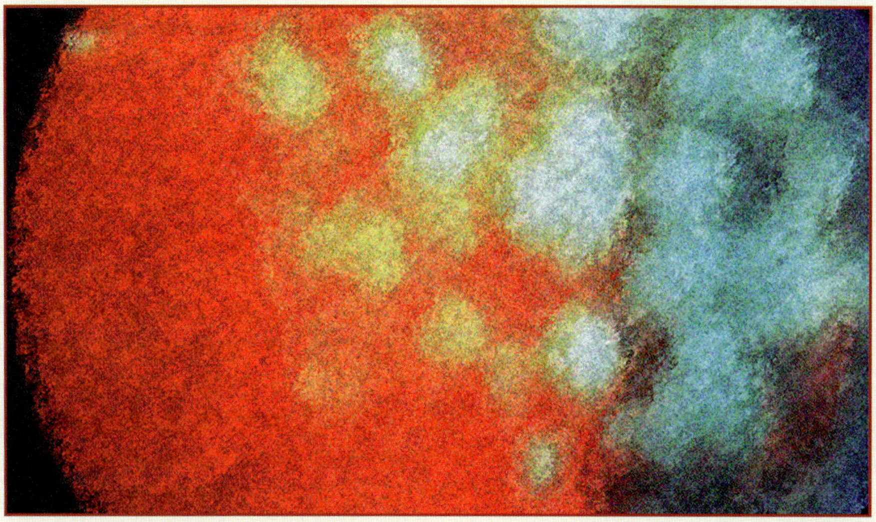

Laser Management of Branch and Central Retinal Vein Occlusions

HERNANDO ZEGARRA
DANIEL FINKELSTEIN
LAWRENCE J. SINGERMAN
JOHN H. NIFFENEGGER
SCOTT D. PENDERGAST

Branch and central retinal vein occlusions are common retinal vascular disturbances. Together, they are the second most frequent cause of retinal vascular disturbance, after diabetic retinopathy. They share the vision-limiting problems of macular edema and neovascularization.

BRANCH RETINAL VEIN OCCLUSION

Guidelines for the laser management of macular edema and neovascularization in branch retinal vein occlusion (BRVO) have been provided by the Branch Vein Occlusion Study Group [1,2] and were published in the 1980s.

Macular edema

Diagnosis of macular edema in the acute phase of BRVO can be difficult because of overlying intraretinal hemorrhage that may not permit appreciation of retinal thickening or cystoid spaces and evaluation of potential visual acuity. Hemorrhage alone can reduce visual acuity significantly, and this decreased acuity can return to normal if no other macular disease is present when the hemorrhage resorbs.

We have found it helpful to distinguish four types of macular edema because different laser management techniques apply to each type: perfused macular edema, nonperfused (ischemic) macular edema, mixed (perfused and nonperfused) macular edema, and macular edema from a distant BRVO. The distinction among these four types of edema depends on high-quality fluorescein angiography of the macula after there is sufficient absorption of intraretinal hemorrhage so that capillary detail can be appreciated.

In perfused macular edema, one sees intact perifoveal retinal capillaries on the transit of the fluorescein angiogram with late accumulation of fluorescein dye in a central cyst involving the center of the fovea (Fig. 6-1). In nonperfused macular edema, fluorescein angiography demonstrates a loss of capillary perfusion in the macular region with no late accumulation of fluorescein dye in the center of the fovea (Fig. 6-2). In the

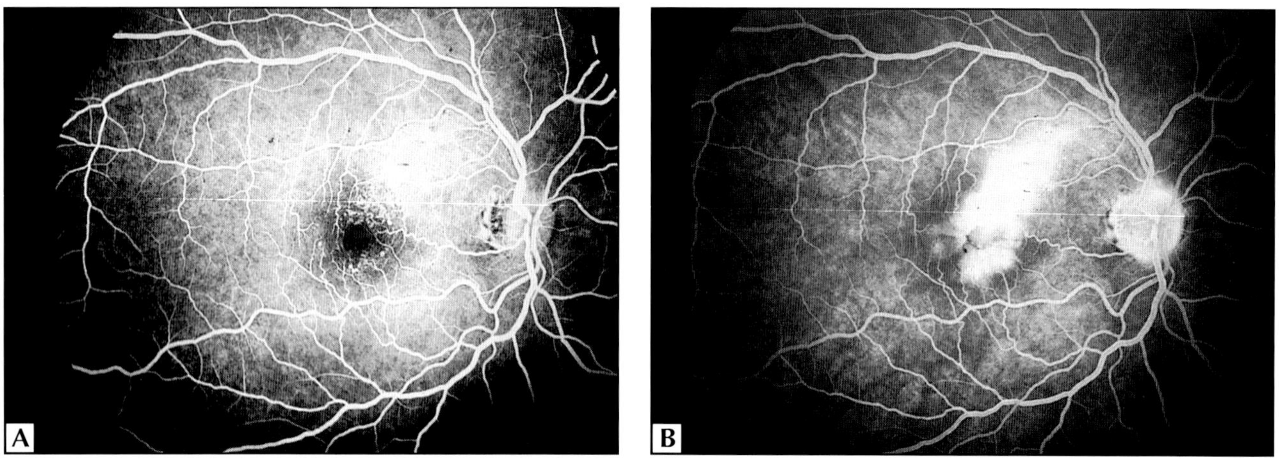

FIGURE 6-1. A, Fluorescein angiogram, transit phase, demonstrating perfused capillary circulation. **B**, Fluorescein angiogram, late phase, same case as *panel A*, demonstrating leakage into central foveal cyst.

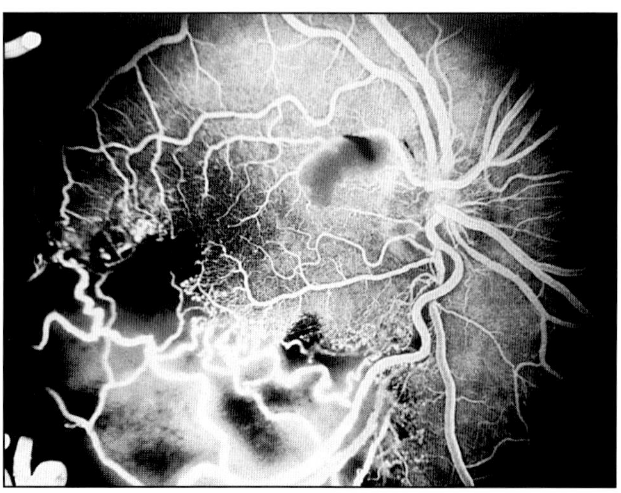

FIGURE 6-2. Fluorescein angiogram, transit phase, demonstrating partial macular nonperfusion.

acute phase of the BRVO that causes ischemic macular edema, however, the appearance is clinically similar to perfused edema, demonstrating a thickened fovea and macula with cystoid spaces present. When fluorescein angiography is performed in ischemic vein occlusion, there is often some fluorescein leakage at the border zone between the perfused and nonperfused retina during the acute phase (the first 6 months), but this leakage is not sufficient to produce accumulation of fluorescein in the center of the fovea.

A mixture of perfused and nonperfused edema is frequently seen in the acute phase of BRVO. There is some dilatation and leakage from perifoveal capillaries along with nonperfusion and a suggestion of leakage of fluorescein dye from the late fluorescein angiogram into the center of the fovea. It is unclear how much of the foveal cystoid edema is from perfused edema and how much is from nonperfused edema. Therefore, wait 6 to 12 months for spontaneous involution of the nonperfused edema and then reevaluate the situation.

In distant edema involving macular edema and a peripheral BRVO in which the blocked segment does not involve the macula, the cause of the macular edema remains obscure. This is a rare type of macular edema in BRVO.

The natural history of vision change without therapy has been described to some degree. For perfused edema, the type predominantly studied in the Branch Vein Occlusion Study [1,2], about one third of patients showed spontaneous improvement without laser photocoagulation. For the nonperfused and mixed forms of macular edema, a small pilot study suggested that the spontaneous improvement rate was far higher, about 90% [3]. Because the macular edema from distant BRVO is so uncommon, the natural history of vision loss in this form of edema is uncertain. However, in our limited experience, we have seen some patients' conditions spontaneously improve [4].

Laser management

After the acute phase of BRVO has resolved so that there has been sufficient intraretinal hemorrhage absorption to obtain high quality fluorescein angiography, the type of macular edema may be ascertained. If the macular edema is a perfused type, with intact capillaries and leakage of fluorescein dye into the center of the fovea, one may next assess the status of visual acuity. If visual acuity has been gradually improving, the patient may be one who has spontaneous improvement. Laser photocoagulation should not be considered until it is clearly demonstrated that visual acuity has stabilized. If visual acuity stabilizes (at a somewhat arbitrary level of 20/40 or worse), grid laser photocoagulation may be considered. The patient must understand that, statistically, the likelihood of improvement is only one to two lines of visual acuity; some patients improve far more and some patients do not improve at all. Of course, the patient should be told that if the vision in the fellow eye is good, improvement in visual acuity is not likely to benefit visual function if the fellow eye maintains better acuity.

Grid laser photocoagulation treatment includes the segment of leaking and dilated capillaries as seen on a high quality fluorescein angiogram and may extend from the vascular arcade to the border of the foveal avascular zone, if those areas are dilated and leaking. As a general guideline, the grid laser photocoagulation is applied using 100-μm spots for 0.1 seconds about one burn width apart, with a light to medium white burn seen at the level of the pigment epithelium (Fig. 6-3). Although treatment is usually performed under topical anesthesia at one sitting, it seems reasonable to avoid treating near the foveal avascular zone at the first sitting, particularly if the foveal landmarks are unclear. In such a circumstance, examination and fluorescein angiography can be repeated 2 months after treatment. Based on the pigmentation from the previous treat-

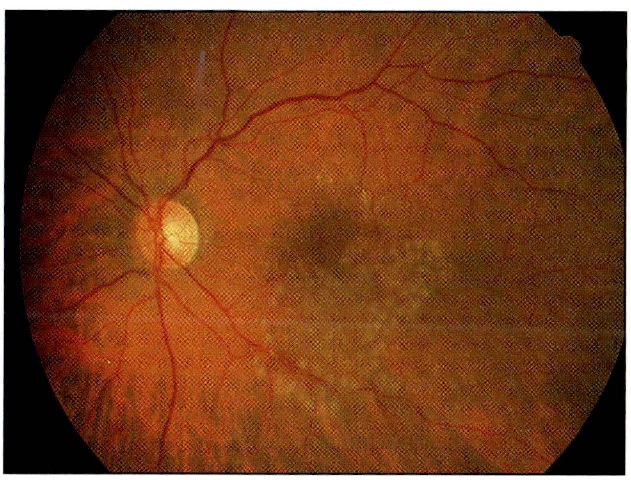

Figure 6-3. Posttreatment color photograph demonstrating pattern of grid laser photocoagulation for the management of macular edema secondary to branch retinal vein occlusion.

ment, any continued leakage, and vision loss the clinician can better evaluate the need for additional laser treatment closer to the fovea. Laser photocoagulation probably can be performed satisfactorily with any wavelength if the laser produces a light to medium light burn. There was no evidence from the Branch Vein Occlusion Study that laser photocoagulation needed to be performed early in the course of macular edema [1]. Consequently, we emphasize waiting for good resorption of intraretinal hemorrhage and sufficient follow-up to ensure that visual acuity has stabilized and is not spontaneously improving before considering laser photocoagulation.

Complications of grid laser photocoagulation are rare when the procedure is performed by an experienced surgeon, but patients must understand that visual acuity may be reduced by complications, including paracentral scotomas or preretinal fibrosis. Macular edema responds to grid laser photocoagulation within 4 to 8 weeks, although its temporal response has never been definitively studied. Visual acuity may respond quickly to grid laser photocoagulation but may also continue to improve slowly over months to years after edema has lessened.

Neovascularization

Retinal neovascularization is a frequent complication of BRVO, occurring in about 50% of patients who have large BRVOs (one quadrant or more of the fundus) associated with capillary nonperfusion (retinal ischemia) of significant extent (defined as 5 disc-diameters in diameter or more). Because about 50% of large BRVOs are associated with ischemia, it would be expected that about 25% of large BRVOs will develop neovascularization. Well-perfused BRVOs will not develop neovascularization. (Remember that ischemic retina may be present only in the far periphery). Neovascularization may occur at the optic nerve head (neovascularization of the disc) or in the peripheral retina (neovascularization elsewhere).

Iris neovascularization is a rare complication of BRVO. It seems to be associated with only very large areas of nonperfusion (greater than one quadrant of the fundus) and is more frequent in patients with diabetes.

Retinal neovascularization usually begins to appear between 4 and 12 months after an ischemic BRVO has occurred. Infrequently, the neovascularization may be noted to develop only after the first year of the occlusion. Although the neovascularization is usually apparent, it must be carefully distinguished from collateral vessels that can form in BRVO and that can mimic the appearance of neovascularization. If it is unclear whether abnormal blood vessels represent collateral vessels or neovascularization, fluorescein angiography may be helpful to demonstrate either profuse leakage from neovascularization or no leakage and minimal staining from collateral vessels.

About 50% of patients with neovascularization develop significant traction or vitreous hemorrhage as vision-limiting complications. The Branch Vein Occlusion Study [1,2] demonstrated that scatter laser photocoagulation placed over the ischemic segment of the fundus from beyond the vascular arcade to the far periphery can reduce by 50% the onset of neovascularization in ischemic occlusions and can reduce by 50% the occurrence of vitreous hemorrhage when neovascularization is already present. Because prophylactic treatment of all ischemic BRVO would lead to twice as many treatments as necessary (because 50% of patients with ischemia do not develop neovascularization), the Branch Vein Occlusion Study [1,2] suggested that laser photocoagulation be applied only after neovascularization begins to develop. However, patients must be monitored closely for development of neovascularization; if a patient cannot be followed every 4 months for the first 2 years after an ischemic occlusion, then the

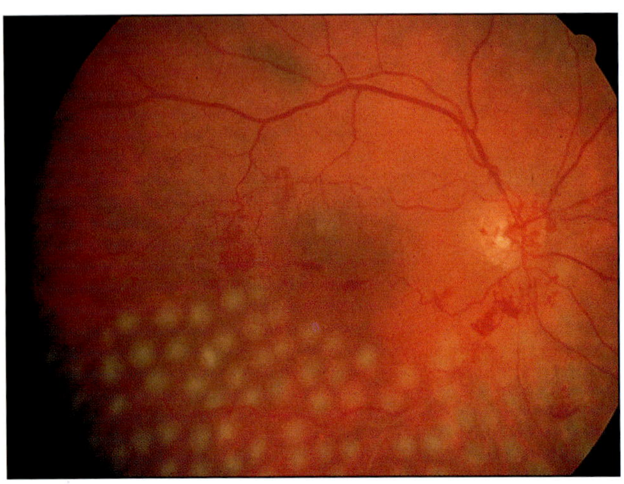

FIGURE 6-4. Posttreatment color photograph demonstrating pattern of scatter laser photocoagulation for the management of neovascularization secondary to branch retinal vein occlusion.

clinician could consider scatter laser photocoagulation before the development of neovascularization.

Scatter laser photocoagulation is applied in the same general manner as it is for the management of proliferative diabetic retinopathy, with 200- to 500-μm medium white burns at 0.1 to 0.2 seconds, absorbed at the level of the retinal pigment epithelium (Fig. 6-4). One should not attempt to close the neovascularization directly with focal treatment either on the disc or in the peripheral retina. Although topical anesthesia is often adequate, some patients suffer significant discomfort and may require peribulbar or retrobulbar anesthesia.

Complications of laser photocoagulation

When performed by an experienced surgeon, laser photocoagulation is remarkably safe for both macular treatment for macular edema and peripheral scatter treatment for the management of neovascularization. However, side effects and complications can occur. Patients must be thoroughly informed of the important benefits and risks of photocoagulation when deciding with the physician whether laser photocoagulation should be performed.

The patient being treated for macular edema should understand that grid laser photocoagulation will produce a noticeable scotoma pattern resembling a "cluster of grapes" or black dots that will gradually fade over a period of weeks to months. However, some patients find the persistence of these scotomas to be an annoying disability. If laser photocoagulation leads to confluent spots, a resulting larger scotoma could be disabling for reading vision or other fine visual tasks, even if the visual acuity is improved by the treatment. Other complications and side effects of macular photocoagulation include inadvertent foveal treatment, preretinal fibrosis, and subretinal fibrosis. Particular care should be taken to avoid photocoagulation over sheets of intraretinal hemorrhage, because the resultant heating of the retinal surface may cause preretinal fibrosis. In addition, laser photocoagulation with sufficient power to puncture Bruch's membrane may be expected to be associated with macular fibrosis. Laser photocoagulation for the management of neovascularization also can produce side effects and complications. Scatter photocoagulation can reduce the visual field extent in the quadrant being treated. Photocoagulation over sheets of intraretinal hemorrhage should be avoided because it can produce preretinal traction that could extend to macular distortion. Other vision-limiting complications and side effects can occur, but are less frequent.

Conclusions

Laser photocoagulation has been shown to be beneficial for management of BRVO complications including macular edema and neovascularization.

CENTRAL RETINAL VEIN OCCLUSION

Central retinal vein occlusion (CRVO) is a relatively common condition that affects older people. It has different forms of presentation and evolution and can resolve spontaneously, but it frequently leads to severe visual loss as a result of severe macular edema and neovascular glaucoma. Less commonly, patients with CRVO may develop retinal neovascularization and vitreous hemorrhage.

The role of laser therapy in the treatment and prevention of the complications of CRVO has been controversial for many years. The Central Vein Occlusion Study [5–8] resolved some of the controversy and provided recommendations for the use of laser therapy in this condition. This study included 725 patients enrolled by eight clinics throughout the United States and one clinic in France. The study patients, who were followed at 4-month intervals for 3 years, were categorized into four groups: nonischemic or perfused (Fig. 6-5), ischemic or

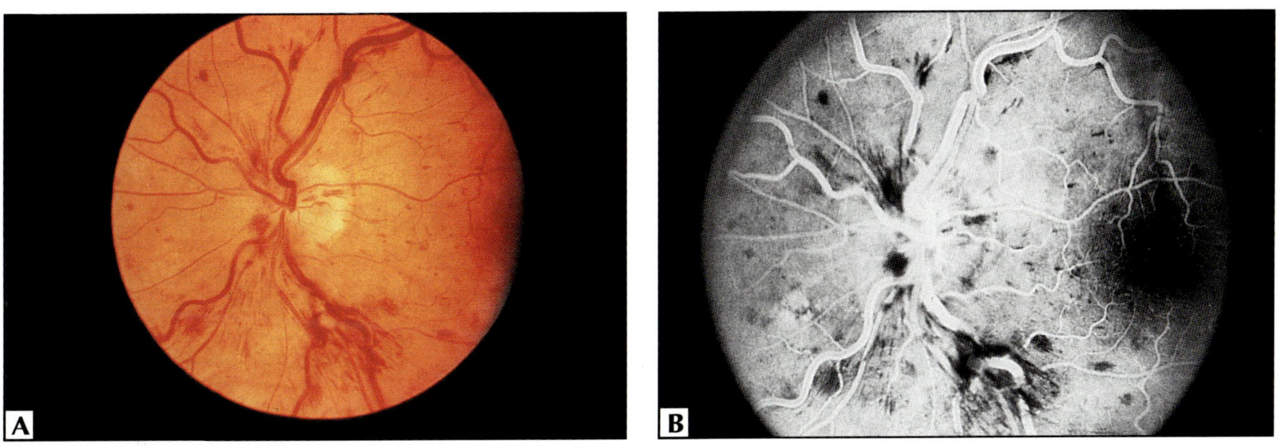

FIGURE 6-5. Nonischemic central retinal vein occlusion. Color photograph (**A**) and full venous phase angiogram (**B**) showing no areas of capillary closure.

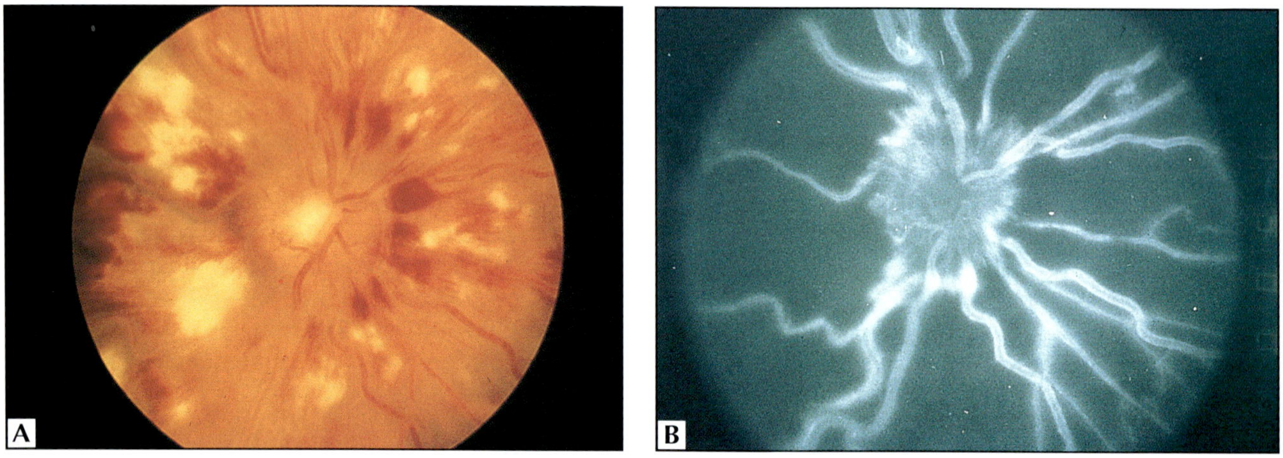

FIGURE 6-6. Ischemic central retinal vein occlusion. Color photograph (**A**) shows multiple microinfarcts. The corresponding angiogram (**B**) shows extensive capillary closure.

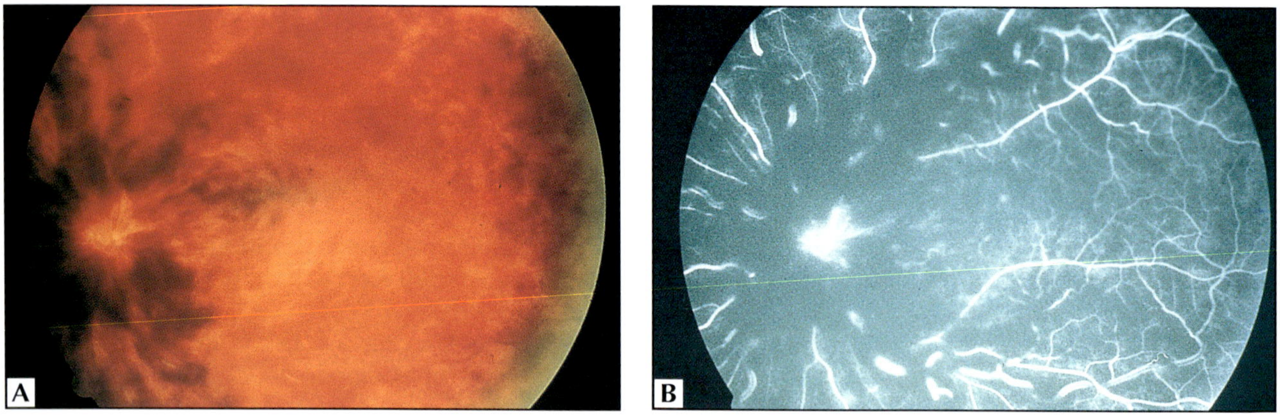

FIGURE 6-7. Indeterminate central retinal vein occlusion. **A**, Confluent retinal hemorrhages in four quadrants. **B**, Corresponding angiogram shows blocked visualization of retinal capillaries.

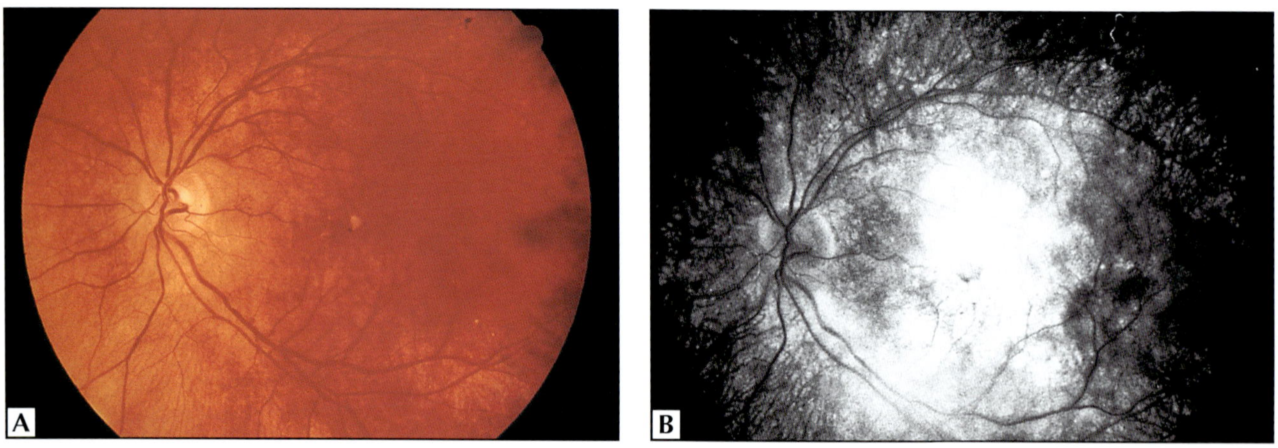

FIGURE 6-8. **A**, Central retinal vein occlusion with macular edema. **B**, Late-phase angiogram corresponding to the color picture shows characteristic cystoid pattern of macular edema.

nonperfused (Fig. 6-6), indeterminate perfusion (Fig. 6-7), and macular edema (Fig. 6-8). The characteristics of each group are listed in Table 6-1. Patients in the ischemic group were randomized to laser therapy or observation to determine whether laser treatment could prevent iris neovascularization. Patients in the macular edema group were randomized to laser therapy or observation to determine whether laser treatment could reduce macular edema and improve vision.

Following the guidelines of the Central Vein Occlusion Study [5–8], laser therapy is currently considered for treatment of the following complications of CRVO: neovascular glaucoma, iris and angle neovascularization (INV-ANV), retinal neovascularization and vitreous hemorrhage, and macular edema.

Neovascular glaucoma

This form of glaucoma is the most severe complication of CRVO and can be its initial presentation. It is characterized by the relatively sudden onset of ocular pain associated with elevated intraocular pressure (IOP) and a history of visual loss of several weeks' to months' duration. Vision is severely decreased, and INV-ANV occurs, obstructing the trabecular meshwork. Treatment includes the use of topical steroids, cycloplegics, and agents to lower IOP. Extensive panretinal photocoagulation will be effective if the angle is only partially compromised. Usually, three to four sessions of panretinal photocoagulation are required, using at least 2000 to 3000 burns of at least 500 µm. Retrobulbar anesthesia often is required, as are topical hyperosmotic agents to clear corneal edema at the time of treatment. Panretinal photocoagulation should be continued until the INV-ANV regresses.

If IOP remains elevated despite resolution of INV-ANV, filtering procedures should be considered. Otherwise, cyclodestructive treatments or enucleation may ultimately be required. The Central Vein Occlusion Study [5–8] showed that panretinal photocoagulation does not always prevent neovascularization; however, neovascular glaucoma could be treated or prevented in most cases if panretinal photocoagulation were applied at the earliest signs of INV-ANV [7]. Therefore, in patients with CRVO, it is critical to have an adequate follow-up schedule to detect early INV-ANV.

TABLE 6-1 CENTRAL RETINAL VEIN OCCLUSION

Nonischemic or perfused CRVO (Fig. 6-5)
Intraretinal hemorrhage present in all four quadrants
Retinal capillary nonperfusion absent or less than 10 disc areas demonstrated on fluorescein angiography
Ischemic or nonperfused CRVO (Fig. 6-6)
Intraretinal hemorrhage present in all four quadrants
Retinal capillary nonperfusion in at least 10 disc areas demonstrated on fluorescein angiography
Indeterminate perfusion CRVO (Fig. 6-7)
Confluent intraretinal hemorrhage present in all four quadrants and preventing evaluation of the retinal capillaries by fluorescein angiography
Macular edema with CRVO (Fig. 6-8)
Nonischemic or ischemic CRVO with clinically significant perfused macular edema demonstrated on fluorescein angiography

CRVO—central retinal vein occlusion.

Iris neovascularization and angle neovascularization

Iris neovascularization and angle neovascularization are essential components of neovascular glaucoma and appear before elevation of IOP. The Central Vein Occlusion Study [7] was designed to determine whether prophylactic panretinal photocoagulation prevents the development of neovascularization in patients with nonperfused CRVO. The study showed that prophylactic panretinal photocoagulation does *not* always prevent the development of INV-ANV. It is the role of the clinician to examine all CRVO patients thoroughly for INV-ANV. In the study, 16% of the overall group, 10% of eyes initially categorized as perfused, and 35% of eyes initially classified as nonperfused or indeterminate had INV-ANV. Therefore, patients with any form of CRVO are at risk for anterior segment neovascularization. Factors that increased the risks for development of INV-ANV included poor visual acuity, more than 30 disc areas of nonperfusion, moderate to severe retinal tortuosity, retinal hemorrhage, and shorter disease duration (less than 1 month).

The guidelines for early detection of INV-ANV are based on the finding that these complications are more likely to occur in the first 6 months of the disease and are strongly correlated with the initial level of visual acuity [8••].

Patients with CRVO and visual acuity of 20/40 or better should be examined every 1 to 2 months for the first 6 months and yearly thereafter. If visual acuity is less than 20/200, monthly evaluations should be done for 6 months to 1 year. If visual acuity is from 20/50 to 20/200, the patient should be examined every 1 to 2 months for 6 months, depending on changes in vision. If at any point during follow-up the visual acuity drops to 20/200 or worse, the clinician should assume that the vein occlusion has become nonperfused, and close follow-up should be extended for several months. Follow-up examinations in patients with CRVO should include a careful examination of the undilated pupil with high magnification under the slit lamp to detect early neovascularization at the pupillary border. Because neovascularization can first appear on angular structures, gonioscopy should always be performed.

As soon as neovascularization is recognized in either the angle or the iris, panretinal photocoagulation should be applied following the parameters listed in Table 6-2. Treatment should be continued until neovascularization resolves.

If a patient is not available for close follow-up, the clinician should carefully consider all risk factors for development of INV-ANV before recommending prophylactic panretinal photocoagulation. Many patients with ischemic CRVO do not develop INV-ANV. Consequently, panretinal photocoagulation applied only when INV-ANV develops appears to save many patients from unnecessary prophylactic treatment.

Retinal neovascularization and vitreous hemorrhage

Retinal neovascularization at the disc or elsewhere occurs in approximately 15% of patients with CRVO. In half these patients, the retinal neovascularization is associated with anterior segment neovascularization. To prevent vitreous hemorrhage, panretinal photocoagulation should be applied at the first signs of retinal neovascularization [7].

The significance of vitreous hemorrhage associated with ANV CRVO is illustrated by the following case. A woman aged 68 years presented with decreased vision in the right eye for several months that had been followed by sudden further decreased vision a few days before presentation. Visual acuity was decreased to hand-motions in the right eye and was 20/15 in the left. In the right eye, an afferent pupillary defect and dense vitreous hemorrhage with no visualization of the fundus were present. The left fundus was unremarkable. Anterior segment evaluation of the right eye showed no evidence of iris neovascularization, but gonioscopy revealed extensive neovascularization throughout the angle structures. IOP was 20 in the right eye and 19 in the left. The patient underwent vitrectomy and endophotocoagulation with the presumptive diagnosis of CRVO complicated by ANV and vitreous hemorrhage. The diagnosis was confirmed at the time of surgery. Gonioscopy should be performed routinely in all patients with vitreous hemorrhage in one eye and a history suggestive of long-standing visual loss with recent worsening.

TABLE 6-2 PANRETINAL PHOTOCOAGULATION FOR CENTRAL RETINAL VEIN OCCLUSION

- 1000 to 2000 treatment spots, 0.5 to 1.0 burn width apart
- Treatment to or beyond the equator in all quadrants
- Treatment no closer than 2 disc diameters temporal to the fovea and 500 μm nasal to the disc
- Spot size 500 or 1000 μm
- Duration 0.2 seconds
- Moderately intense whitening of the retina

Macular edema

Macular edema is common in CRVO and accounts for decreased vision in a substantial number of patients. Some beneficial effects of laser treatment were suggested by small nonrandomized studies [9,10]. The Central Vein Occlusion Study [7] evaluated the effect of grid laser therapy in a group of 155 patients with CRVO associated with macular edema. Of these patients, 77 were randomized to treatment and 78 to observation only. Although macular edema was significantly reduced angiographically in treated patients, final visual acuity was similar in the treated and untreated groups. Therefore, laser therapy is not indicated in cases of macular edema associated with CRVO.

In the study, treated patients under age 60 showed a trend toward improved vision. However, the small number of patients in this age group did not allow a statistically significant result. Individualized clinical

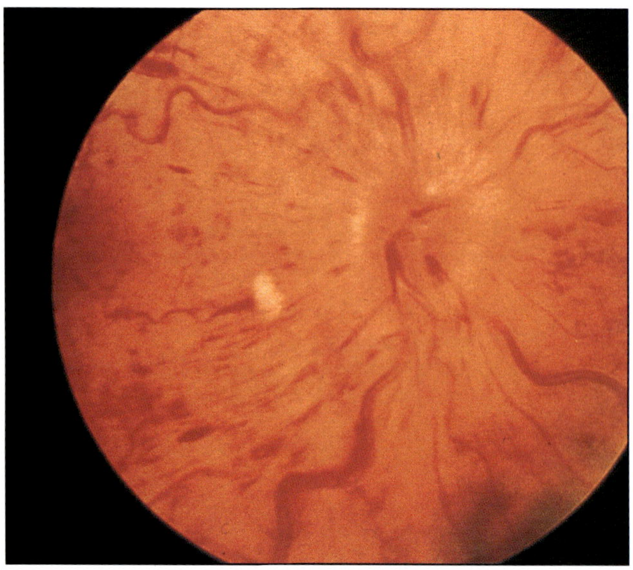

FIGURE 6-9. Right fundus showing characteristic features of central retinal vein occlusion of recent onset.

judgment should be used in patients under age 60 with macular edema and CRVO. The following example illustrates this point.

CRVO was diagnosed in man aged 55 years whose vision was 20/100 (Fig. 6-9). A year later, the hemorrhagic component of the vein occlusion had resolved; however, visual acuity remained decreased at 20/60 secondary to macular edema involving the temporal aspect of the macula (Fig. 6-10). Laser therapy directed to the area of leakage that was identified on angiography caused resolution of the edema with improvement of vision to 20/20 level (Fig. 6-11).

The beneficial effect of laser therapy in this patient may have resulted from his relatively younger age compared with the majority of CRVO patients and perhaps to the localized nature of the edema, which resembled the type of edema seen in branch vein occlusions.

Conclusions

Prophylactic panretinal photocoagulation in CRVO does not always prevent anterior segment neovascularization and should be applied only at the first sign of INV-ANV to prevent development of neovascular glaucoma.

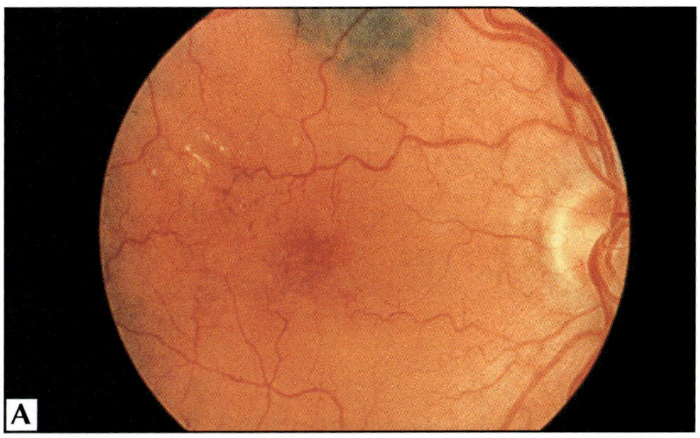

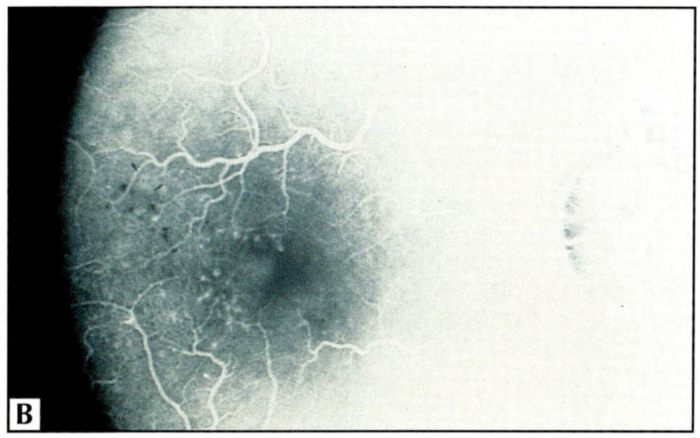

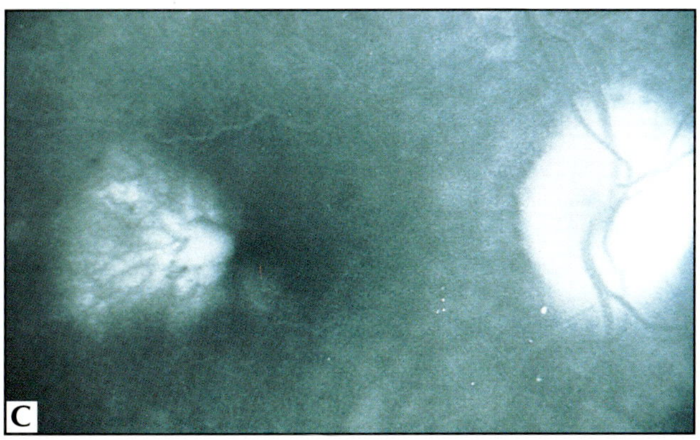

FIGURE 6-10. **A**, Same eye as in Figure 6-5, years later, showing resolution of hemorrhage. Corresponding angiograms showing, **B**, capillary abnormalities temporal to fovea and **C**, sector cystoid macular edema.

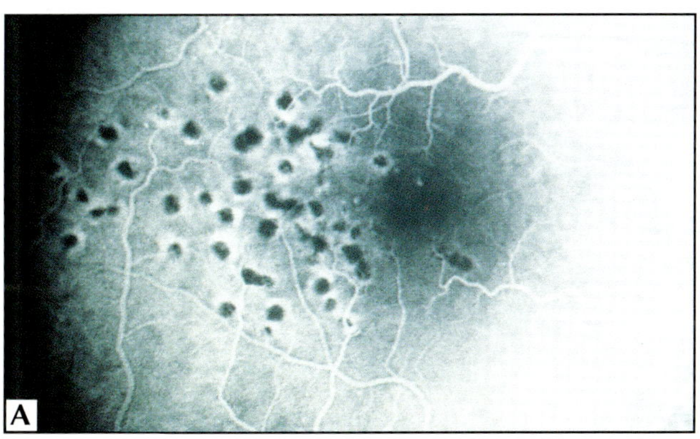

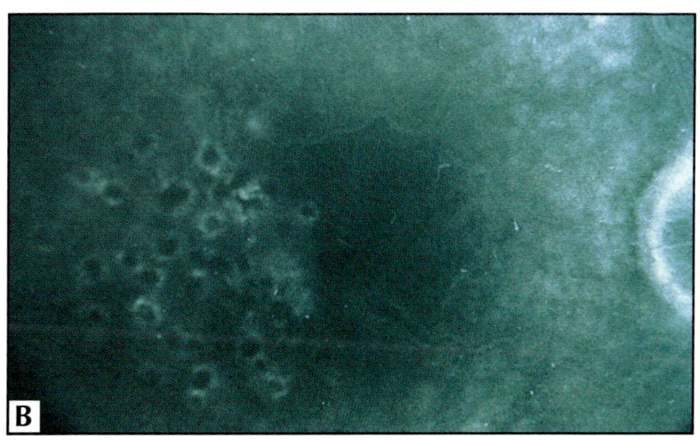

FIGURE 6-11. Early- and late-phase angiogram, same eye as shown in Figures 6-5 and 6-6, a few months after laser treatment. **A**, Angiogram of laser scars temporal to the fovea. **B**, No macular edema in the late phase.

Because perfused and indeterminate CRVOs frequently become ischemic early in their course, careful evaluation of the iris and angle should be done in all patients with CRVO, especially in the first 6 months. Laser therapy is not indicated in macular edema associated with CRVO, but it may be considered in patients under age 60.

Investigational Chorioretinal Venous Anastomosis for the Management of Branch and Central Retinal Vein Occlusion

McAllister and Constable [11] popularized the use of laser to effect a chorioretinal anastomosis to bypass the venous occlusion in CRVO. They showed that this treatment could result in improvement in visual acuity. Fekrat *et al.* [12] showed similar evidence strongly suggesting that, at least occasionally, macular edema can be lessened and visual acuity improved in perfused CRVO with macular edema and vision loss. These investigations and others [13–15] have emphasized that vision-limiting complications can occur and that there is no reason to expect that the procedure would be useful in ischemic vein occlusion.

Further studies are under way to evaluate the potential of this investigative procedure.

References and Recommended Reading

Recently published papers of particular interest have been highlighted as:

- • Of interest
- •• Of outstanding interest

1. Branch Vein Occlusion Study Group: Argon laser photocoagulation for macular edema in branch vein occlusion. *Am J Opthalmol* 1984, 98:271–282.

2. Branch Vein Occlusion Study Group: Argon laser scatter photocoagulation for prevention of neovascularization and vitreous hemorrhage in branch vein occlusion. *Arch Opthalmol* 1986, 104:34–41.

3. Finkelstein D: Ischemic macular edema: recognition and favorable natural history in branch vein occlusion. *Arch Opthalmol* 1992, 110:1427–1434.

4. Finkelstein D, Patz A: Distant effect of peripheral branch vein occlusion on the macula. *Tr Am Ophthalmol Soc* 1988, LXXXVI:380–388.

5. Central Vein Occlusion Study Group: Baseline and early natural history report. The Central Vein Occlusion Study. *Arch Ophthalmol* 1993, 115:486–491.

6. Central Vein Occlusion Study Group: Evaluation of grid pattern photocoagulation for macular edema in central vein occlusion. The Central Vein Occlusion Study Group M report. *Ophthalmology* 1995,102:1425–1433.

7. Central Vein Occlusion Study Group: A randomized clinical trial of early panretinal photocoagulation for ischemic central vein occlusion. The Central Vein Occlusion Study Group N report. *Ophthalmology* 1995, 102:1434–1444.

8.•• Central Vein Occlusion Study Group: Natural history and clinical management of central retinal vein occlusion. *Arch Ophthalmol* 1997, 1154:486–491.

This report summarizes the guidelines for the management of CRVO.

9. Gutman FA, Zegarra H: Macular edema secondary to occlusion of the retinal veins. *Surv Ophthalmol* 1984, 28(Suppl):462–470.

10. Klein ML, Finkelstein D: Macular grid photocoagulation for macular edema in central retinal vein occlusion. *Arch Ophthalmol* 1989, 107:1297–1302.

11. McAllister IL, Constable J: Laser-induced chorioretinal anastomosis for treatment of nonischemic central retinal vein occlusion. *Arch Ophthalmol* 1995, 113:456–462.

12. Fekrat S, Goldberg FM, Finkelstein D: Laser-induced chorioretinal venous anastomosis for nonischemic central or branch retinal vein occlusion. *Arch Ophthalmol* 1998, 116:43–52.

13. Browning DJ, Antoszyk AN: Laser chorioretinal venous anastomosis for nonischemic central retinal vein occlusion. *Ophthalmology* 1998, 105:670–677.

14. Luttrull JK: Epiretinal membrane and traction retinal detachment complicating laser-induced chorioretinal venous anastomosis. *Am J Ophthalmol* 1997, 123:698–699.

15. Eccarius SG, Moran MJ, Slingsby JG: Choroidal neovascular membrane after laser-induced chorioretinal anastomosis. *Am J Ophthalmol* 1996, 122:590–591.

Selected Bibliography

Coscas G, Dhermy P: Occlusions veineuses rétiniennes. In *Socíetíe Francaise D'Ophtalmologie* Paris: Masson; 1978.

Orth DH, Patz A: Retinal branch vein occlusion. *Surv Ophthalmol* 1978, 22:357–376.

CHAPTER **7**

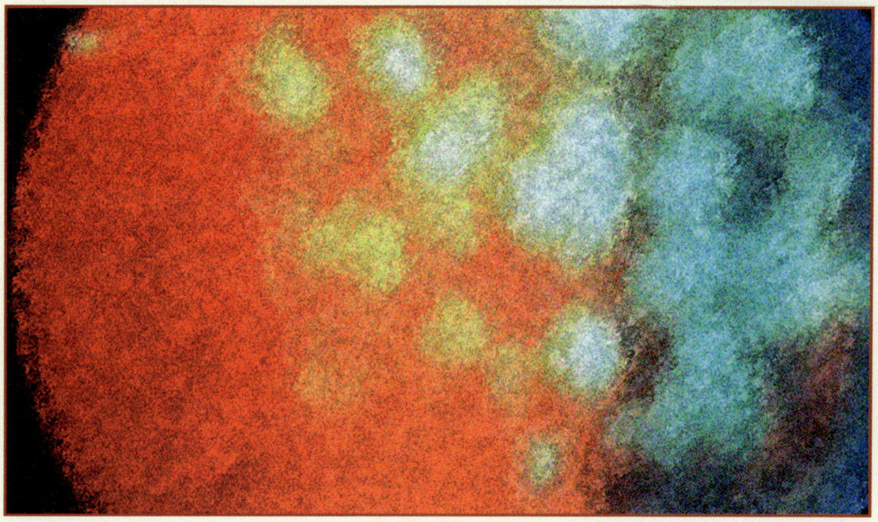

Laser Treatment of Choroidal Neovascular Membrane in Age-Related Maculopathy

Gisèle Soubrane
Gabriel Coscas

In developed countries, age-related maculopathy (ARM) is the leading cause of severe and irreversible central visual loss in people aged more than 50 years. The neovascular form is estimated to develop in approximately 8% of patients with ARM. However, this form accounts for 88% of the legal blindness associated with ARM, because the condition affects both eyes over time. Risk factors for development of choroidal neovascular membrane (CNV) in the fellow eye include central macular characteristics and systemic hypertension [1••].

The neovascular form of ARM often occurs as sudden or recent subacute visual loss with a relative central or paracentral scotoma and accompanying metamorphopsia. Biomicroscopic signs of CNV include the presence of subretinal fluid, retinal or subretinal hemorrhages and lipids, elevation of the retinal pigment epithelium (RPE), cystic changes in the sensory retina, and discoloration of the RPE. Fluorescein angiography has been the standard imaging modality used in evaluation and treatment of CNV. Stereoangiographic interpretation of neovascular ARM remains invaluable in identifying the type, location, and extent of CNV. At present, indocyanine green (ICG) angiography is providing additional clues that are frequently useful and may be essential.

Recognition of the different lesion components has been an evolving process as a result of refinement of our knowledge [2]. CNV associated with ARM may have various complex angiographic manifestations. It can be classified into two major types on the basis of fluorescein angiography: well-defined (classic) CNV and ill-defined (occult) CNV. At first examination, 13% to 30% of patients present with well-defined CNV and the rest with occult or associated CNV components [3,4]. The boundaries of CNV can be obscured by a pigment epithelium detachment (PED), a thick layer of blood or other material, and elevated blocked fluorescence. On ICG angiography, CNV can manifest as localized active CNV, or diffuse dormant areas.

Information obtained in long-term follow-up with fluorescein angiography constitutes the foundation for photocoagulation treatment guidance. According to this classification, different treatment approaches may be considered, but randomized clinical trials have demonstrated the efficacy of laser photocoagulation only for well-defined CNV on fluorescein angiography.

TREATMENT OF WELL-DEFINED CHOROIDAL NEOVASCULAR MEMBRANES

Well-defined CNV is characterized on fluorescein angiography by early bright choroidal hyperfluorescence with well-demarcated boundaries with or without a lacy or vascular pattern. The area of hyperfluorescence is often underlined with a hypofluorescent rim. With progressive dye transit, the boundaries of well-defined CNV become obscured by the rapid and extensive leakage of dye. During recirculation, the dye progressively pools into the overlying subsensory retinal space and into the cystic retinal spaces. On ICG angiography, one third to one half of the well-defined CNV can be identified as an early hyperfluorescent lacy pattern depending on the instrument used.

Three categories of well-defined CNV are distinguished according to their distance from the fovea: extrafoveal, juxtafoveal, and subfoveal. Extrafoveal CNV is located 200 µm or more from the center of the xanthophyll pigment and the foveal avascular zone. The posterior boundary of juxtafoveal CNV falls from 1 to 199 µm from the fovea. Subfoveal CNV is present within the center of the fovea.

Because the treatment technique of well-defined CNV relates to its distance from the fovea, determination of its precise location is crucial. The fovea is considered to be the anatomic center of both the xanthophyll pigment area and the foveal avascular zone [5,6]. Xanthophyll pigment is delineated on a blue light frame (shot before injection, without the barrier filter) and its geometric center is defined as the fovea. The foveal avascular zone is most clearly visible on an early frame of the stereoangiographic film. Moreover, the exact location and the extent of the CNV (including the dark rim) in relation to the fovea are determined on a frame from the arteriovenous phase, in which the neovascularization has not yet begun to leak. These landmarks are drawn either directly onto transparent paper [6] or drawn with the help of a viewer (Documentor D1-2 microfilm reader, Zeiss, Jena, Germany) [7] or, as is currently possible, automatically mapped using digitized imaging systems [8,9]. If the fovea is obscured by blood, the area of fixation can be determined with the projection of a fixation cross on the patient's retina or more accurately with the scanning laser ophthalmoscope (SLO) (Rodenstock Instrument GmBH, Munich, Germany) [10].

The efficacy of the different laser wavelengths available has been compared in several studies. For extrafoveal CNV, krypton laser has been shown to be as effective as argon green on visual acuity outcome and rate of recurrence [11]. Small differences were evidenced by the Macular Photocoagulation Study Group [12] in the photocoagulation of subfoveal CNV with either argon green or krypton red. Diode, dye red, and yttrium-aluminum-garnet (YAG) double frequency lasers have been evaluated in pilot studies. Specific situations might require use of the optimal wavelength to avoid iatrogenic complications. Red wavelengths are well transmitted through opalescent media, justifying their use in elderly patients with ARM. Furthermore, there is minimal uptake by macular xanthophyll and by a thin layer of blood that is often contiguous to the peripheral neovascular arcade on the foveal border or to a major retinal vessel overlying the membrane. Small true differences may exist between different wavelengths, but this would require a large number of patients in order to be verified.

Photocoagulation

This treatment modality, evaluated in various trials, involves the complete destruction of the neovascular net with confluent, overlapping, intense laser burns. Argon green laser photocoagulation of extrafoveal CNV has been reported to influence visual outcome favorably as much as 3 to 5 years after treatment. Krypton red laser photocoagulation has been shown to be efficient for juxtafoveal CNV [13].

Direct laser treatment of subfoveal CNV—new or recurrent lesions—has been demonstrated to result in less severe visual loss when compared with the natural course of this disease [14, 15]. The Macular Photocoagulation Study's (MPS) [14] subfoveal trials found that laser treatment was effective in reducing severe visual loss in treated eyes over 42 months of follow-up study. Treated eyes also retained a stable level of contrast threshold scores and a greater reading speed than those that did not receive treatment. However, laser-treated eyes experienced an immediate decline in visual acuity. Treatment benefit depended on the size of the membrane and the initial acuity. Eyes with small lesions (≤1 MPS disc area) and poor (20/200 or worse) or moderate (20/125 to 20/160) vision derived the greatest benefit from laser therapy, as did eyes with intermediate-size lesions (>1 to ≤2 MPS disc areas) and poor vision. Eyes with larger lesions (>2 MPS disc areas) with good or poor initial visual acuity did not benefit substantially from photocoagulation [15].

Treatment for recurrent subfoveal CNV also showed positive results with respect to severe visual acuity loss, average visual acuity, and average change in visual acuity at 2 years' follow-up [16]. Reading speed and contrast threshold levels supported the use of photocoagulation treatment.

The Macular Photocoagulation Study [14] recommends extensive education to prepare patients for an immediate and possibly profound decrease in visual acuity after direct treatment of subfoveal CNV in exchange for a better long-term level of visual function. Patients should be monitored closely for spontaneous decline of visual acuity before direct photocoagulation is applied.

Reluctance to ablate the foveal center that results in immediate and permanent decline in visual acuity has led to consideration of the use of an alternative technique of laser photocoagulation. The technique of the Perifoveal Laser Photocoagulation of Créteil group [17] for larger subfoveal CNV consists of a "doughnut" of confluent burns applied to the periphery of the choroidal neovascular lesion with sparing of the central foveal avascular zone (400 μm in diameter). In a randomized clinical trial, this technique was applied to well-defined and occult CNV. A lifetable analysis demonstrated a six-line loss of vision in 17% of treated eyes compared with 48% of untreated eyes at 2 years' follow-up. A final reading visual acuity of J4 or better was attained with the assistance of low-vision aids in 73% of the treated eyes and in 47% of the untreated eyes. Persistent subretinal fluid and fluorescein leakage inside the foveal avascular zone, which resolved with time, were common in treated eyes because this area was not photocoagulated. Finally, morphologic success, defined as resolution of fluorescein leakage in the area ablated by laser treatment, was achieved in 53 of 68 treated eyes compared with 19 of 59 untreated eyes that progressed to an atrophic scar. A parallel pilot study found an even better visual outcome [18]. Perifoveal treatment may be helpful in preserving visual acuity and pretreatment central fixation [19] and in providing low-vision rehabilitation, particularly for near-vision tasks. Progressive expansion of RPE atrophy results eventually in the development of an eccentric fixation point.

The technique of the Créteil group [17] is a useful alternative for treatment of CNV extending beyond the foveal avascular zone without immediate decline in visual acuity. Eventually, the functional results of the subfoveal or the perifoveal techniques become similar.

Postoperative management

Laser treatment is performed with the objective to coagulate and obliterate the entire area of CNV and to prevent the eye from developing recurrences. The high rate of recurrences after photocoagulation in eyes with ARM (from 48% to 76%) necessitates that complete treatment of the proliferating membrane be performed.

The first step is to determine the precise area to be treated. It is essential to completely and uniformly cover the entire neovascular membrane as well as the peripheral dark rim with intense confluent burns. Postoperative laser fundus photographs must be carefully compared with preoperative tracing. Manual or digitized techniques ensure that complete treatment of CNV is performed. Adequacy of treatment reduces the high rate of recurrence and avoids severe visual acuity loss [20].

The depth and quality of treatment can be assessed with an immediate post-treatment ICG angiogram. ICG dye can disclose the perfusion of the remaining new vessels still perfused within the treated area as a result of limited leakage of the dye. A late leakage (*eg,* at 20 minutes) may occur on the border of the area, thus demonstrating the thermal damage to choroidal vessels [21].

Approximately 60% of treated eyes will experience persistent and possibly recurrent CNV within the first 3 months after treatment, but will also manifest recurrences after that time. Various risk factors have been identified that affect the frequency of recurrences, especially characteristics of the fellow eye.

A biomicroscopic and an angiographic examination must, in any case, be performed at 2 weeks to rule out any persistent CNV. Earlier evaluation with fluorescein angiography is not informative because of profuse leakage of the dye within the photocoagulation scar. ICG angiography performed 1 to 5 days after treatment can image persistent CNV more precisely than fluoresoein angiography can in that period [22]. Follow-up visits must be performed at 1, 2, and 3 months postoperatively and every trimester thereafter to identify recurrences as early as possible.

Identification of a recurrence is often a challenge. Symptoms are not always perceived by the patient. Fluorescein angiography, for the most part, requires comparative, careful analysis of all available fluorescein angiograms to identify an area of discrete late leakage. ICG angiography will, in many cases, be an efficient adjunct test to discern the exact area of recurrence [23]. Early and immediate re-treatment of any well-defined CNV recurrence is recommended, especially when the intention is to spare the fovea.

In experimental models, ingrowth of new choroidal vessels after laser photocoagulation could explain the high recurrence rate observed in clinical experience. An ultrastructural study of the choroidal vascular repair following krypton laser injury in rats showed that three processes occur: initial recanalization of the damaged vessels, neovascularization at the periphery of large lesions, and, at 2 weeks, atrophy of both recanalized and newly formed capillaries [24]. This observation parallels the timing and the location of recurrences following laser photocoagulation in humans. Furthermore, photocoagulation does not eliminate retinal production of angiogenic activity [25]. The factors playing a role in new vessels' ingrowth—as with their scarring and exact sequence—remain unknown, even in experimental models.

Randomized clinical trials have demonstrated the efficacy of using laser photocoagulation to treat well-defined CNV in any location compared with allowing the disease to pursue its natural course. The resulting visual function is related to the location of the membrane, the quality of the initial photocoagulation treatment, and the absence of associated occult new vessels, which need to be ruled out.

TREATMENT OF ISOLATED OCCULT CHOROIDAL NEOVASCULAR MEMBRANES

Features of occult CNV may be subdivided into isolated occult CNV or fibrovascular PEDs based on fluorescein angiography [2]. In isolated occult CNV (or late leakage of undetermined source), the early phase of the angiogram does not identify a discrete and discernible source of leakage. Frames from the middle and late phases show diffuse leakage into the overlying subsensory retinal space, often with punctate or stippled hyperfluorescence in the outer retina. The boundaries of this form of occult CNV are poorly demarcated on fluorescein angiography.

Fibrovascular PED is an area of irregular elevation of the RPE, consisting of speckled hyperfluorescence within 1 to 2 minutes after fluorescein injection and persistence of staining or leaking of fluorescein dye within 10 minutes after injection. This type of occult CNV will be considered together with vascularized PED later in this chapter.

Direct photocoagulation treatment

Complete coagulation of isolated occult CNV that does not extend through the center of the foveal avascular zone on fluorescein angiography has been suggested as beneficial in the prevention of additional severe visual acuity loss. However, it has only been shown to be successful in one third of eyes and therefore cannot be recommended [26]. Failure of treatment is clearly related to imprecise delineation of the boundaries of the CNV, which results in a high rate of subfoveal recurrence.

Angiography with ICG has been shown not only to confirm but also to delineate occult CNV better in a large number of eyes using SLO systems or digital imaging instruments. Conversion of isolated occult CNV to an early well-defined lacy pattern or to a late well-delineated staining plaque results in treatment eligibility in 15% to as much as 34% [27–31].

In terms of extrafoveal or juxtafoveal occult CNV, preliminary data suggest that ICG angiography–guided laser photocoagulation can obtain at least short-term resolution of the exudative manifestation in 56% to 63% of eyes [28,29,30]. In some of these selected cases, visual function stabilizes or even improves during follow-up.

Subfoveal occult CNV has a poor long-term natural history, but this is not invariable. Moreover, most occult CNV involves the entire macular area at presentation. Although at presentation 60% of eyes with subfoveal membranes had 20/50 or better visual acuity, 36% retained the same level after 12 to 95 months' follow-up [26].

Subfoveal occult CNV was not considered in the protocols of the Macular Photocoagulation Study's [14] subfoveal trials. In the Créteil group [17], final visual results did not differ according to the type of new vessels included. Direct photocoagulation was shown to be effective in preservation of visual acuity but only if initial baseline acuity was 20/100 or worse.

In a pilot study, only focal spots at the edge of the plaque of neovascularization on ICG study were photocoagulated [32]. Preliminary results suggest that this approach may improve the visual prognosis of eyes with lesions that cannot presently be treated.

The benefit of ICG-guided laser photocoagulation has not been evaluated in a prospective randomized controlled clinical trial. No treatment approach has yet been considered for eyes with subfoveal occult CNV retaining a visual acuity of 20/100 or better.

Indirect scatter laser photocoagulation

This alternative treatment was considered to avoid the destructive effects of confluent laser photocoagulation in symptomatic eyes that presented with subfoveal occult CNV and retain some useful visual acuity. This ... eovascular process ... RPE.

... e designed to test ... eatment study, the ... ciated with visible ... ray) photocoagula- ... seline visual acuity ... 'indirect grid" laser ... id to occupy at least ... leaving a visual acu- ... burns were applied ... avoiding the area of ... atter laser treatment ... or long term for visu- ... angiographic pattern. ... ed eyes had lost 6 or ... 4% had become legal-

... eyes with occult CNV ... . In addition, patients ... at significant risk for ... second eye [35], thus ... iopment of new treat-

...NED CHOROIDAL ... ASSOCIATED ...L NEOVASCULAR MEMBRANE

The combination of well-defined and occult CNV is not uncommon in symptomatic eyes. This association may occur during the follow-up of isolated occult CNV [26]. Within a short period of time (9 to 12 months), well-defined CNV developed in 52% of eyes, resulting in a median loss of visual acuity of 2.5 lines [36•].

If the entire lesion spares the center of the foveal avascular zone on fluorescein angiography, laser treatment to the entire area may be considered. Treatment of only the well-defined CNV is probably not to be recommended. Furthermore, even when the entire area of well-defined and occult CNV is managed with dense treatment, there is a very high likelihood of persistence or recurrence, for which additional treatment through the foveola may be indicated [37•]. Frequent follow-up with fluorescein and ICG angiography is of paramount importance in these borderline cases to reduce the risk of additional severe visual acuity loss resulting from recurrences.

If the occult lesion extends into the center of the foveal avascular zone and the well-defined CNV is juxtafoveal, visual outcome results of complete coverage of the well-defined component are almost equivalent to those of no treatment at 36 months' follow-up [37•]. Fluorescein angiography in this group of eyes suggests the need for caution when considering treating only part of a neovascular membrane with laser treatment. ICG angiography has produced limited data on the result of photocoagulation of a hot spot on the border of a late-staining plaque of occult CNV [32].

Information on management of lesions with well-defined and occult CNV extending under the geometric center of the foveal avascular zone has been provided by the Macular Photocoagulation Study's subfoveal trials [14,16] and the Créteil trial [17]. Specifically, the initial size of the lesion, the location of the peripheral neovascular border, and the initial visual acuity are factors that determine the treatment strategy.

In the absence of definitive treatment possibilities and guidelines, clinical evaluation of well-defined CNV associated with occult CNV should be carefully performed at presentation with all available diagnostic tools, including ICG angiography. These examinations should also be performed during the immediate follow-up period if photocoagulation has been selected as part of the therapeutic regimen.

Treatment of Vascularized Pigment Epithelium Detachment

The inability to delineate serous PED from vascularized PED accurately made the results of numerous studies on the natural course and treatment of PED secondary to ARM unreliable. The Moorfields' clinical trial [38] showed a greater visual loss in eyes in which avascular PED was treated as opposed to untreated. The grid laser photocoagulation does not improve the visual prognosis in "avascular" retinal PED; these results, however, do not apply to "vascularized" PED [39].

Notches at the edge of PEDs are believed to indicate the site of occult choroidal new vessels. Treatment directed to this ill-defined hyperfluorescence and the contiguous edge of the PED induced resolution or decreased PED in eight of the 14 eyes treated [40] but has not been shown to be predictable in other locations. However, with the use of fluorescein angiography, the leakage due to CNV located within the PED merges in late staining of the PED.

Enhanced imaging with ICG angiography appears to be of particular value in patients with serous and hemorrhagic macular detachments, which occur in 22% [31] to 31% [41] of ARM patients at presentation. Since 1992, Yannuzzi *et al.* [42] have worked specifically to characterize and classify occult CNV with an overlying PED. ICG can localize the neovascularization by segregating the serous component, which remains isofluorescent or hypofluorescent during the sequence, from the vascularized component, which presents as an early and late hyperfluorescence [41].

The most frequent finding at presentation in Yannuzi's study [42] is neovascularized plaque (62% of vascularized PED), defined as CNV larger than one disc area in the late phase, with variable delineation. Focal CNV, solitary (Fig. 7-1) or multiple, present as a well-delineated bright area no larger than one disc diameter on ICG videoangiography. Focal CNV was identified in 38% of vascularized PED. The use of SLO videoangiog-

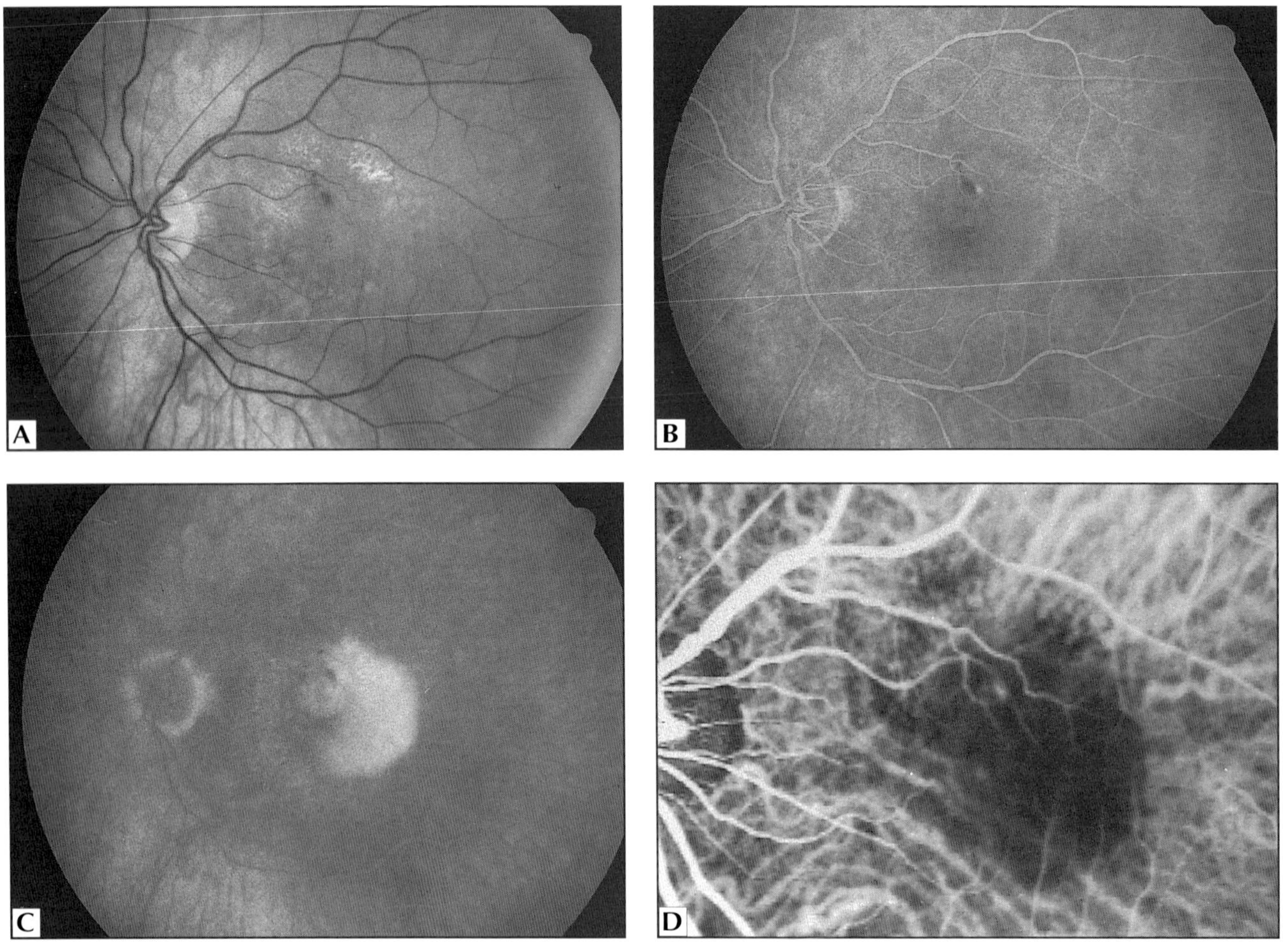

FIGURE 7-1. Vascularized pigment epithelium detachment (PED) in a man aged 80 years. **A**, Red-free frame: PED involving the entire macular area and underlined by hard exudates superiorly. Within the detachment, small retinal hemorrhages are obvious. **B**, Venous phase of fluorescein angiography. Uneven and delayed filling of the PED, only the temporal border of which presents some hyperfluorescence. Within the detachment, superior to the macular area, a small hyperfluorescent spot is adajcent to the larger retinal hemorrhage, suggesting ingrowth of new vessels. **C**, Late phase of fluorescein angiography. The irregular PED is now totally filled with dye. The nearly even hyperfluorescence does not allow identification of the exact site of the new vessels. **D**, Early phase of indocyanine green (ICG) angiography. The PED is deeply hypofluorescent (Scanning Laser Ophthalmoscope, Heidelberg Engineering, Heidelberg). In this hypofluorescent zone, one limited area is hyperfluorescent.

(Continued)

raphy also allowed identification of anastomosis between the deep choroidal vascular component and one or more retinal vessels (Fig. 7-2) [43••]. This observation has established a high-risk group with a very unfavorable outcome after photocoagulation therapy as well as in natural history.

The well-circumscribed focus must be precisely located in relation to the fovea and the retinal vessels used as landmarks for photocoagulation treatment. A small reinjection of ICG will fill the retinal vessels in the late phase [44]. Mapping the location of the "hot-spot" to the fovea on digitized images of the early-phase fluorescein and of the late-phase ICG angiography at the time of reinjection was found to be very helpful in our clinic.

Limited pilot studies by Slaker *et al.* [29], Regillo *et al.* [28], and Lim *et al.* [45] have assessed the value of ICG angiography–guided laser photocoagulation of vascularized PED. For the most part, only well-defined hyperfluorescent focal lesions located outside of the fovea were considered eligible for laser photocoagulation with ICG guidance (*see* Fig 7-1). No immediate deleterious effect, such as a tear in the RPE, was observed after laser photocoagulation. Vascularized PED showed complete or partial resolution after one or multiple laser treatments in 43% [29], 63% [28], and 76% of eyes [45] respectively. Recurrences were common, occurring in 45% of eyes after 6 months' follow-up [45] and 51% of eyes after 12 months' follow-up [29]. Visual acuity was stabilized in 51% [29] and 18% of eyes [45] respectively. Transient stabilization of visual acuity may be possible, but the benefit diminishes with time. The small sample size in these studies (21 eyes [28], 35 eyes [29], and 20 eyes [45]) must be emphasized as well as the lack of a control group.

Combined with fluorescein angiography, ICG angiography may offer the possibility of broadening the eligibility guidelines for treatment of eyes with vascularized PED. However, the eligibility criteria may be inappropriate when using ICG imaging as a guide for laser therapy. It has been shown that the type of occult

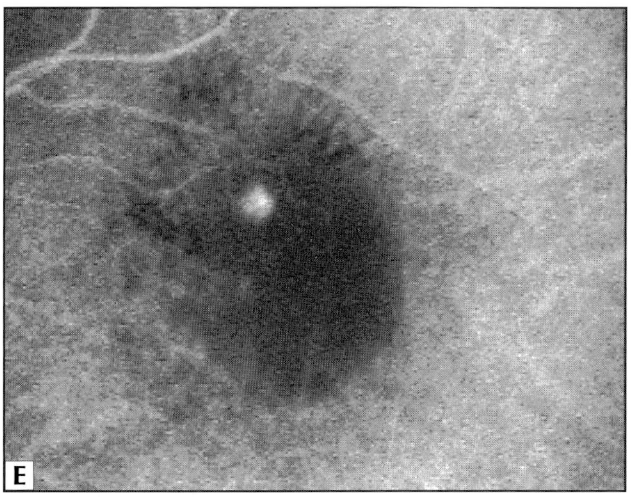
E

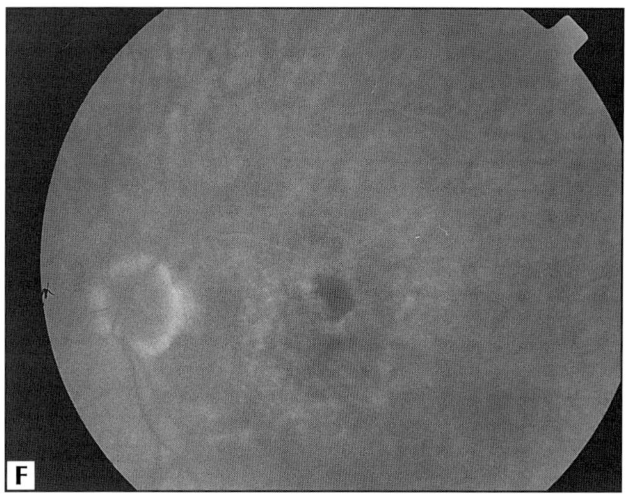
F

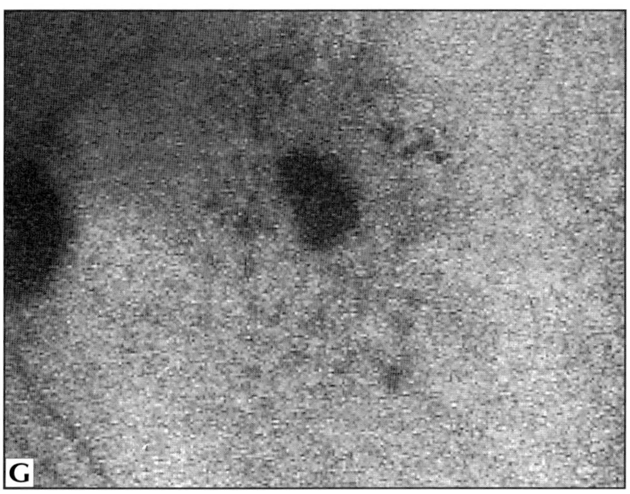
G

FIGURE 7-1. (*CONTINUED*) **E**, Late phase of ICG angiography. The PED remains totally dark, beyond the limit of the increased hyperfluorescence of the new vessels. The location of the focal hyperfluorescence, outside of the central avascular zone, allowed for an attempt at direct photocoagulation. **F**, Posttreatment fluorescein angiography. Limits of the photocoagulation scar are well-defined and without leakage. The PED does not fill with fluorescein. **G**, Late phase of ICG angiography. Disappearance of the blockage caused by settling of the PED. The border of the photocoagulation area is perfectly outlined. No recurrence is identifiable.

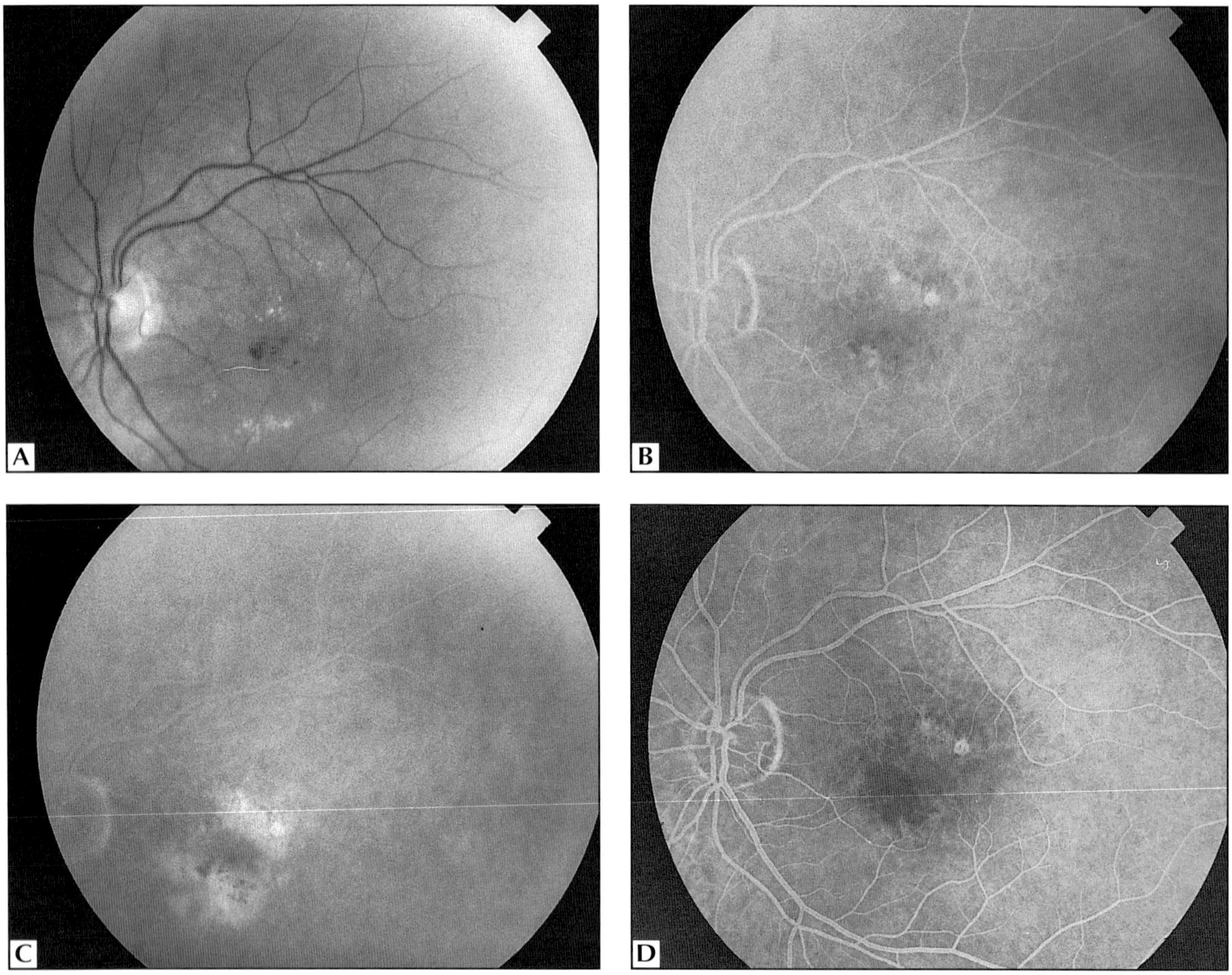

FIGURE 7-2. Vascularized pigment epithelium detachment (PED) in a woman aged 83 years. **A**, Red-free photograph. PED in the inferior temporal part of the avascular zone surrounded by limited hard exudates. Within the area of the PED numerous small dot hemorrhages can be found. **B**, Late fluorescein angiogram. The PED is not filled at this relatively late phase. Conversely, two hyperfluorescent focal areas are visible, one at the 1-o'clock position of the foveal avascular zone (without surrounding hemorrhages) and one at the 7-o'clock position of the avascular zone, associated with small hemorrhages. **C**, Very late fluorescein angiogram. Leakage of dye is apparent in the surrounding area of the two previously noted hyperfluorescent spots. **D**, After photocoagulation of the inferior hyperfluorescent spot, the chorioretinal anastomosis is much more clearly evident within the photocoagulation scar.

CNV present in the first eye is highly predictive of the type of neovascularized disease to be found in the second eye [35]. A definitive answer to establish the benefit of laser treatment for occult CNV associated with PED requires a prospective multicenter randomized clinical trial.

TREATMENT OF OBSCURED CHOROIDAL NEOVASCULAR MEMBRANE

Different components, such as thick blood and accumulation of whitish material, can block the angiographic detection of CNV. In these cases, the type of CNV present cannot be identified through the use of fluorescein angiography.

Hemorrhagic disciform

Thick blood that is contiguous or overlying an area of well-defined or occult CNV may obscure fluorescence from the choroid and from the CNV located directly beneath it. In fluorescein angiography, late leakage of dye may be observed within the blockage of subretinal blood, probably corresponding to a part of the CNV that is located more anteriorly. In general, the therapeutic approach for most CNV obscured by hemorrhage is observation. Waiting until the hemorrhage clears may eventually result in localization of the CNV through fluorescein angiography

Hayashi and De Laey [46] were the first to demonstrate that ICG videoangiography was better at delineating neovascularization under this condition. Destro and Puliafito [47] also noted that ICG videoangiography was useful in the study of CNV if hemorrhage was overlying the neovascularization. Both studies reported isolated positive results of photocoagulation guided by videoangiography.

A prospective study of 20 patients showed that ICG angiography was able to detect CNV [48]. The extent of CNV was identified in 60% of eyes that had ICG angiography. However, thick subretinal hemorrhage still partially obscured CNV in 40% of eyes. At the time of this writing, no large series have been published concerning findings on such patients after laser treatment.

Expanding gas injection in very recent subretinal hemorrhages associated with face-down positioning the day following surgery can displace subretinal blood from the fovea. In a small pilot study, we are currently assessing this technique to improve detection of CNV with both fluorescein and ICG angiography. Improved detection of CNV obscured by hemorrhage may allow earlier treatment and ultimately result in improved preservation of central vision.

Accumulation of material

In addition to blood, white-yellow material can mask underlying CNV on fluorescein angiograms. This material includes fibrin resulting from a subretinal hemorrhage, hard exudates, and pseudovitelliform material, which can totally hide the leakage of dye. In addition, on ICG angiograms this material may also block underlying choroidal fluorescence. However, our experience has shown that ICG videoangiography allows identification of the associated CNV in pseudovitelliform macular lesions.

ALTERNATIVE PHOTOCOAGULATION TECHNIQUES

Laser treatment of CNV is performed with the objective of destroying the CNV and preventing the eye from developing recurrences. Although randomized prospective controlled clinical trials have improved our ability to treat CNV associated with ARM, the ability to treat this disease with attendant preservation of visual acuity remains unsatisfactory. As a result, various alternative techniques, including surgical excision of CNV membranes (occasionally associated with endophotocoagulation), radiotherapy, use of antiangiogenic pharmacologic therapeutic agents, and preventive photocoagulation of drusen have begun to emerge. Attempts to minimize the overlying photoreceptor damage aim at preserving central visual function. It is important to emphasize that these alternative techniques remain investigational.

Reduction of photoreceptor damage

Use of the continuous-wave neodymium (Nd):YAG laser to successfully treat CNV while attempting to minimize overlying photoreceptor damage has been studied. In 17 of 19 eyes with ARM and juxtafoveal well-defined CNV, the Nd:YAG laser obliterated the membrane; visual acuity remained stable or improved. These results, however, concern only a small sample with a lack of control subjects and a limited follow-up period [49].

The extent of retinal damage is related to the passage of temperature gradient in the RPE. Among the different hypotheses of biophysical factors that might be used to localize damage, repetitive-pulse photocoagulation seems to be the most promising technique. In one study, multiple short (514 nm) argon laser pulses applied to rabbit retina resulted in the healing of the RPE in a single sheet of cells, showing clear signs of viability, and the directly adjacent neural retina was not damaged [50]. Similar experimentation has been performed with diode laser (810 nm) [51]. These techniques are presently under clinical evaluation.

Dye-enhanced photocoagulation (*ie*, supravital dyes) has been suggested for use since 1984. The light absorption characteristics of the vital tissues can be modified by exogenous dyes. The absorption peak of ICG is similar to the emission peak of the diode laser (805 nm). Therefore, ICG dye–enhanced diode laser photocoagulation can be performed, which may allow for the selective destruction of ICG-containing CNV with relative sparing of RPE and normal neighboring neurosensory retina. Experimental CNV membranes were successfully closed. Preliminary results in occult CNV are encouraging [52]. Randomized, prospective controlled clinical trials of ICG dye–enhanced laser photocoagulation are still pending.

Photodynamic therapy

In the past, photosensitizers have been applied in attempted photodynamic therapy of ocular diseases. Photodynamic therapy is a developing modality in which selective destruction of tissues is achieved. The photosensitizer dye is taken up by the proliferating cells, such as leukemic cells, malignant cells, targeted T lymphocytes, and endothelial cells. These tissues are then exposed to light at the absorption maximum of the dye, leading to formation of singlet oxygen and reactive intermediates, which can react directly with cellular component and lead to auto-oxidation and direct damage to cell membrane, mitochondria, lysosomes, and the nucleus. This results in cell death of the targeted neovascular and tumor tissues. An effective closure has been demonstrated in experimental CNV [53,54]. The efficiency of liposomal benzoporphyrin derivative and tin ethyl etiopurpurin [55] is currently being tested in clinical trials (*see* Chapter 10, "Photodynamic Therapy for Ocular Tumors and Neovascularization").

Preventive photocoagulation of high-risk drusen

Large or soft drusen have been shown to be strong risk factors for development of exudative ARM in fellow eyes of patients with one affected eye. In the past, several laser treatment strategies have been shown to eliminate drusen. Several pilot studies have investigated whether laser treatment of drusen within the second eye reduces the incidence of neovascularization and accompanying loss of vision. The treatment protocol involves application of relatively light laser burns to the drusen area at least 500 μm from the center of the foveal avascular zone. However, the number, location (either directly targeting drusen or scattering the laser in the posterior pole), size, and intensity of the burns as well as whether drusen were targeted specifically for treatment have varied among the studies.

Recent reports from two randomized pilot studies [56,57] have supported the beneficial effect of drusen photocoagulation treatment. In one eye of 22 patients with bilateral drusen and 16 fellow eyes in which 50% of the eyes were assigned randomly to laser treatment [56], an average of 100 grayish burns configured in a horseshoe pattern temporal to the fovea were placed on and between drusen. The mean area of the drusen was reduced by 50% at 12 months after treatment. By 36 months, untreated eyes had significantly worse vision from baseline, whereas treated eyes remained stable. Five untreated eyes—four eyes of patients with bilateral drusen and one fellow eye—developed CNV, whereas none of the treated eyes did so.

In the second study, 27 patients with bilateral large symmetric drusen were randomized to an average of 132 laser burns in one eye [57]. Endpoint for photocoagulation was a "slightly visible lightening of the retinal pigment epithelium or outer retina overlying the drusen." Total disappearance of drusen was observed by 6 months in 63% of the 27 treated eyes. After an average follow-up of 3 years, the visual improvement of two or more lines occurred in six treated eyes versus no control eyes. Two (7%) patients had CNV develop in both eyes and two (7%) patients had CNV develop in their untreated eyes only.

Results from these two small clinical trials involving mostly eyes of patients with bilateral drusen provide evidence that the long-term effects of laser treatment in patients with bilateral drusen may be beneficial.

Recently however, the short-term effects of low-intensity laser treatment were published from a multicentered, randomized clinical trial [58••]. Twenty laser burns, 100 μm in diameter in a pattern of 3 rows placed between the 12- and 6-o'clock positions beyond the temporal perimeter of the foveal avascular zone, were applied to a group of 156 eyes with bilateral drusen and a group of 120 second eyes. The intended intensity of the burns was light to moderate. In the bilateral drusen group, CNV developed in four of 156 treated eyes and in two of the 156 observed eyes with no change in visual acuity over 18 months. However, in the second-eye group, 10 of 59 treated eyes and two of 61 observed eyes developed CNV by 18 months.

Although the potential risk for geographic atrophy might be a threat for central vision, the high rate of predominantly occult CNV in fellow eyes during the year after initial treatment with laser and the proximity of the CNV to the area of laser treatment point to a causal role for laser treatment in fellow eyes. Because occult CNV typically has a slower course than well-defined CNV, however, no significant loss of visual acuity has been noted to date.

Indocyanine green angiography was not performed in this study. It may be that some of the fellow eyes had a plaque-like lesion that would have been visible on ICG angiography despite the absence of signs of occult CNV on clinical examination and fluorescein angiography. Low-intensity laser photocoagulation may temporarily regulate vascular endothelial growth factor or another angiogenic agent and thus stimulate proliferation of endothelial cells or promote leakage from preexisting endothelial cell proliferation.

At present, "preventive" laser treatment, both focal (direct) of drusen and scatter (nondirect) in areas near drusen, cannot be recommended until the long-term results of this ongoing trial are obtained.

CONCLUSIONS

Fluorescein angiography has been and remains the standard imaging modality used in evaluation and treatment of CNV in ARM. The use of ICG angiography in clinical evaluation of CNV has made numerous technologic improvements in recent years, and further advancement in resolution and sensitivity are to be expected in the future. The greatest utility of ICG angiography appears to be in identifying areas of presumed (or undetected) occult CNV and must be performed if fluorescein angiography leaves any doubt of CNV type.

Indeed, recognition of the types of CNV is crucial in determining eligibility for use of laser photocoagulation. Randomized, prospective clinical trials with long-term fo low-up have demonstrated that laser treatment is beneficial in terms of visual acuity in well-defined extrafoveal and juxtafoveal CNV. Immediate postlaser photographic control and overlay will help to ensure adequate coverage and reduce the incidence of recurrence and persistence.

Two techniques are used for subfoveal CNV. Complete ablation, as recommended by the Macular Photocoagulation Study [14], shows a stable benefit in small and intermediate subfoveal CNV with low initial visual acuity. For larger lesions, the perifoveal technique of the Créteil group [17] seems more appropriate because patients do not experience an immediate and definitive visual loss but instead may benefit from treatment—especially for near-vision tasks. However, photocoagulation treatment is not a treatment for ARM but only for its neovascular complication.

For other types of CNV, no treatment approach can currently be recommended. Limited pilot studies have suggested some beneficial effect of direct photocoagulation based on fluorescein or ICG angiography for occult CNV with or without PED. Dye-enhanced photocoagulation and photodynamic therapy are presently being evaluated in randomized clinical trials. Investigators continue to search for angiostatic alternative forms of treatment to control the neovascularization when this complication of ARM is found.

Much research remains to be done to reduce the frequency of severe visual loss. Risk factors might possibly be modified in an attempt to prevent development of CNV. Basic research continues in the identification of stimulators and inhibitors of CNV and in their interaction in the hope of understanding these mechanisms and eventually achieving pharmacologic control of the entity.

Because the underlying cause of ARM remains unknown, the most important future goal would be the treatment of ARM itself before the onset of its clinical complications, whether atrophic or neovascular. Basic research studies on the nature of chorioretinal disease may uncover fruitful new lines of investigation.

References and Recommended Reading

Recently published papers of particular interest have been highlighted as:
- • Of interest
- •• Of outstanding interest

1.•• Macular Photocoagulation Study Group: Risk factors for choroidal neovascularization in the second eye of patients with juxtafoveal or subfoveal choroidal neovascularization secondary to age-related macular degeneration. *Arch Ophthalmol* 1997, 115:741–747.

The prognosis of the fellow eye is affected strongly by the presence in the central macula of five or more drusen, focal hyperpigmentation, one or more large drusen, and systemic hypertension. These factors should be considered when counseling patients with unilateral neovascular ARM and when targeting patients for preventive intervention.

2. Macular Photocoagulation Study: Subfoveal neovascular lesions in age-related macular degeneration: guidelines for evaluation and treatment in the macular photocoagulation study. *Arch Ophthalmol* 1991, 109:1242–1257.

3. Freund KB, Yannuzzi LA, Sorenson JA: Age-related macular degeneration and choroidal neovascularization. *Am J Ophthalmol* 1993, 115:786–791.

4. Gelfand YA, Linn S, Miller B: The application of the Macular Photocoagulation Study eligibility criteria for laser treatment in age-related macular degeneration. *Ophthalm Surg Lasers* 1997, 28:823–827.

5. Quentel G, Coscas G: Intérêt des rétinographies en lumière monochromatique (verte, rouge et bleue) lors de la photocoagulation des membranes néovasculaires juxtafovéolaires. *Bull Mem Soc Fr Ophtalmol* 1981, 81:1047–1050.

6. Coscas G, Glaser G, Green WR, *et al.*: Dégénérescences maculaires acquisés liées à l'âge et néovaisseaux sous-rétiniens. In *Rapport à la Société Française d'Ophtalmologie*. Paris: Masson, 1991:486.

7. Chamberlain JA, Bressler NM, Bressler SB, *et al.*: Photographs and fluorescein angiograms in the identification and treatment of choroidal neovascularization in the Macular Photocoagulation Study. *Ophthalmology* 1989, 96:1526–1534.

8. Clark FM, Freeman WR, Goldbaum MH: Digital overlay of fluorescein angiograms and fundus images for treatment of subretinal neovascularization. *Retina* 1992, 12:118–126.

9. Mimoun G, Soubrane G, Bunel P, *et al.*: Calque automatique des néovaisseaux sous-rétiniens : un nouvel outil pour la photocoagulation maculaire. *Ophtalmologie* 1991, 5:29–32.

10. Mimoun G, Meunier I, Quaranta M, *et al.*: Intérêt du SLO pour la détermination de la fixation avant photocoagulation des néovaisseaux sous-rétiniens maculaires. *Ophtalmologie* 1995, 9:197–199.

11. William AR, Cruess AF, Ballantyne M, *et al.*: Argon green vs. krypton red laser photocoagulation for extrafoveal choroidal neovascularization secondary to age-related macular degeneration: 3-year results of a multicentre randomized trial. *Can J Ophthalmol* 1996, 31:11–17.

12. Macular Photocoagulation Study Group: Evaluation of argon green vs. krypton red laser for photocoagulation of subfoveal choroidal neovascularization in the Macular Photocoagulation Study. *Arch Ophthalmol* 1994, 112:1176–1184.

13. Macular Photocoagulation Study Group: Laser photocoagulation for juxtafoveal choroidal neovascularization: five-year results from randomized clinical trials. *Arch Ophthalmol* 1994, 112:500–509.

14. Macular Photocoagulation Study Group: Laser photocoagulation of subfoveal neovascular lesions in age-related macular degeneration: results of a randomized clinical trial. *Arch Ophthalmol* 1991, 109:1220–1241.

15. Macular Photocoagulation Study: Visual outcome after laser photocoagulation for subfoveal choroidal neovascularization secondary to age-related macular degeneration: the influence of initial lesion size and initial visual acuity. *Arch Ophthalmol* 1994, 112:480–488.

16. Macular Photocoagulation Study Group: Laser photocoagulation of subfoveal recurrent neovascular lesions in age-related macular degeneration: results of a randomized clinical trial. *Arch Ophthalmol* 1991, 109:1232–1241.

17. Coscas G, Soubrane G, Ramahefasolo C, *et al.*: Perifoveal laser treatment for subfoveal choroidal new vessels in age-related macular degeneration: results of a randomized clinical trial. *Arch Ophthalmol* 1991, 109:1253–1265.

18. Orth D, Rosculet JP, De Bustros S: Foveal sparing photocoagulation for exudative age-related macular degeneration. *Retina* 1994, 14:153–159.

19. Schneider U, Kuck H, Kreissig I: Fixation and central visual field after perifoveal krypton laser treatment of subfoveal neovascularizations. *Eur J Ophthalmol* 1993, 3:193–200.

20. Macular Photocoagulation Study Group: The influence of treatment extent on the visual acuity of eyes treated with krypton laser for juxtafoveal choroidal neovascularization. *Arch Ophthalmol* 1995, 113:190–194.

21. Quaranta M, Wolf S, Soubrane G, *et al.*: Immediate and delayed ICG angiography control post-laser treatment for visible choroidal new vessels. *Invest Ophthalmol Vis Sci* 1994, 35(Suppl):1564.

22. Wolf S, Wald KJ: Detection of persistent choroidal neovascularization using indocyanine green choroidal angiography. *Retina* 1993, 13:81–82.

23. Sorenson JA, Yannuzzi LA, Slakter JS, *et al.*: A pilot study of digital indocyanine green videoangiography for recurrent occult choroidal neovascularization in age-related macular degeneration. *Arch Ophthalmol* 1994, 112:473–479.

24. Pollak A, Korte GE: Vascular remodeling after laser photocoagulation: concurrent regeneration and atrophy. *Acta Anatomica* 1992, 143:151–159.

25. Campochiaro PA, Blaydes SH: Photocoagulation does not ablate angiogenic markers in rabbit retina. *Arch Ophthalmol* 1988, 106:676–679.

26. Soubrane G, Coscas G, Francais C, *et al.*: Occult subretinal new vessels in age-related macular degeneration: natural history and early laser treatment. *Ophthalmology* 1990, 97:649–657.

27. Guyer DR, Yannuzzi LA, Slakter JS, *et al.*: Digital indocyanine-green videoangiography of occult choroidal neovascularization. *Ophthalmology* 1994, 101:1727–1737.

28. Bischoff P, Speiser P: Indocyanine green angiography and laser treatment of subretinal neovascular membranes in age-related macular degeneration. *Klin Monatsbl Augenheilkd* 1994, 204:298–301.

29. Regillo CD, Benson WE, Maguire JI, *et al.*: Indocyanine green angiography and occult choroidal neovascularization. *Ophthalmology* 1994, 101:280–288.

30. Slakter JS, Yannuzzi LA, Sorenson JA, *et al.*: A pilot study of indocyanine green videoangiography-guided laser photocoagulation of occult choroidal neovascularization in age-related macular degeneration. *Arch Ophthalmol* 1994, 112:465–472.

31. Krott R, Quaranta M, Coscas G: Choroidal circulation and indocyanine green videoangiography in eyes presenting occult subretinal neovascularization. *Invest Ophthalmol Vis Sci* 1993, 34(Suppl):1164.

32. Guyer DR, Yannuzzi LA, Ladas I, *et al.*: Indocyanine green–guided laser photocoagulation of focal spots at the edge of plaques of choroidal neovascularization. *Arch Ophthalmol* 1996, 114:693–697.

33. Bressler NM, Maguire MG, Murphy PL, Alexander J: Macular scatter ("grid") laser treatment of poorly demarcated subfoveal choroidal neovascularization in age-related macular degeneration. *Arch Ophthalmol* 1996, 114:1456–1464.

34. Arnold J, Algan M, Soubrane G, *et al.*: Indirect scatter laser photocoagulation to subfoveal choroidal neovascularization in age-related macular degeneration. *Graefe's Arch Clin Exp Ophthalmol* 1997, 235:208–216.

35. Chang B, Yannuzzi LA, Ladas ID, *et al.*: Choroidal neovascularization in second eyes of patients with unilateral exudative age-related macular degeneration. *Ophthalmology* 1995, 102:1380–1386.

36.• Stevens TS, Bressler NM, Maguire MG, *et al.*: Occult choroidal neovascularization in age-related macular degeneration. A natural history study. *Arch Ophthalmol* 1997, 115:345–350.

Data were obtained from 52 observed eyes with subfoveal occult CNV with poorly demarcated boundaries during a 9- to 12-month follow-up. The morphologic analyses of changes on fluorescein angiography showed that 32% of the occult CNV more than doubled their original size. Well-defined CNV developed in 52% of eyes that had previously been without it. The median loss of visual acuity of 2.5 lines was directly related with the anatomic aspect.

37.• Macular Photocoagulation Study Group: Occult choroidal neovascularization. Influence on visual outcome in patients with age-related macular degeneration. *Arch Ophthalmol* 1996, 114:400–411.

Analysis of the influence of the presence of occult CNV in the krypton red laser photocoagulation study on anatomic and visual acuity outcomes. Classic CNV have a clear benefit from photocoagulation even though more than 50% of eyes develop a recurrence. Laser treatment of classic CNV only when occult CNV was associated was not beneficial. The limited sample number of eyes with isolated occult CNV precluded wider conclusions about the value of treatment. Thus, identification of occult CNV *before* considering laser treatment is of crucial importance.

38. Moorfield Macular Study Group: Retinal pigment epithelial in the elderly: a controlled trial of argon laser photocoagulation. *Br J Ophthalmol* 1982, 66:1–16.

39. Singerman LJ: Laser photocoagulation for choroidal new vessel membrane complicating age-related macular degeneration associated with pigment epithelial detachment. *Retina* 1988, 8:115–121.

40. Maguire JI, Benson WE, Brown GC: Treatment of foveal pigment epithelial detachments with contiguous extrafoveal choroidal neovascular membranes. *Am J Ophthamol* 1989, 109:523–529.

41. Yannuzzi LA, Slakter JS, Sorenson JA, *et al.*: Digital indocyanine green videoangiography and choroidal neovascularization. *Retina* 1992, 12:191–223.

42. Yannuzzi LA, Hope-Ross M, Slakter JS, *et al.*: Analysis of vascularized pigment epithelial detachments using indocyanine green videoangiography. *Retina* 1994, 14:99–113.

43.•• Kuhn D, Meunier I, Soubrane G, *et al.*: Imaging of chorioretinal anastomoses in vascularized retinal pigment epithelium detachments. *Arch Ophthalmol* 1995, 113:1392–1398.

Continuous recording of the early phases of fluorescein and ICG angiography identified chorioretinal anastomoses in 93% of vascularized PED with hot spots at an early stage of ARM. Failure of laser photocoagulation of the hot spots might be related to their double vascular supply.

44. Brucker AJ, Brant A, Nyberg W: "Landmark injection" for localization of choroidal lesions using indocyanine green angiography. *Retina* 1993, 13:169–171.

45. Lim JI, Aaberg TM, Capone A, *et al.*: Indocyanine green angiography-guided photocoagulation of choroidal neovascularization associated with retinal pigment epithelial detachment. *Am J Ophthalmol* 1997, 123:524–532.

46. Hayashi K, De Laey JJ: Indocyanine green angiography of neovascular membranes. *Ophthalmologica* 1985, 190:30–39.

47. Destro M, Puliafito CA: Indocyanine green videoangiography of neovascular membranes. *Ophthalmology* 1989, 96:846–853.

48. Reichel E, Ducker JS, Puliafito CA: Indocyanine green angiography and choroidal neovascularization obscured by hemorrhage. *Ophthalmology* 1995, 102:1871–1876.

49. Nishikawa S, Okisaka S: Photocoagulation with continuous wave Nd:YAG laser for neovascular maculopathy. *Jpn J Ophthalmol* 1992, 36:44–55.

50. Roider J, Michaud NA, Flotte TJ, *et al.*: Response of the retinal pigment epithelium to selective photocoagulation. *Arch Ophthalmol* 1992, 110:1786–1792.

51. Trivino A, Ramirez JM, Andres MV, *et al.*: Comparison between chorioretinal effects of the single-pulse versus micropulsed diode laser in pigmented rabbits. *Lasers Light Ophthalmol* 1997, 8:31–38.

52. Reichel E, Puliafito CA, Duker JS, *et al.*: Indocyanine green dye-enhanced diode laser photocoagulation of poorly defined subfoveal choroidal neovascularization. *Ophthalmic Surg* 1994, 25:195–201.

53. Miller JW, Walsh AW, Kramer M, *et al.*: Photodynamic therapy of experimental choroidal neovascularization using lipoprotein-delivered benzoporphyrin. *Arch Ophthalmol* 1995, 113:810–818.

54. Kramer M, Miller JW, Michaud N, *et al.*: Liposomal benzoporphyrin derivative verteporfin photodynamic therapy. Selective treatment of choroidal neovascularization in monkeys. *Ophthalmology* 1996, 103:427–438.

55. Peyman GA, Moshfeghi DM, Moshfeghi A, *et al.*: Photodynamic therapy for choriocapillaris using tin ethyl etiopurpurin ($SnET_2$). *Ophthalm Surg Lasers* 1997, 28:409–417.

56. Frennesson IC, Nilsson SEG: Laser photocoagulation of soft drusen in early age-related maculopathy (ARM). The one-year results of a prospective, randomized trial. *Eur J Ophthalmol* 1996, 6:307–314.

57. Little HL, Showman JM, Brown BW: A pilot randomized controlled study on the effect of laser photocoagulation of confluent soft macular drusen. *Ophthalmology* 1997, 104:623–631.

58.•• The Choroidal Neovascularization Prevention Trial Research Group: Laser treatment in eyes with large drusen. Short-term effects seen in a pilot randomized clinical trial. *Ophthalmology* 1998, 105:11–23.

The short-term results of laser photocoagulation to high-risk drusen in a randomized clinical trial show that to date the patients with bilateral drusen do not present changes in visual acuity whether treated or simply observed. Conversely, in second eyes of patients already having exudative ARM in the first eye occult choroidal neovascular membrane developed significantly more frequently in treated than observed eyes ($P = 0.02$).

CHAPTER 8

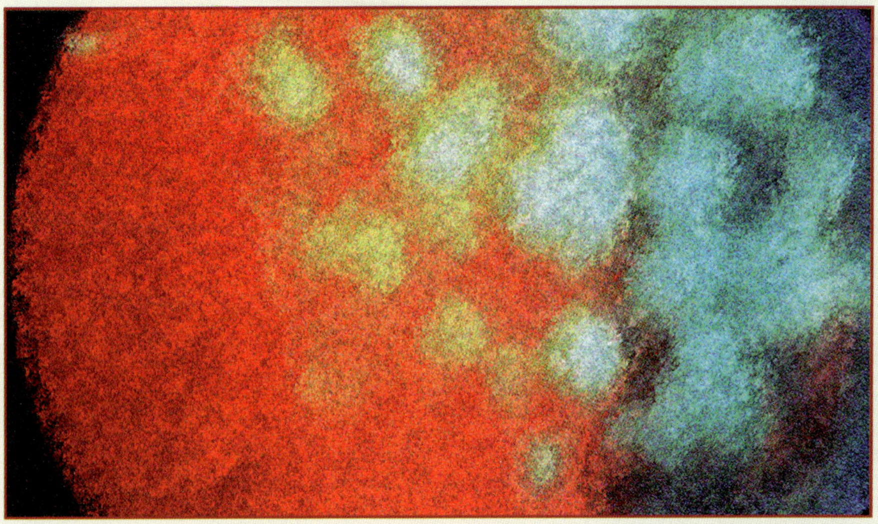

Photocoagulation of Other Causes of Choroidal Neovascular Membranes

JOHN H. NIFFENEGGER
LAWRENCE J. SINGERMAN
HERNANDO ZEGARRA
SCOTT D. PENDERGAST

Photocoagulation is the major form of treatment of choroidal neovascularization (CNV) in macular diseases. This chapter reviews the clinical characteristics and treatment of CNV in diseases other than age-related macular degeneration (AMD), which are important diseases, although much less common than AMD [1•]. Knowledge of the pathology, natural history, and response of non-AMD diseases to treatment remains incomplete. In many situations, management of these disorders is influenced by extrapolation from the results of the Macular Photocoagulation Study (MPS) [2].

Almost any pathologic process that disturbs the retinal pigment epithelium (RPE) and Bruch's membrane can be associated with CNV. Ocular histoplasmosis syndrome, idiopathic CNV, pathologic myopia, angioid streaks, multifocal choroiditis, serpiginous choroidopathy, choroidal osteoma, choroidal rupture, hereditary dystrophies, and many other conditions have been reported.

Pathologic investigation has not been possible for all of these diseases. Understanding of the basic mechanisms of CNV has been derived from histopathologic studies of AMD [3]. Because of the common characteristics of a break in Bruch's membrane in the early stages of CNV and the common occurrence of a disciform lesion late in the process, it is hypothesized that the pathogenesis of CNV has important similarities regardless of the specific associated disease.

CNV has been divided histopathologically into two types according to the location of the new vessels [4]. In type I CNV, initial growth of these new vessels appears to be between the inner and outer aspects of Bruch's membrane. Extension occurs within the subpigment epithelial space, which is the typical situation in AMD. In type II CNV, the growth pattern of CNV in young patients tends to be in the subsensory retinal space. This suggests that removal of CNV, in conditions in which growth is anterior to the RPE, has some chance of restoring useful visual function in these patients. Removal of CNV in AMD typically results in removal of native RPE, which reduces the likelihood of useful central vision after subretinal surgery [5].

The two forms of treatment most commonly employed for CNV are laser photocoagulation and surgical removal of the neovascular membrane. Laser has been proven to be the most effective treatment available and is the subject of this chapter. Prognosis largely depends on the location of the CNV (Fig. 8-1). The Macular Photocoagulation Study [7–9] proved the efficacy of argon laser photocoagulation for extrafoveal CNV secondary to AMD, ocular histoplasmosis syndrome (OHS), and idiopathic CNV. Krypton laser photocoagulation has been shown to be efficacious in juxtafoveal CNV [10–12]. The benefit of photocoagulation of subfoveal CNV has been demonstrated in select cases of AMD [13–15]. A pilot randomized trial of photocoagulation of subfoveal CNV in ocular histoplasmosis by Fine *et al.* [16] did not yield a definitive recommendation. In general, foveal treatment is avoided in CNV not secondary to AMD.

The value of photocoagulation in less common causes of CNV has not been studied thoroughly, and results of the Macular Photocoagulation Study must be cautiously considered. Differences as well as similarities between these disorders and those specifically observed in the study must be examined.

In some patients who are not eligible for photocoagulation treatment, submacular surgery may offer the possibility of improved outcome. To date, no prospective randomized clinical trials have been completed comparing submacular surgery with either laser treatment or natural history. Uncontrolled series of subfoveal surgery for histoplasmosis CNV suggest that impressive improvement in visual acuity is possible [17]. The Submacular Surgery Trial (a National Eye

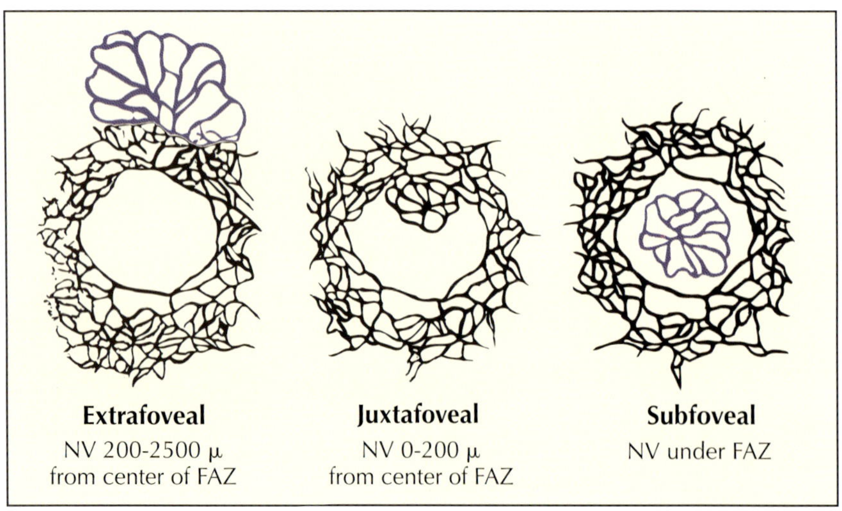

FIGURE 8-1. An important prognostic and therapeutic factor in choroidal neovascularization is its location in relation to the center of the foveal avascular zone. Proper assessment of location requires high-quality fluorescein angiography. FAZ—foveal avascular zone; NV—neovascularization. (*From* Singerman [6]; with permission.)

Institute-sponsored, prospective, randomized, controlled, multicenter trial) is evaluating submacular surgery compared with natural history or laser in subfoveal CNV in OHS, and a similar study of submacular surgery for subfoveal CNV in AMD is to begin in 1998. Little is known regarding the response to surgery of less common forms of CNV.

OTHER CAUSES OF CHOROIDAL NEOVASCULARIZATION

Ocular histoplasmosis syndrome

Ocular histoplasmosis syndrome is one of the more common causes of CNV not associated with AMD. It is endemic in areas bordering the Ohio and Mississippi river valleys, where a relatively high proportion of young lifelong residents react positively to histoplasmin skin testing [18]. Positive reactions to skin testing are more common in patients with disciform lesions [19]. Reactivation of apparently inactive lesions has been reported with skin testing [20]. Most patients suffer a subclinical infection or mild flu-like illness [21]. Epidemic infection, however, has been reported to be associated with cleaning chicken coops, demolition of old buildings, or exposure to sites inhabited by bats. Similar disease outside of endemic areas, such as in Europe, has been reported, and the etiology of this disorder is only presumed in most cases.

The fundus findings in OHS are described as a triad of macular scar or hemorrhage associated with peripapillary chorioretinal atrophy and punched-out peripheral chorioretinal lesions ("histo spots") [22]. CNV may arise at a chorioretinal scar and cause loss of central vision [23]. End-stage lesions appear similar to the disciform scars found in AMD. CNV in OHS, however, is not associated with drusen [3]. The CNV associated with OHS tends to be subretinal and anterior to the plane of the RPE more frequently than is CNV associated with AMD [4].

Hypothetically, focal choroiditis damages Bruch's membrane, RPE, and choriocapillaris, thus causing an exudative detachment of the retina or subretinal hemorrhage. Resolution of the choroiditis leaves a focal area of atrophy. Choroidal vessels associated with the chorioretinal atrophy may decompensate, causing serous exudation, CNV, and transient serous detachment of the retina. A hemorrhagic detachment may occur that later resolves to form a disciform scar. Analysis of five choroidal neovascular membranes from patients with OHS showed growth in the subretinal space. The vessels tended to be engulfed by a monolayer of proliferating pigment epithelial cells. Surgical excision of subfoveal CNV theoretically allows reapproximation of the retinal photoreceptors with the native RPE and subsequent improvement in vision [5].

Differentiation of inactive scars from active CNV is essential in the management of patients with OHS. Fluorescein angiography of chorioretinal scars demonstrates hyperfluorescence, beginning first in the periphery, adjacent to normal choroid, with later spread to the center of the scar. In neovascularization, hyperfluorescence begins in the area of CNV and then spreads more peripherally. The late phase shows hyperfluorescence of the entire lesion in either case. The scar will show staining. The lesion with active CNV will have hyperfluorescence of the overlying serous subretinal detachment (Fig. 8-2). Recurrence must be recognized and treated promptly to reduce the risk of vision loss from foveal involvement.

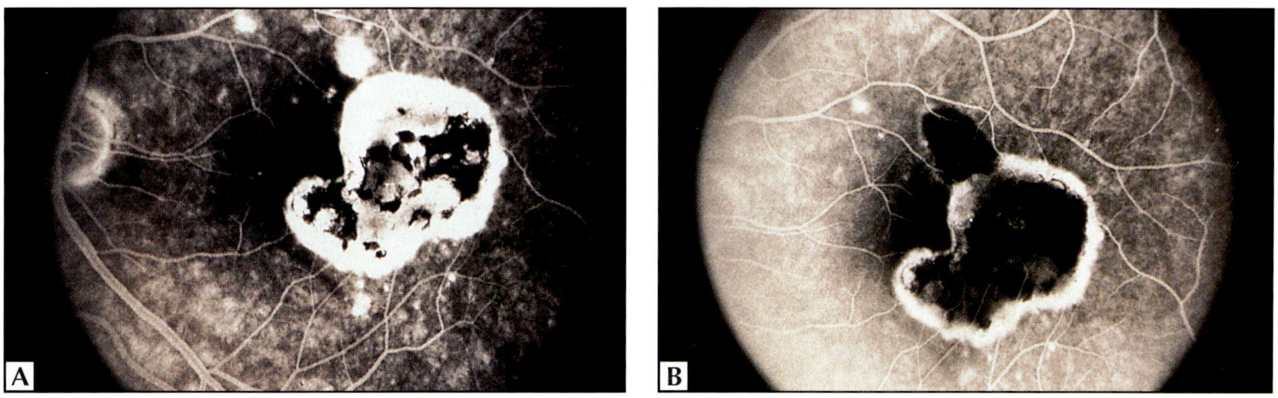

FIGURE 8-2. Laser photocoagulation of choroidal neovascularization (CNV) in ocular histoplasmosis syndrome. **A,** One year after laser to two adjacent areas of CNV, there is increased hyperfluorescence at the superonasal margin of the previous treatment, contiguous with the previously inactive scar. Clinical examination revealed a small serous/hemorrhagic retinal detachment in this area (note the hypofluorescence corresponding to hemorrhage inferonasal to the upper lesion, highlighting probable CNV). **B,** One week following the second laser treatment to the area of reactivation, there is resolution of the detachment with no residual hyperfluorescence. Acuity improved to 20/30. (*From* Singerman and Novak [24]; with permission.)

The pathophysiology of recurrence is not well understood. Histopathology of subfoveal membranes suggests a nonuniform distribution of blood vessels and large areas of avascular membrane that would not likely be imaged adequately by angiography, which could contribute to incomplete treatment and thus to recurrence [25].

Natural history studies have demonstrated a significant risk of vision loss from CNV in OHS, but at a rate lower than that seen in AMD, with a substantial number of eyes maintaining good vision [26]. Spontaneous improvement has been observed [27]. The Macular Photocoagulation Study [8] evaluated the efficacy of laser photocoagulation in extrafoveal and juxtafoveal CNV. Argon laser photocoagulation was demonstrated to reduce the risk of severe visual loss in eyes with extrafoveal choroidal neovascular membranes associated with OHS. Krypton laser photocoagulation was found to be beneficial in OHS-related juxtafoveal CNV [10].

In the study of argon laser photocoagulation in extrafoveal CNV, 48% of eyes in the observation group, compared with 9% in the laser treatment group, lost six or more lines of visual acuity after 3 years of follow-up [28]. Visual acuity was worse than 20/200 in 39% of the untreated eyes, compared with 5% of treated eyes. Of treated eyes, 66% had visual acuity of 20/40 or better, compared with 38% in the untreated group.

In the study of krypton laser photocoagulation in juxtafoveal CNV, after 3 years of follow-up 25% of eyes in the observation group versus 5% in the treatment group lost six or more lines of vision. Data on visual acuity, reading vision, and anatomic outcomes during 5 years of follow-up were available for 236 (92%) of the 256 study patients [29]. Untreated eyes with OHS were at much greater risk of a six-line decrease in visual acuity from the 1-year through the 5-year examination than were treated eyes (unadjusted risk ratio, 2.60; risk ratio, 4.26 after adjustment for visual acuity and hypertension at baseline; $P < 0.001$ for both).

The argon laser photocoagulation study of extrafoveal CNV and the krypton laser photocoagulation study of juxtafoveal CNV had similar treatment protocols. The treatment technique, discussed later in this chapter, is routinely employed in the photocoagulation of well-defined nonsubfoveal CNV regardless of the associated disease. The Macular Photocoagulation Study [7–10] protocol called for photocoagulation of the entire area of hyperfluorescence in an effort to obliterate the CNV completely.

The treatment of subfoveal CNV associated with OHS was not specifically addressed by the Macular Photocoagulation Study. The natural history is guarded, with more than 75% of patients developing 20/200 or worse visual acuity over a 2- to 3-year period [30]. A pilot randomized study by Fine *et al.* [16] of photocoagulation for the treatment of subfoveal CNV secondary to OHS did not demonstrate either benefit or detriment from laser treatment in 25 patients enrolled over a 2-year period.

Favorable results from subfoveal surgery have encouraged some investigators [31]. Thomas *et al.* [31] reported a retrospective series of 117 consecutive patients with a mean follow-up of 13 months. Improvement of three or more Snellen lines occurred in 40% of patients. Postoperative visual acuity improved to 20/40 or better in 35% [32•]. A more favorable surgical prognosis appears to be positively related to extrafoveal location of the CNV ingrowth site [33]. In patients with extrafoveal ingrowth sites, 60% obtained 20/40 vision. Only 7% of patients with juxtafoveal or subfoveal ingrowth site had final visual acuity of 20/40.

Regardless of the method of treatment, the fellow eye needs to be observed carefully. A 5-year prospective follow-up of the Macular Photocoagulation Study [34] OHS patients in the extrafoveal and juxtafoveal studies determined that 35 (9%) of 394 eyes initially free of neovascularization developed CNV in the fellow eye. Histo spots of any type in the macula tripled the risk for later development of CNV. CNV was preceded by an atypical histo spot in the same location in 32 of the 35 eyes that developed CNV.

Idiopathic neovascularization

Choroidal neovascularization in the absence of atrophic retinal scars, drusen, or other retinal abnormality is termed *idiopathic*. This is an important category of CNV, especially in younger patients. In a retrospective study in Western Europe, 17% of CNV found in patients younger than 50 years of age was idiopathic [35].

The Macular Photocoagulation Study's [9,28] clinical trial of argon laser photocoagulation in extrafoveal CNV found a substantial reduction in the risk of losing six or more lines of vision in the treated group (16%) compared with the observation group (34%). In 5-year follow-up data, 38 (97%) of 39 patients with juxtafoveal idiopathic CNV in the krypton laser photocoagulation study demonstrated that treatment was associated with a significant reduction in risk of developing six or more lines of vision loss [29].

The natural history of idiopathic subfoveal CNV was retrospectively studied in 19 consecutive patients [36]. The prognosis appears to be significantly better than in AMD and some other causes of CNV. Over a median follow-up of 87 months, 95% of the patients had stable or improved visual acuity. Patients with initial lesions one disc area or smaller were more likely to have a final vision of 20/60 or better and less likely to have a final visual acuity of 20/200 or worse. This relatively favorable natural history must be considered when considering treatment of subfoveal lesions.

Eyes with idiopathic CNV have been included in reports of subfoveal surgery for CNV [31,37]. The visual results are less impressive than in patients with OHS but better than in reports of surgery for subfoveal CNV associated with AMD. In a series of eight eyes undergoing surgery for idiopathic subfoveal CNV, a mean improvement of three Snellen lines and final acuity of 20/40 or better in two eyes were obtained [31]. Recurrence occurred in 50% (four of eight eyes).

Pathologic myopia

Choroidal neovascularization occurs in between 5% to 10% of myopes and is more common in those with more than five diopters (D) of myopia. Bilateral involvement is not uncommon [38,39]; it is a frequent cause of CNV in patients less than 50 years of age, accounting for over 60% of CNV in a review of young patients in Western Europe [35].

Fuchs' spot is the term commonly used to describe a dark macular lesion from hemorrhage or RPE hyperplasia thought to represent changes secondary to or associated with the development of CNV in myopic patients [40]. Lacquer cracks, or linear breaks in Bruch's membrane, may develop in association with choroidal thinning and atrophy accompanying elongation of the globe in pathologic myopia. CNV may extend through these breaks, causing hemorrhage and disciform scarring [3, 23]. Subretinal hemorrhage not associated with CNV is more common in younger patients and tends to resolve spontaneously in a few months. Vision usually remains stable or improves over several months [41].

Choroidal neovascular membranes associated with myopia often appear as grayish circumscribed lesions near the fovea. Subretinal fluid tends to be minimal, hemorrhage is limited, and subretinal exudation is not common. Hyperfluorescence on fluorescein angiography occurs early but does not leak profusely (Fig. 8-3). Hyperfluorescence may be confined to the borders of the choroidal neovascular membrane. CNV may occur at the border of atrophic areas of RPE, which cause window defect, thus requiring careful attention to the angiographic results to find any areas of discrete leakage. CNV may arise in the fovea in a large proportion of myopic eyes developing CNV [42].

Indocyanine green (ICG) angiography is a useful diagnostic tool to differentiate lacquer cracks from CNV in retinal and subretinal hemorrhages [43•,44]. Lacquer cracks appear as hypofluorescent lines in the late phases of the ICG angiography, in contrast to hyperfluorescent leakage or staining seen in CNV.

The natural history of CNV in pathologic myopia is variable and complicates recommendations for laser treatment. Some authors report a poor prognosis. Hotchkiss and Fine [38] found that 14 of 27 eyes lost two or more lines of vision during 2 years of follow-up. Twelve patients became legally blind. Other studies report a less severe prognosis. Two thirds of patients observed by Fried *et al.* [39] had stable or improved vision without treatment, although in 50% the CNV involved the fovea during a 5-year follow-up period.

Photocoagulation of extrafoveal CNV in high myopia may be effective in preventing or limiting severe and irreversible loss of vision. Pece *et al.* [45] followed 133 consecutively treated eyes prospectively for at least 12 months. Posttreatment mean visual acuity was stable compared with pretreatment visual acuity. Recurrent CNV developed in 58% of eyes at the end of the 5-year follow-up period. At final evaluation, complete destruction of CNV was achieved in 100 eyes (75%).

Soubrane and Pisan [46] randomized 38 eyes to photocoagulation and 28 eyes to observation. The eyes not receiving treatment generally had a marked decline

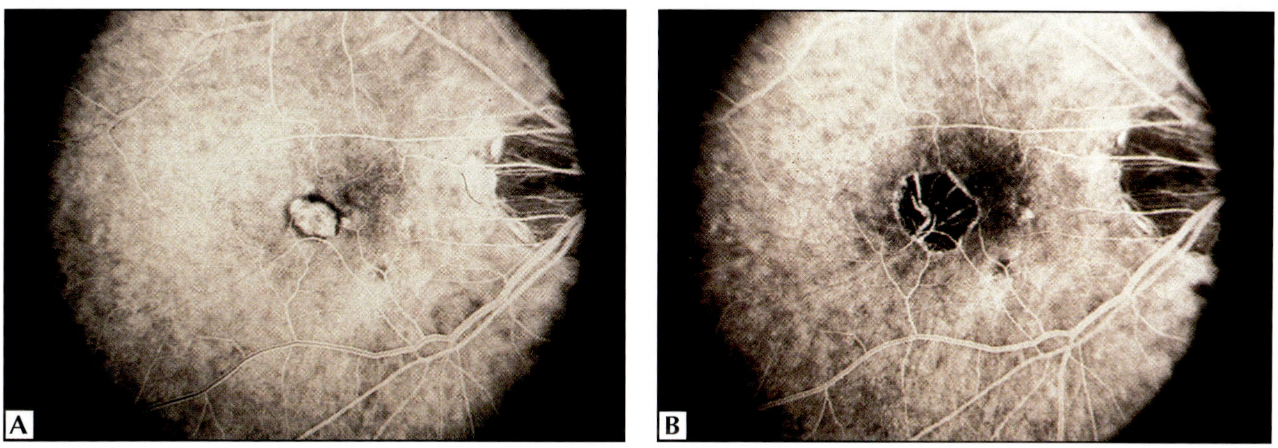

FIGURE 8-3. Choroidal neovascularization (CNV) secondary to pathologic myopia. **A,** Fluorescein angiogram shows a circumscribed lacy CNV inferior to the fovea. **B,** Two months after photocoagulation, the CNV is quiescent and acuity has improved to 20/200.

in vision, with 80% having final visual acuity of less than 20/100. Treated eyes were remarkably stable but did not have any statistical improvement in vision compared with untreated eyes. The authors concluded that laser therapy for CNV in degenerative myopia probably is efficacious, although it is also difficult and associated with significant risks and potential for complications. Progressive enlargement of atrophic laser scars has been reported [47]. Extension of atrophic treatment scars to the fovea, however, is not usually associated with a serious increase in vision loss.

Photocoagulation technique in high myopia includes exact determination of foveola location to avoid inadvertent foveal ablation [48]. Risk of this complication can be reduced using red-free photographs to determine the center of xanthophyll pigmentation or mapping the foveal avascular zone onto the digital angiogram [49]. Large spot size (200 µm or greater), long duration (0.2 to 0.5 seconds or longer), and, possibly, the use of yellow or green wavelengths to close CNV visible in areas of atrophic RPE may reduce the risk of choroidal hemorrhage [50].

Laser treatment in patients with subfoveal CNV associated with pathologic myopia may offer no improvement over the natural course. Surgical removal of the CNV has been performed in some cases. Outcome data remain preliminary, but hope exists that improvement over the natural history may be possible. Five eyes with CNV associated with pathologic myopia (more than 6 D of myopia and stigmata of myopic degeneration) were included in a report of subfoveal surgery [37]. Visual acuity improved two lines or more in two eyes and was stable or declined less than two lines in three eyes. One recurrence took place during the follow-up period of 6 to 15 months. In a series of ten myopic eyes undergoing surgical removal of CNV by Thomas *et al.* [31], mean visual acuity declined by one line and recurrent CNV developed in two eyes.

Angioid streaks

Angioid streaks are irregular radiating lines that appear similar to blood vessels in size and color, thus the term *angioid*. Histopathologic examination reveals that these lines are actually calcified breaks in Bruch's membrane. Various systemic disorders have been associated with angioid streaks, including pseudoxanthoma elasticum, Paget's disease of bone, Ehlers-Danlos syndrome, sickle cell disease, thalassemia, and other blood dyscrasias (Fig. 8-4) [23,24,51–54]. In a series of 50 patients, Clarkson and Altman [55] found that 50% had an identifiable systemic diagnosis. Skin biopsy specimens have exhibited changes suggestive of pseudoxanthoma elasticum in some patients with angioid streaks who did not have clinically evident skin changes [56].

Choroidal neovascularization may grow through the breaks in Bruch's membrane to cause serous or hemorrhage detachment of the RPE. Minor injury can cause traumatic rupture of the fragile calcified Bruch's membrane, thus resulting in sudden loss of central vision [23]. Deterioration in visual acuity may occur in the absence of CNV by subtle, progressive atrophic degeneration. Visual acuity can drop to the 20/200 level, often in the absence of marked atrophy of the RPE.

Most CNV associated with angioid streaks occurs in the papillomacular bundle, nasal to the fovea. Laser treatment in this region may cause visual field defects. In addition, a risk exists of damaging major vessels when treating near the optic disc. In Paget's disease, CNV may be large and thus may increase the difficulty of treatment. Prompt laser treatment may be considered in selected cases because it has been found to reduce the rate of visual loss.

The fluorescein angiographic features of angioid streaks are variable, typically appearing as hyperfluorescent lines. The angioid streaks and their main complication, CNV, can sometimes be difficult to visualize in the presence of diffuse pigment migration, diffuse atrophy of the RPE, or hemorrhage. ICG angiography displays angioid streaks in the form of hyperfluorescent lines with numerous associated hyperfluorescent foci. The angioid streaks are clearly visualized, appearing more numerous and larger with ICG angiography than with red-free images or fluorescein angiography. ICG angiography may allow more precise localization of CNV than fluorescein angiography does [57•].

The visual prognosis in eyes with angioid streaks and CNV is poor. Typically, the CNV progresses to cause severe vision loss. Frequently, CNV occurs in the fellow eye. CNV has been treated with both argon and krypton laser photocoagulation [54,58,59]. Although untreated eyes cannot be considered adequate controls in these studies, treated eyes had better visual outcome than untreated eyes.

Laser photocoagulation of CNV in angioid streaks may end CNV and help stabilize visual acuity or slow down visual loss. Pece *et al.* [60] recently reported a study of 66 consecutive eyes of 52 patients with extrafoveal, well-defined CNV secondary to angioid streaks who underwent direct laser photocoagulation and were observed for 3 to 108 months (mean, 34.5 months; median, 20 months). Pretreatment mean visual acuity was 20/40 (range, 20/200 to 20/20); posttreatment mean visual acuity was 20/80 at 2 years. During the first year after treatment, visual acuity decreased significantly ($P < 0.01$) but manifested no significant change thereafter. CNV recurred one or more times in 77% of the eyes, but by the time of final examination, CNV had been eliminated completely in 31 eyes (47%).

Fellow eyes with natural progression of CNV were considered control eyes. Final visual acuity in treated eyes was better than that in untreated eyes ($P < 0.01$). Considering the very high frequency of recurrences (77% of the eyes studied), an intense clinical and fluorangiographic follow-up period is strongly recommended.

Gelisken *et al.* [61] also reported long-term follow-up of patients treated with laser photocoagulation. Patients received follow-up for 2 months to 16 years (mean, 3.4 years). The authors concluded that laser treatment was beneficial and allowed maintenance of useful vision longer.

Five eyes with subfoveal CNV associated with angioid streaks were included in a report of subretinal surgery [37]. One patient had improvement from 20/300 to 20/50. Visual acuity was stable in three eyes and declined in one. No recurrences happened during the follow-up period, which ranged from 6.5 to 32 months. Thomas *et al.* [31] reported results in four patients undergoing subfoveal removal of choroidal neovascular membranes. Final visual acuity was 20/200 or worse in all eyes.

Multifocal choroiditis

Several groups of investigators have reported multifocal choroiditis not related to OHS but with similar end-stage findings [62–68]. Unlike eyes with OHS, these eyes often have evidence of vitreous inflammation, although this finding is variable [69]. Anterior segment inflammation occurs in about 50% of eyes. Acute lesions appear as yellow or gray choroidal lesions, which may initially block and later stain with fluorescein [23]. Inactive lesions typically are smaller than those seen in OHS. Most patients are from geographic areas where OHS is not endemic. In 25% of unilateral cases, severe inflammation may occur in the second eye months or years later. Females and young patients in their 30s and 40s are more commonly affected. The disorder has been reported in children. Multifocal choroiditis and CNV have been associated with multiple evanescent white dot syndrome and acute idiopathic blind spot enlargement syndrome in one series [69].

CNV similar to that seen in OHS often develops (Fig. 8-5). The final scar appears similar to scars seen in

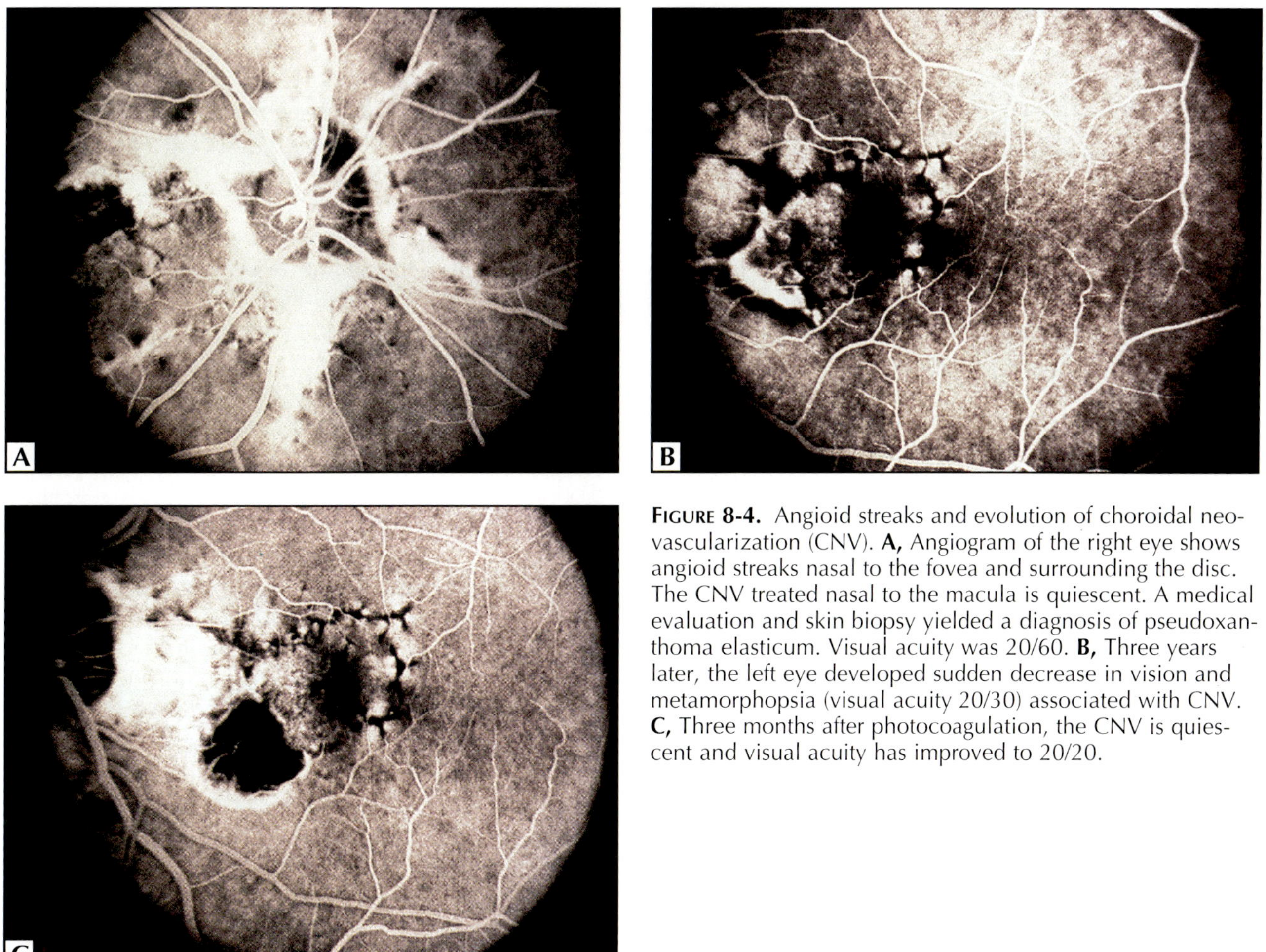

FIGURE 8-4. Angioid streaks and evolution of choroidal neovascularization (CNV). **A,** Angiogram of the right eye shows angioid streaks nasal to the fovea and surrounding the disc. The CNV treated nasal to the macula is quiescent. A medical evaluation and skin biopsy yielded a diagnosis of pseudoxanthoma elasticum. Visual acuity was 20/60. **B,** Three years later, the left eye developed sudden decrease in vision and metamorphopsia (visual acuity 20/30) associated with CNV. **C,** Three months after photocoagulation, the CNV is quiescent and visual acuity has improved to 20/20.

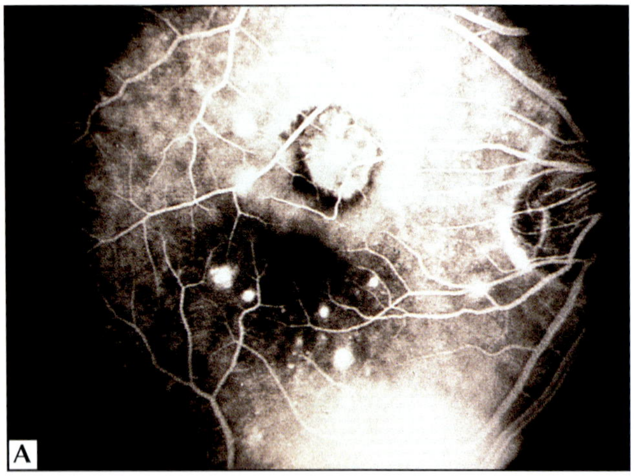
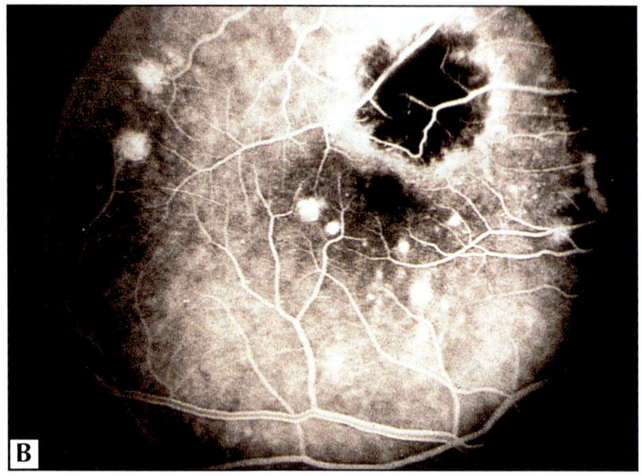

FIGURE 8-5. Multifocal choroiditis and choroidal neovascularization (CNV). **A,** Angiogram reveals well-defined hyperfluorescence superior to the fovea representing CNV. Scattered round hyperfluorescent lesions correspond to areas of choroiditis. **B,** Two weeks following photocoagulation, the CNV is quiescent and the areas of choroiditis are stable.

OHS, but the acute and subacute lesions in multifocal choroiditis have a significantly different appearance. Acute and subacute lesions, although observed in OHS, are rare. These lesions are more commonly found in multifocal choroiditis and panuveitis. Chronic, subacute, and acute lesions may be present in the same eye. Subretinal fibrosis and scarring may become extensive and confluent.

Multifocal choroiditis and panuveitis (MCP), punctate inner choroidopathy (PIC), and diffuse subretinal fibrosis (DSF) syndrome can be considered to comprise a spectrum of choroiditis syndromes [70]. CNV develops in nearly one third of patients with MCP and PIC. Severe visual loss in these diseases usually result from subfoveal CNV. Brown *et al.* [70] studied 41 patients with MCP, 16 with PIC, and five with DSF. The mean follow-up was more than 38 months. CNV developed within choroiditis lesions in 22 of the eyes (19 patients) with MCP, causing visual acuity worse than 20/50 in 14 eyes. Thirty eyes had PIC. Six of seven eyes with 20/50 or poorer vision had CNV. Six other eyes had macular CNV that regressed spontaneously with good resultant vision. Seven of 10 eyes with DSF had 20/200 vision or worse caused by fibrosis and atrophy in the macula.

Inflammatory lesions and some CNV may respond to steroid therapy [67] (Fig. 8-6). Photocoagulation may also be effective for CNV [67,71] (Fig. 8-5). In our experience, recurrent as well as new CNV may occur more commonly in multifocal choroiditis than in other causes of CNV. We recommend oral corticosteroid therapy for any active inflammation threatening the macula or optic nerve. Laser treatment is recommended for any CNV not under the center of the fovea. Active inflammation often accompanies CNV, so that concurrent steroid therapy and laser treatment are often required. Subfoveal CNV might be considered for surgical removal, but to date no proof of the benefit of this approach in this disease or in other diseases has been demonstrated.

Serpiginous choroiditis

Serpiginous choroiditis is a chronic, recurring inflammation of the RPE and choroid that is of unknown etiology. Lesions typically begin in the peripapillary region, extending in a radial or curvilinear pattern [72]. Patchy lesions may begin in the macula or periphery. Serpiginous choroiditis usually affects otherwise healthy young or middle-aged patients. The disease typically begins in one eye, eventually becoming bilateral months or years later [73]. Recurrent attacks can occur weeks or years after the initial onset, involving larger areas of the fundus [74]. Visual field defects correspond to the affected fundus lesions and can be followed by use of the Amsler grid. Often the asymptomatic eye has an area of chorioretinal scarring near the optic nerve.

Onset of paracentral and central scotoma tends to be sudden. Within weeks of onset of symptoms, during the active phase of inflammation, examination reveals discrete gray-white discoloration of the RPE and inner choroid. Anterior chamber reaction occasionally is present [75]. After a few weeks, the grayish lesions pale and later atrophy. A fibrous scar may be present in older lesions. Hyperplasia of the RPE often borders the atrophic areas [76]. In addition to inflammation of the RPE and choriocapillaris, retinal vasculitis and branch vein occlusion have been associated with serpiginous choroiditis [77]. RPE detachment and neovascularization of the disc and retina have been reported [78].

Approximately 25% develop CNV near the border of atrophic scars [23]. In a series of 54 patients reviewed by Blumenkranz *et al.* [79], 14 (26%) had either active CNV or disciform macular scarring.

Clinicopathologic findings include a diffuse and focal infiltrate of lymphocytes in the choroid, with larger aggregations of lymphocytes at the margin of serpiginous lesions [80]. Lesions are characterized by a loss of RPE and photoreceptors and variable amounts of RPE hyperplasia. Breaks in Bruch's membrane through which fibroglial scar tissue extends from the choroid are present in areas of CNV.

Patients may become symptomatic with recurrent inflammation at the margin of previous chorioretinal scarring [81]. On fluorescein angiography, hyperfluorescence from recurrent inflammation must be distinguished from leakage associated with CNV. Inflammatory lesions tend to have subtle hyperfluorescence and leakage late in the angiogram. Blocked fluorescence is seen on ICG angiography. CNV has earlier and more dramatic leakage. Subretinal hemorrhage or lipid indicates CNV.

Treatment with oral or periocular steroids should be considered when inflammation threatens the fovea [73,76]. Hooper and Kaplan [82] have advocated combination therapy of azathioprine, cyclosporine, and prednisone for patients unresponsive to steroids alone. It is advisable to prescribe a systemic steroid for the patient to use at home for the first day or two after symptoms recur, until complete eye examination and fluorescein angiography can be performed. Laser photocoagulation can be beneficial in treating CNV in selected patients and should be considered in patients with active CNV.

Choroidal rupture

Choroidal rupture is a fairly common complication of blunt ocular trauma. Direct choroidal ruptures are uncommon and tend to occur anterior to the equator, where direct contusion of the globe occurred. Indirect choroidal rupture is more common and in one series was found to occur in 5% to 10% of blunt trauma [83]. In indirect choroidal rupture, breaks in the choriocapillaris, RPE, and Bruch's membrane occur posterior to the equator and tend to be concentric to the disc. Hemorrhage in the choroid, subretinal space, and retina often accompany choroidal rupture. CNV may develop, usually at the foveal margin of the choroidal

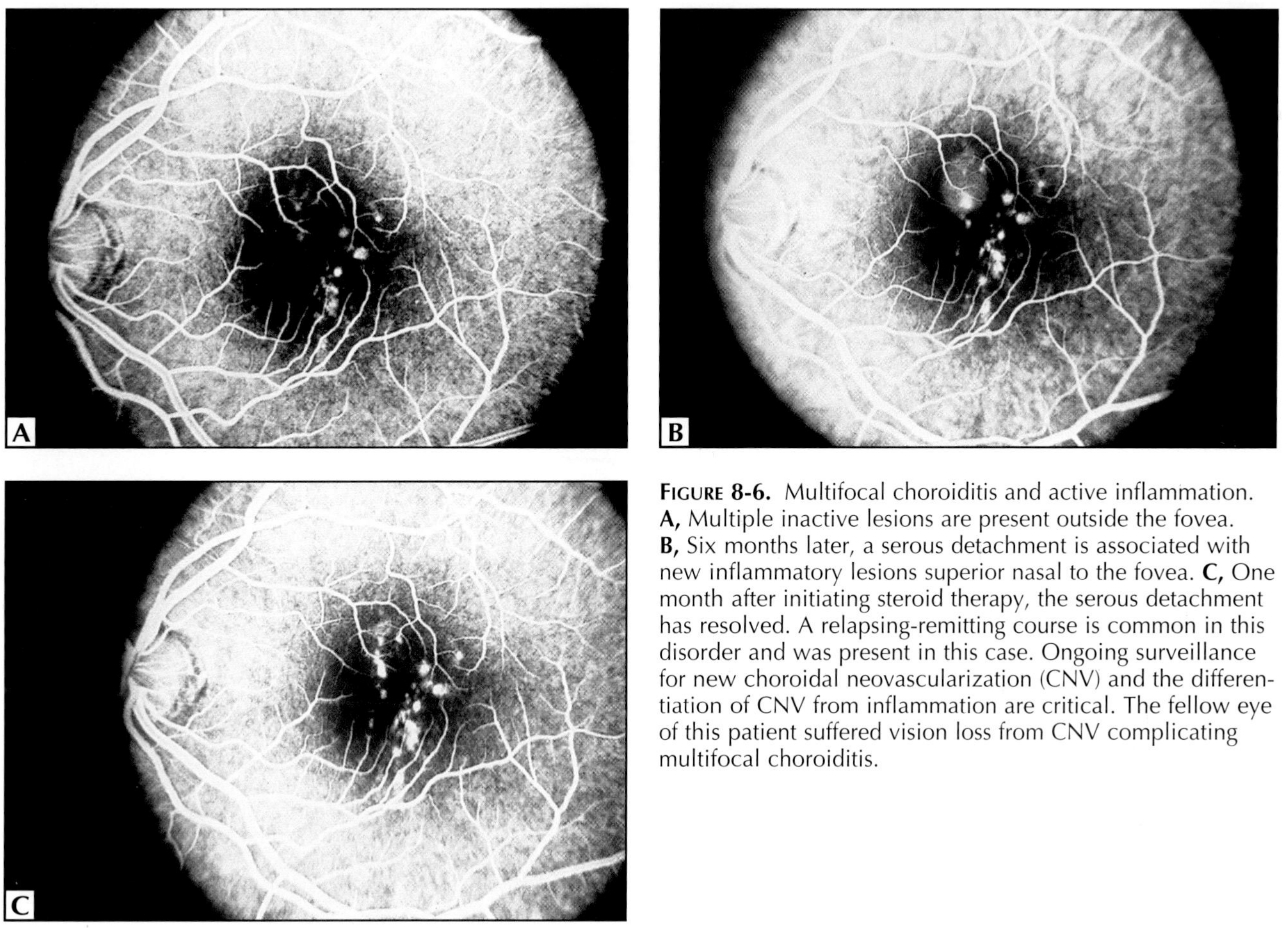

FIGURE 8-6. Multifocal choroiditis and active inflammation. **A,** Multiple inactive lesions are present outside the fovea. **B,** Six months later, a serous detachment is associated with new inflammatory lesions superior nasal to the fovea. **C,** One month after initiating steroid therapy, the serous detachment has resolved. A relapsing-remitting course is common in this disorder and was present in this case. Ongoing surveillance for new choroidal neovascularization (CNV) and the differentiation of CNV from inflammation are critical. The fellow eye of this patient suffered vision loss from CNV complicating multifocal choroiditis.

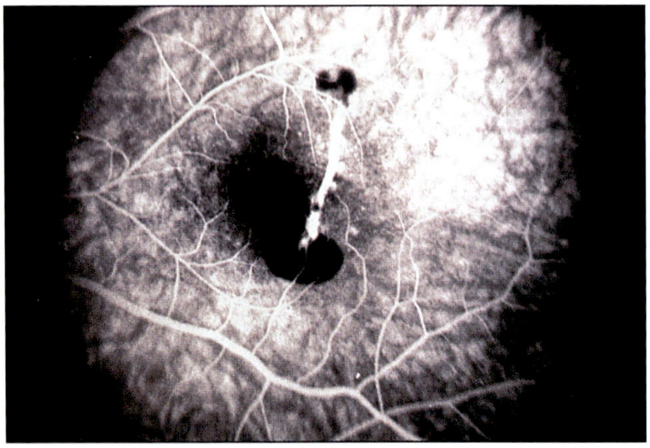

FIGURE 8-7. Choroidal rupture and choroidal neovascularization (CNV). Angiogram of patient with acute loss of vision from 20/20 to 20/80. Examination revealed serous hemorrhagic detachment of the temporal macula. Active CNV is obscured by hemorrhage at each end of the choroidal rupture. (*From* Singerman and Novak [24]; with permission.)

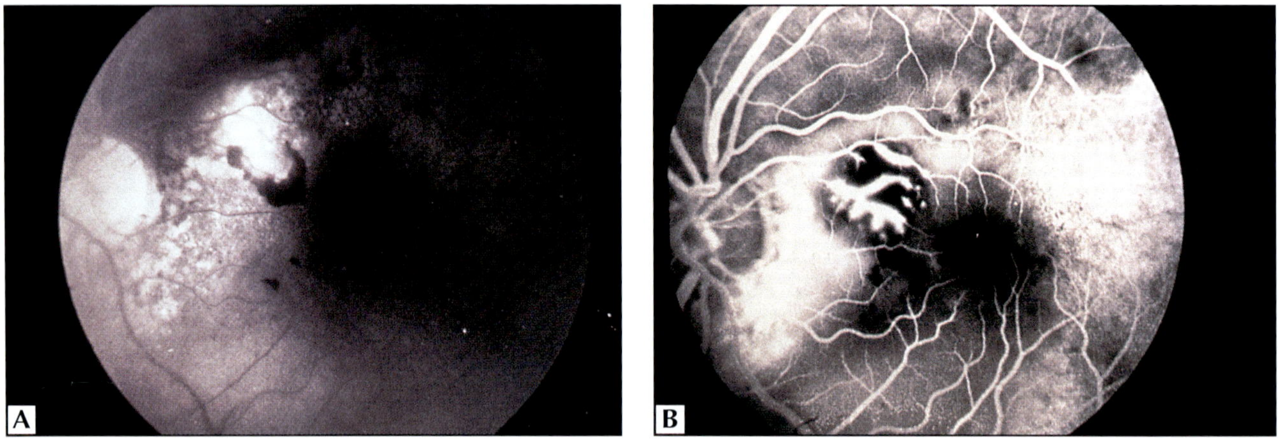

FIGURE 8-8. Choroidal osteoma and neovascularization. **A,** Angiogram from a woman aged 24 years with a choroidal osteoma. Superonasal to the fovea is a focus of intense hyperfluorescence surrounded by hemorrhage. Acuity is 20/30. **B,** Two days after treatment (with blue-green laser in 1975), all new vessels have been obliterated; however, there is hyperfluorescence from thermal vasculitis. (*From* Singerman and Novak [24]; with permission.)

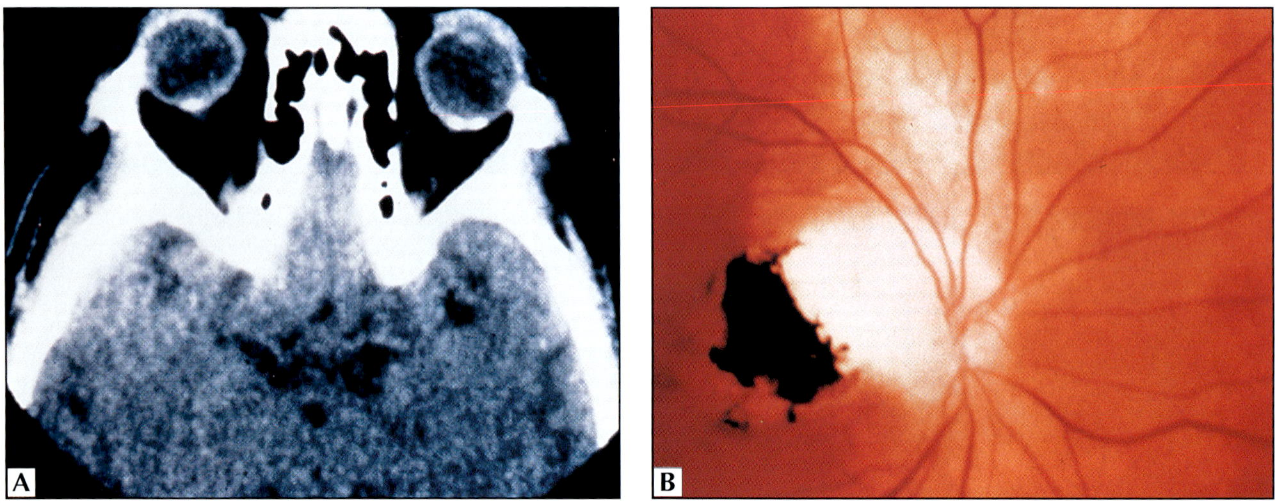

FIGURE 8-9. Bilateral choroidal osteoma in a man aged 34 years. **A,** Computed tomography of the head reveals bilateral calcification of the posterior pole. **B,** Fundus photograph from the same patient 18 years after photocoagulation in the superior papillomacular bundle. The hyperpigmentation at the temporal edge of the treated area is due to heavy blue-green absorption of laser administered in 1974. The hypopigmentation superior to the superotemporal arcade is residual osteoma and overlying retinal pigment epithelial change. (*From* Singerman *et al.* [104]; with permission.)

rupture (Fig. 8-7). Visual loss resulting from serous exudation or hemorrhage from CNV can occur months or years after the original trauma. Laser photocoagulation may be helpful in cases of CNV [84]. Neovascularization may involute without treatment [85]. Submacular surgery may allow improved vision in patients with subfoveal CNV [86].

Choroidal osteoma

Choroidal osteoma was first described in detail by Gass *et al.* [87] in 1978. Most patients with this rare, benign tumor of cancellous bone are white females. In 10% to 25% of patients the osteoma is bilateral [88,89]. Lesions typically occur in the juxtapapillary region and macula. The majority of eyes maintain good visual acuity of 20/30 or better [90]. Osteoblasts grow in the choroid and may organize in haversian systems. Slow growth of the tumor occurs in approximately 50% of patients. Choroidal vasculature may intermix with the compact bone of the osteoma, forming vascular tufts distinct from CNV.

Up to one third of patients with choroidal osteoma may develop CNV [91]. Symptoms are associated with CNV and serous or hemorrhagic detachment of the macula. Little experience with the treatment of CNV in these tumors has been noted (Fig. 8-8) [92,93] . Several treatments may be necessary to obliterate the CNV, but useful vision can be salvaged (Fig. 8-9).

Infectious choroiditis

Infectious diseases have been associated with CNV. Focal choroiditis may play a role in the pathogenesis of these diseases. CNV has been reported in endocarditis with metastatic choroidal abscess [94,95] and in miliary choroidal tuberculosis [96]. Subretinal neovascularization with disciform scar formation is an uncommon but reported complication of rubella retinopathy [97].

Hereditary dystrophies

Several hereditary dystrophies may be associated with CNV. Best's vitelliform dystrophy is an autosomal dominant disease that usually has its onset in children 3 to 10 years of age. Affected patients may develop CNV and macular detachment with subsequent disciform scarring and loss of vision to 20/100 or worse, but this is uncommon [23, 98].

Fundus flavimaculatus is characterized by yellowish flecks that resemble drusen but are more irregular and, on fluorescein angiography, either do not fluoresce or fluoresce irregularly [23]. Patients with this disease generally begin losing central vision in childhood or early adulthood. CNV and disciform macular detachment occur uncommonly [99].

Choroideremia is an X-linked recessive chorioretinal degenerative disease, characterized by progressive atrophy of the choroid and RPE. Until recently, it was believed that vision was unaffected until the macula became involved late in the course of the disease. However, CNV may develop in association with choroideremia, although this occurs rarely [100]. Increased awareness by ophthalmologists of this complication may reveal more cases of neovascularization in choroideremia and other hereditary dystrophies, and some cases, if diagnosed early enough, may be treatable.

Patients with autosomal dominant Sorsby's fundus dystrophy are at a high risk for CNV and severe vision loss. In a retrospective study, 10 eyes with well-defined extrafoveal CNV were treated with laser. All 10 developed recurrent CNV and severe vision loss due to recurrent or persistent CNV on the foveal side of the laser scar [101].

Idiopathic polypoidal choroidal vasculopathy

Idiopathic polypoidal choroidal vasculopathy is an unusual hemorrhagic disorder of the posterior pole, first described in middle-aged black women [102,103]. Clinical findings include irregularly round serous and hemorrhagic RPE detachments, apparently derived from large vascular channels. The lesions cluster around the optic nerve, and drusen and macular RPE changes are conspicuously absent (Fig. 8-10) [104].

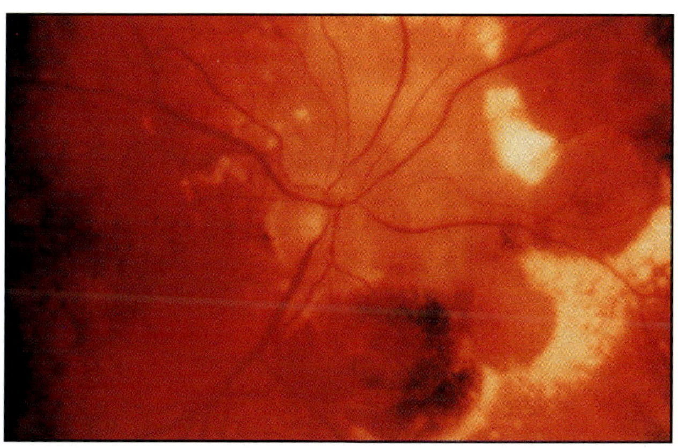

FIGURE 8-10. Idiopathic polypoidal choroidal vasculopathy. Note the several irregular and indistinct areas of serosanguineous retinal pigment epithelium elevation with exudate at their margins. A polypoid vascular channel can be seen under the superior papillomacular bundle. (*From* Singerman *et al.* [104]; with permission.)

Digital pressure on the globe does not collapse these lesions. Vitreous hemorrhage occurs commonly and is a significant cause of visual loss. In a minority of cases, fluorescein angiography discloses CNV. In the majority, however, the lesions appear smaller on angiography and do not leak. Spontaneous regression typically leaves subretinal scarring. Choroidal inflammation has been suggested as a possible etiology based on ICG angiography findings [105]. The disorder follows a remitting–relapsing course. Laser photocoagulation to the polypoidal "feeding" vessels has led to resolution. In many cases, vitrectomy is required to clear the media and to regain vision.

Idiopathic juxtafoveal telangiectasis

Irregular dilation and beading of the parafoveal capillary bed not associated with known predisposing conditions are termed *idiopathic juxtafoveal telangiectasis*. Various subgroups have been described [106–108]. Type 1A is unilateral, most commonly affecting middle-aged men. Type 1B is unilateral but occurs in older men, typically with less edema and visual loss. Type 2 is bilateral, affects women as well as men, and involves small areas of the inferior temporal parafoveal capillaries. Multiple yellow refractile opacities may be present near the inner retinal surface. Black pigment may be present in the retina temporal to the fovea. In type 3, bilateral cystic atrophy and foveal capillary nonperfusion are present.

The dilated capillaries may become incompetent, resulting in edema, exudate, and RPE changes accounting for mild to moderate visual loss. Because the disease may be self-limited, continued observation is probably warranted. Moderate grid laser photocoagulation for persistent or progressive visual loss can be performed in an effort to reduce macular edema [104]. CNV is uncommon but is a well-recognized cause of more severe loss of vision. Subretinal exudation or hemorrhage should prompt angiography to search for CNV. The ophthalmologist should consider photocoagulation if the CNV is outside the foveal avascular zone.

Miscellaneous disorders

Probably any disease that affects the RPE may eventually be associated with CNV. The list of diseases reported to be associated with CNV is constantly growing [1,23]. These include *Toxocara canis* infection, ocular toxoplasmosis, sarcoidosis, Harada's disease, central serous chorioretinopathy, choroidal melanocytic nevus, demarcation lines caused by rhegmatogenous retinal detachment, chorioretinal folds, photocoagulation, focal treatment of diabetic maculopathy, optic nerve drusen, chronic papilledema, and many, many more.

INDOCYANINE GREEN ANGIOGRAPHY

Indocyanine green is a tricarbocyanine dye with a peak absorbance (805 nm) and fluorescence (835 nm) in the near-infrared range. Light in the near-infrared range penetrates opaque media better than shorter-wavelength light does [109]. The molecular weight is higher than that of fluorescein, and ICG is highly protein bound. ICG tends to accumulate in the neovascular membrane and tends not to leak progressively, as in fluorescein angiography [110]. These properties make ICG angiography a useful imaging technique when CNV is not well-defined by fluorescein angiography, or in lesions that are obscured by hemorrhage or turbid fluid. A clinicopathologic correlation of CNV has demonstrated fibrovascular choroidal neovascular membrane corresponding to ICG imaging of occult CNV not well-defined by fluorescein angiography [111].

ICG angiography can add clinically useful information by identifying well-defined areas of hyperfluorescence in CNV poorly defined by fluorescein angiography, in eyes with pigment epithelial detachments, and in recurrent occult CNV [112,113]. The angiographic appearance of CNV, although well-defined by fluorescein angiography, may be variable, in some instances showing only poorly demarcated leakage on ICG angiography, in others showing well-demarcated leakage in areas defined as occult by fluorescein angiography [114]. ICG is also helpful to image disorders that disturb the RPE, Bruch's membrane, and choriocapillaris, such as angioid streaks [115].

TREATMENT TECHNIQUES

Laser

Fundamental aspects of the evaluation, laser treatment, and follow-up of patients with CNV have been described [6]. Prompt identification of CNV and timely treatment are essential to provide optimal management of these patients. When CNV is suspected, referral to an experienced laser surgeon is preferable to obtaining a fluorescein angiogram that may take days or weeks to be developed and interpreted. Even a short delay in treatment may allow an extrafoveal lesion to progress into the fovea or require a larger treatment area, increasing scotoma size [116,117]. Optimally treatable lesions are more likely in patients who have good visual acuity, examined within a month of the onset of symptoms [118]. Patients who have had symptoms for several months or present with poor visual acuity have a lower probability of having an extrafoveal or juxtafoveal lesion treatable with laser, with potential for good central vision. Some subfoveal lesions may benefit from laser treatment, as recommended by the Macular Photocoagulation Study [13–15] subfoveal photocoagulation study, but not with the expectation of good central vision.

Optimal treatment depends on adequate patient education, recent angiography illustrating the area requiring treatment, proper laser technique, and rigorous follow-up. Once the decision to treat the CNV has been made, the patient should be informed that the goal of therapy is to reduce the risk of future vision loss, not to regain vision already lost. The high risk of recurrence and the importance of daily monitoring of the Amsler grid should be emphasized. Office staff and receptionists must be trained to recognize symptoms of recurrence reported by the patient and to arrange prompt reexamination.

A recent, high-quality, readily visible angiogram is used to guide precise localization and treatment of the CNV [119]. In certain cases, ICG angiography may provide information supplemental to fluorescein angiography. Because of the potential for rapid growth of the CNV, the angiogram should be less than 72 hours old. Before laser therapy, retrobulbar anesthesia can be used for analgesia and akinesia, thus reducing the chance of inadvertent laser damage of the fovea or macula not involved by the CNV. Topical anesthetic may be adequate in cooperative patients.

Laser wavelength can be selected to improve the ease of treatment and may theoretically improve efficacy of treatment. Commonly employed laser sources include argon green, krypton red, and dye yellow or red. Diode laser sources are less commonly used. Blue-green wavelengths should be avoided because of their greater absorbance by foveal xanthophyll (Fig. 8-11). Red sources have the advantage of greater transmission through corneal and lens opacities, turbid subretinal fluid, or hemorrhage. Less lenticular scatter and lower absorbance by hemoglobin allow more precise laser placement with red wavelengths. Yellow laser is better absorbed by hemoglobin, which may provide better absorption of laser directly in the CNV. This can be particularly useful in areas of atrophic RPE, which have poor absorption of the red wavelengths.

In the Macular Photocoagulation Study's [120] subfoveal photocoagulation study, no consistent clinically or statistically significant difference between argon green or krypton red laser was found. Focal retinal vascular narrowing was more common in eyes treated with green laser. In a Canadian study of extrafoveal CNV secondary to histoplasmosis, krypton red was no better than argon green [121]. The important point is for the laser surgeon to obtain an adequately intense burn to destroy the CNV reliably.

The initial stage of laser treatment involves outlining the CNV and blocked fluorescence with light, noncontiguous, 100-mm to 200-mm, 0.1-second to 0.2-second burns placed 100 mm outside its margins. More intense burns are then placed contiguously on the perimeter closest to the fovea using 200-mm spots of 0.2 to 0.5 seconds duration. The power is adjusted to obtain a uniform white burn. The remainder of the perimeter is treated when appropriate burn intensity is reached. Finally, the internal portion of the membrane is treated with overlapping 200-mm, 0.5- to 1.0-second burns. Complete treatment requires dense whitening of the entire CNV plus a 100-mm margin beyond the angiographically evident lesion (except blood).

During photocoagulation, care is taken to avoid retinal vessels. Feeder vessels are treated directly, 100 mm beyond their lateral borders and 300 mm radially beyond their visible base. Thermal papillitis and nerve fiber layer defect field loss are potential complications of treatment of peripapillary CNV and large lesions nasal to the fovea [122,123]. Treatment of peripapillary

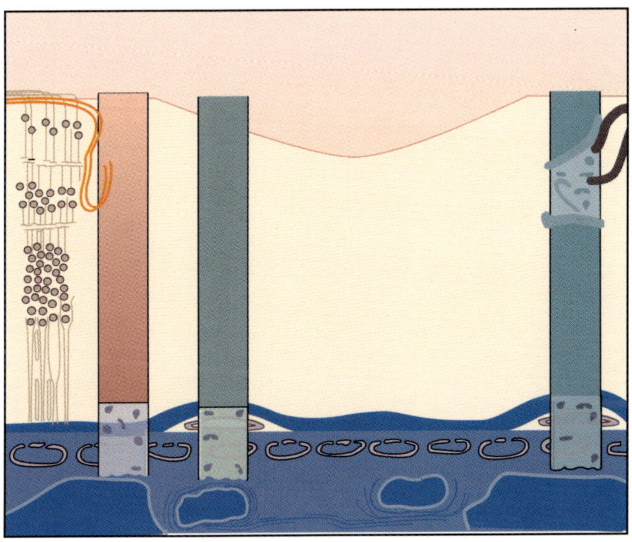

FIGURE 8-11. Absorption characteristics for the various laser modalities commonly used in the treatment of choroidal neovascularization must be kept in mind. Argon blue-green was the laser used in the early versions of the Macular Photocoagulation Study but is rarely used for macular treatment due to absorption by foveal xanthophyll. Argon green and dye yellow are minimally absorbed by xanthophyll and are more commonly used for these treatments. Krypton or dye red sources penetrate media opacities and blood far more effectively than argon green. (*From* Singerman [6]; with permission.)

lesions should spare 1.5 to 2 hours of the papillomacular bundle and not extend within 100 mm of the disc margin. Recurrent areas of CNV should have a treatment margin extending 300 mm into previously treated areas. The Macular Photocoagulation Study [124] studied the effect of treatment of peripapillary and large lesions nasal to the fovea and found beneficial results consistent with those observed in the entire study group (nasal and nonnasal lesions).

The need for accuracy in treatment of juxtafoveal CNV was emphasized by a Macular Photocoagulation Study report [125]. In the group with OHS and CNV within 200 mm of the fovea, only 5% of eyes with adequate laser treatment covering the foveal side of the CNV had severe visual acuity loss, compared with 25% of eyes with either some of the foveal side remaining untreated or a wide border of treatment on the foveal side.

The objective of photocoagulation is to destroy the CNV while preserving as much of the fovea as possible. The Macular Photocoagulation Study [7–15] has established argon and krypton laser photocoagulation as standard methods of treatment. Sequential treatment of the CNV with red and yellow wavelengths with the dye laser offers theoretical advantages and may allow improved results (Fig. 8-12) [50]. Whitening behind the CNV is accomplished first with the red wavelength (630 nm to 647 nm), which penetrates the deep choroid. The vessels of the CNV may then be visible against the white background. Closure of these vessels may be enhanced by changing to yellow (577 nm), which is highly absorbed by hemoglobin. Although the exact mechanisms of efficacious photocoagulation are not well understood, it seems reasonable that optimal uptake of laser energy in the CNV may increase the ability to obliterate the new vessels. Areas where the CNV is covered by hemorrhage are treated with red wavelengths. Areas of atrophic RPE and visibly red membranes and feeder vessels are treated with yellow wavelength. If a dye or multiwavelength laser is not available, krypton can be used for the red wavelength and argon green substituted for the yellow dye laser [126].

At completion of the laser session, posttreatment fundus photographs should be taken to document the area of treatment, allowing comparison with pretreatment photographs and the appearance at follow-up visits [127]. It is very useful to compare immediately posttreatment red-free photographs, developed while the patient is still at the clinic, to allow re-treatment of missed areas before the patient leaves [128]. If retrobulbar anesthesia has been used, the eye is patched. The patient is reinstructed in the importance of daily mon-

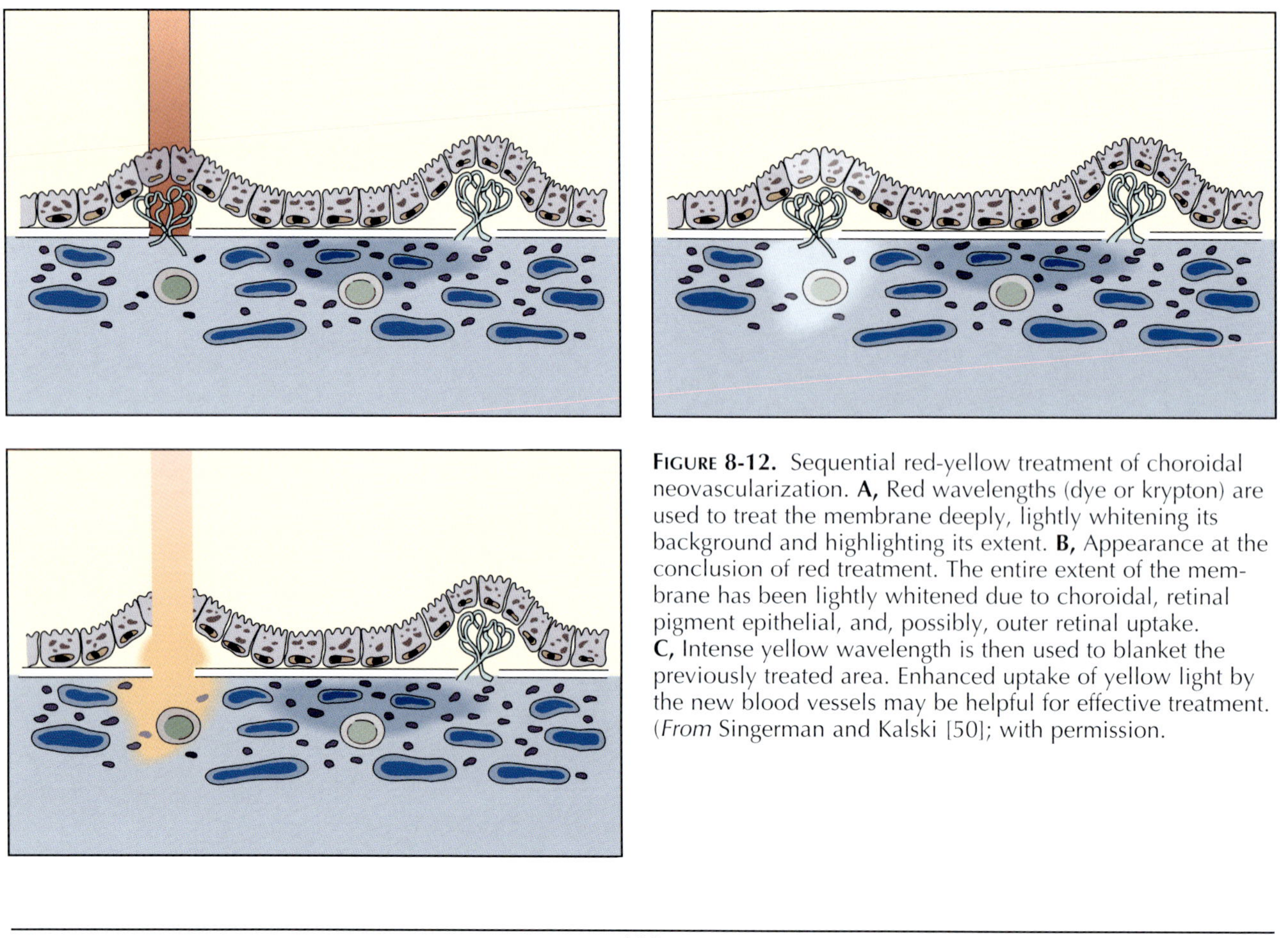

FIGURE 8-12. Sequential red-yellow treatment of choroidal neovascularization. **A,** Red wavelengths (dye or krypton) are used to treat the membrane deeply, lightly whitening its background and highlighting its extent. **B,** Appearance at the conclusion of red treatment. The entire extent of the membrane has been lightly whitened due to choroidal, retinal pigment epithelial, and, possibly, outer retinal uptake. **C,** Intense yellow wavelength is then used to blanket the previously treated area. Enhanced uptake of yellow light by the new blood vessels may be helpful for effective treatment. (*From* Singerman and Kalski [50]; with permission.

itoring of the Amsler grid and prompt reexamination if change in vision occurs.

Exacting follow-up is required to detect and treat persistent or recurrent neovascularization promptly. Fluorescein angiography is routinely repeated during the first several visits. The laser surgeon refers to the projected angiogram while examining the fundus with contact lens biomicroscopy. Fluorescein angiography of adequately treated CNV should show an evenly hyperfluorescent rim of staining adjacent to the area of treatment. Areas of persistence appear as a focal leak, usually at the margin of the treated area. Central leakage of a treatment scar that has a broad rim of surrounding hypofluorescence usually does not signify persistence and tends to resolve spontaneously. Re-treatment is avoided unless enlargement of the hyperfluorescent area is seen on follow-up angiography.

At 1 to 2 weeks after treatment, residual edema and retinal vasculitis may prevent visualization of persistent CNV. During this period, only a positive angiogram is helpful to inform decisions regarding the possible need for additional treatment. A follow-up angiogram must be obtained by 1 month after treatment even if one has been obtained 1 to 2 weeks after treatment. An acceptable follow-up schedule between laser treatment and follow-up visits is shown in Table 8-1.

Follow-up is continued indefinitely because recurrence has been known to occur years after treatment. Any sign of recurrence should be evaluated with prompt angiography and then treated unless the extent of treatment exceeds that suggested by the Macular Photocoagulation Study [7–15] protocol. In cases that do not meet these criteria, treatment must be considered on an individual basis. Visual acuity generally remains stable within 6 months of successful treatment. Late loss of acuity should prompt an evaluation to rule out recurrence but may be secondary to gradual enlargement of atrophy related to the area of treatment [129].

Complications of laser treatment are uncommon. The most serious complication is inadvertent foveal treatment. Projection of a recent, high-quality, magnified angiogram is essential to reduce risk of this complication. Retrobulbar anesthesia may also be helpful. The risk of choroidal hemorrhage can be reduced by employing durations of 0.2 seconds or longer and by avoiding spot sizes smaller than 200 mm. Thermal vasculitis and macular pucker more commonly occur after blue-green laser treatment. Now that blue-green wavelengths are avoided, macular pucker becomes less frequent and tends not to be visually significant.

TABLE 8-1 SUGGESTED POSTLASER FOLLOW-UP SCHEDULE

1 to 2 weeks (optional)
3 to 4 weeks (mandatory)
2 months
4 months
6 to 7 months
9 to 12 months
Every 4 to 6 months in second posttreatment year
Every 6 to 12 months indefinitely

Subfoveal surgery

Recent series of subfoveal surgery have suggested that CNV associated with focal conditions such as ocular histoplasmosis, idiopathic causes, multifocal choroiditis, punctate inner choroidopathy, and traumatic choroidal rupture may be responsive to subretinal surgery. In addition, pathologic myopia CNV may be a diffuse disorder treatable with this approach, although this surgery may be more difficult in high myopes. In many cases, patients tend to be younger than patients with AMD and may be more likely to have CNV in the subretinal space (type II CNV). Visual outcomes are likely to be better than those seen in surgery for CNV in AMD. Candidates for subretinal surgery tend to have subfoveal lesions not eligible for photocoagulation according to Macular Photocoagulation Study [13–15] guidelines, significant thick subretinal hemorrhage, or characteristics preventing extrapolation of the study results. The natural history of the disorder must be considered.

Refinements in surgical techniques have reduced the incidence of complications and simplified the procedure. A standard three-port vitrectomy is employed [31]. The posterior hyaloid is removed in most cases. A small retinotomy is made with a 36-gauge bent sharp spatula. Retinal vessels are avoided. A 33-gauge cannula is then used to inject balanced salt solution into the subretinal space to develop a working space around the CNV. Tissue plasminogen activator has been found useful in evacuation of submacular hemorrhage [130]. Intraocular pressure (IOP) is transiently elevated, and subretinal forceps are used to grasp the CNV.

The retinotomy site is elastic and allows a surprisingly large complex to be extracted. Care must be taken to ensure that all recognizable CNV is removed. Fragmentation and incomplete initial removal of the CNV are not uncommon. Several minutes after completing extraction of the CNV, IOP is normalized. Laser to the retinotomy site is avoided in uncomplicated cases. Partial fluid air exchange is performed, and the eye is left with an air tamponade in uncomplicated cases.

Intraoperative complications include retinal holes near the macula. These tend to be more common in patients with extensive prior photocoagulation and in AMD.

Choroidal hemorrhage is not uncommon but is usually controlled by transiently elevated IOP. The usual risks of vitrectomy surgery such as retinal breaks, retinal detachment, endophthalmitis, and cataract apply in these patients. The most common postoperative complication, as in laser surgery, is recurrence, which occurs in approximately 30% to 50% of cases [31]. Final visual outcomes are limited by recurrences, loss of photoreceptors and subfoveal RPE, and damage to the choriocapillaris.

Investigational therapies

Various new therapies are being investigated in an effort to improve outcomes and to offer treatment to patients with CNV not eligible for photocoagulation or surgery. Pharmacologic approaches to the treatment of CNV are currently under investigation.

A randomized controlled clinical trial of interferon α-2a found that it provided no treatment benefit for CNV secondary to AMD and might even be associated with poorer visual outcome. However, the lack of a clear dose-response relationship suggested that the observed differences might be due to chance [131].

Ionizing radiation may prevent endothelial cell proliferation in newly forming vessels in choroidal neovascular membranes. Two small studies have investigated radiation therapy in AMD [132,133]. Treated eyes appear to have less progression. Results are preliminary and a prospective randomized trial would be helpful to determine the efficacy of this approach.

Photodynamic therapy offers the hope of improving the selectivity and effectiveness of laser therapy by using photochemically active dyes to produce localized tissue damage. Experimental generators of singlet oxygen [134] and lipoprotein-delivered benzoporphyrin [135] have the ability to selectively close choroidal new vessels and may be a promising, selective therapy for CNV.

Techniques for subretinal surgery are improving but damage to the RPE appears to be a limiting factor in visual recovery. Transplantation of RPE cells may allow improved function by repopulating the areas affected by RPE atrophy or damage. This technology remains in its early stages but has been applied in a limited group of patients [136]. Further evaluation will be required before this technique can be considered for wider application.

The Submacular Surgery Trial (Baltimore, MD) is a pilot randomized controlled clinical trial in which we are participating. AMD is being studied in groups 1A to 3. OHS and idiopathic membranes are being studied in group 4. All lesions have subfoveal involvement.

Eligibility criteria include the following: lesions with evidence of classic CNV reducing vision to the 20/100 to 20/800 range are included in groups 1A, 1B, and 2. Patients assigned to group 1A and group 1B have not had prior laser treatment and have lesions with less than 50% of the affected area involved by hemorrhage. In group 1A, new subfoveal lesions with well-demarcated boundaries and moderate size (<2.0 to 3.5 disc areas) are randomized to surgery or laser. Group 1B includes poorly demarcated lesions, or well-demarcated CNV larger than allowed in group 1A. In group 1B, new subfoveal lesions with evidence of classic CNV but poorly demarcated boundaries, less than or equal to 9.0 disc areas in size, are randomized to surgery or observation. Well-demarcated lesions with evidence of classic CNV larger than those included in group 1A (<3.5 to 9.0 disc areas) are also included in group 1B and randomized to surgery or observation.

Recurrent lesions with prior laser treatment, evidence of classic CNV, less than or equal to 9.0 disc areas are eligible for group 2 and are randomized to surgery or laser. New or recurrent larger lesions (CNV less than or equal to 9.0 disc areas) are eligible for group 3 and are randomized to surgery or observation. Visual acuities may range from 20/100 to light perception.

Patients with OHS or idiopathic CNV are included in group 4 and, if eligible, are randomized to surgery or observation. Lesions may be new or recurrent. Scars in OHS with an associated sensory detachment may also be eligible. The lesion must be less than or equal to 9.0 disc areas in size. Visual acuity must be in the range of 20/50 to 20/800.

No results are available from this trial to date. Thus far, the investigators have successfully recruited approximately 250 patients. A full-fledged clinical trial is now being undertaken for patients with OHS. AMD will be the subject of a full-scale trial, which will begin in 1998.

CONCLUSIONS

Even with the significant advances in subfoveal surgery, laser treatment is probably our best tool currently for treating CNV. Ultimately, prevention of CNV is the best approach. Randomized clinical trials of laser treatment have been possible for common diseases associated with CNV, and the basis of modern laser therapy has been derived from these important studies. For less common diseases, such as angioid streaks, randomized trials will require many years and many clinical centers to enroll sufficient patients to render a significant result. The rarity of some disorders precludes the development of such trials. To manage less common disorders associated with CNV, we are compelled to extrapolate from the proven benefit described for more common diseases. Each of these has its own unique clinical setting. Technical advances in surgical management make subretinal surgery a therapeutic consideration in selected cases. Advances in nonsurgical therapies raise hopes of improved outcomes.

Many factors need to be considered, including the patient's age, visual needs, coexistent vision-limiting ocular conditions, and adverse effects of treatment. Each disorder has its own pattern of these factors, which must be considered to manage patients with CNV optimally.

REFERENCES AND RECOMMENDED READING

Recently published papers of particular interest have been highlighted as:
- • Of interest
- •• Of outstanding interest

1.• Niffenegger JH, Singerman LJ: Other causes of choroidal neovascular membranes. In *Retina, Vitreous, Macula*. Edited by Guyer DR, Yannuzzi LA, Green WR. Philadelphia: WB Saunders, 1998: in press.

This chapter summarizes the laser, surgery, and investigational therapies for the treatment of choroidal neovascular membranes.

2. Singerman LJ, Lamkin J, Addiego R, *et al.*: Laser treatment of choroidal neovascularization. In *Lasers in Ophthalmic Surgery*. Edited by Karlin DB. Cambridge, MA: Blackwell Science; 1995:112–139.
3. Green WR: Retina. In *Ophthalmic Pathology: An Atlas and Textbook*. Edited by Spencer WH. Philadelphia: WB Saunders; 1985:589–1292.
4. Gass JDM: Biomicroscopic and histopathologic considerations regarding the feasibility of surgical excision of subfoveal neovascular membranes. *Trans Am Ophthalmol Soc* 1994, 92:91–111.
5. Gass JDM: Biomicroscopic and histopathologic considerations regarding the feasibility of surgical excision of subfoveal neovascular membranes. *Am J Ophthalmol* 1994, 118:285–298.
6. Singerman LJ: Important points in the management of patients with choroidal neovascularization. *Ophthalmology* 1985, 92:610–614.
7. Macular Photocoagulation Study Group: Argon laser photocoagulation for senile macular degeneration: results of a randomized clinical trial. *Arch Ophthalmol* 1983, 100:912–918.
8. Macular Photocoagulation Study Group: Argon laser for ocular histoplasmosis: results of a randomized clinical trial. *Arch Ophthalmol* 1983, 101:1347–1357.
9. Macular Photocoagulation Study Group: Argon laser for idiopathic neovascularization: results of a randomized trial. *Arch Ophthalmol* 1983, 101:1358–1361.
10. Macular Photocoagulation Study Group: Krypton laser photocoagulation for neovascular lesions of ocular histoplasmosis: results of a clinical trial. *Arch Ophthalmol* 1987, 105:1499–1507.
11. Macular Photocoagulation Study Group: Krypton laser photocoagulation for idiopathic neovascular lesions: results of a randomized clinical trial. *Arch Ophthalmol* 1990, 108:832–837.
12. Macular Photocoagulation Study Group: Krypton laser photocoagulation for neovascular lesions of age-related macular degeneration: results of a randomized clinical trial. *Arch Ophthalmol* 1990, 108:816–824.
13. Macular Photocoagulation Study Group: Laser photocoagulation of subfoveal neovascular lesions in age-related macular degeneration: results of a randomized clinical trial. *Arch Ophthalmol* 1991, 109:1220–1231.
14. Macular Photocoagulation Study Group: Laser photocoagulation of subfoveal recurrent neovascular lesions in age-related macular degeneration: results of a randomized clinical trial. *Arch Ophthalmol* 1991, 109:1232–1241.
15. Macular Photocoagulation Study Group: Subfoveal neovascular lesions in age-related macular degeneration: guidelines for evaluation and treatment in the Macular Photocoagulation Study. *Arch Ophthalmol* 1991, 109:1242–1257.
16. Fine SL, Wood WJ, Isernhagen RD, *et al.*: Laser treatment for subfoveal neovascular membranes in ocular histoplasmosis syndrome: results of a pilot randomized clinical trial. *Arch Ophthalmol* 1993, 111:19–20.
17. Thomas MA, Grand G, Williams DF, *et al.*: Surgical management of subfoveal choroidal neovascularization. *Ophthalmology* 1992, 99:952–968.
18. Edwards LB, Acquaviva FA, Livesay VT, *et al.*: An atlas of sensitivity to tuberculin, PPD-B, and histoplasmin in the United States. *Am Rev Respir Dis* 1969, 99:1–32.
19. Schlaegel TF, Weber JC, Helveston E, *et al.*: Presumed histoplasmic choroiditis. *Am J Ophthalmol* 1967, 63:919–925.
20. Krause AC, Hopkins WG: Ocular manifestations of histoplasmosis. *Am J Ophthalmol* 1951, 39:564–566.
21. Goodwin RA, Shapiro JL, Thurman GH, *et al.*: Disseminated histoplasmosis: clinical and pathologic correlations. *Medicine (Baltimore)* 1980, 59:1–33.
22. Woods AC, and Wahlen HE: The probable role of benign histoplasmosis in the etiology of granulomatous uveitis. *Trans Am Ophthalmol Soc* 1959, 57:318–343.
23. Gass JDM: *Stereoscopic Atlas Of Macular Diseases*. St. Louis: CV Mosby; 1987.
24. Singerman LJ, Novak MA: Subretinal neovascularization. In *Laser Photocoagulation of the Retina*. Edited by Yannuzzi LA. Philadelphia: JB Lippincott; 1989:27–46.
25. Bynoe LA, Chang TS, Funata M, *et al.*: Histopathologic examination of vascular patterns in subfoveal neovascular membranes. *Ophthalmology* 1994, 101:1112–1117.
26. Schlaegel TF: Histoplasmic choroiditis. *Ann Ophthalmol* 1974, 6:237–252.
27. Singerman LG, Wong B, Ai E, *et al.*: Spontaneous improvement in the first affected eye of patients with bilateral disciform scars. *Retina* 1985, 5:135–143.
28. Macular Photocoagulation Study Group: Argon laser photocoagulation for neovascular maculopathy: three year results from randomized clinical trials. *Arch Ophthalmol* 1986, 104:694–701.

29. Macular Photocoagulation Study Group: Laser photocoagulation for juxtafoveal choroidal neovascularization: five-year results from randomized clinical trials. *Arch Ophthalmol* 1994, 112: 500–509.

30. Kleiner RC, Ratner CM, Enger C, *et al.*: Subfoveal neovascularization in the ocular histoplasmosis syndrome: a natural history study. *Retina* 1988, 8:225–229.

31. Thomas MA, Dickinson JD, Melberg NS, *et al.*: Visual results after surgical removal of subfoveal choroidal neovascular membranes. *Ophthalmology* 1994, 101:1384–1396.

32.• Holekamp NM, Thomas MA, Dickinson JD, *et al.*: Surgical removal of subfoveal choroidal neovascularization in presumed ocular histoplasmosis: stability of early visual results. *Ophthalmology* 1997, 104:22–26.

Extended follow-up of the surgical removal of suboveal CNV demonstrates stable visual results.

33. Melberg NS, Thomas MA, Burgess DB: The surgical removal of subfoveal choroidal neovascularization: ingrowth site as a predictor of visual outcome. *Retina* 1996, 16:190–195.

34. Macular Photocoaglation Study Group: Five-year follow-up of eyes of individuals with ocular histoplasmosis and unilateral extrafoveal or juxtafoveal choroidal neovascularization. *Arch Ophthalmol* 1996, 114:677–688.

35. Cohen SY, Laroche A, Leguen Y, *et al.*: Etiology of choroidal neovascularization in young patients. *Ophthalmology* 1996, 103:1241–1244.

36. Ho AC, Yannuzzi LA, Pisicano K, *et al.*: The natural history of idiopathic subfoveal choroidal neovascularization. *Ophthalmology* 1995, 102:782–789.

37. Adelberg DA, Del Priore LV, Kaplan HJ: Surgery for subfoveal membranes in myopia, angioid streaks, and other disorders. *Retina* 1995, 15:198–205.

38. Hotchkiss ML, Fine SL: Pathologic myopia and choroidal neovascularization. *Am J Ophthalmol* 1981, 91:177–183.

39. Fried M, Siebert A, Meyer-Schwickerath G, *et al.*: Natural history of Fuch's spot: a long-term follow-up study. *Doc Ophthalmol Proc Ser* 1981, 28:215–221.

40. Gass JDM: Pathogenesis of disciform detachment of the neuroepithelium. VI. Disciform detachment secondary to heredodegenerative, neoplastic and traumatic lesions of the choroid. *Am J Ophthalmol* 1967, 63:689–711.

41. Hayasaka S, Uchida M, Setogawa T: Subretinal hemorrhages with or without choroidal neovascularization in the maculas of patients with pathologic myopia. *Graefes Arch Clin Exp Ophthalmol* 1990, 228:277–280.

42. Hampton GR, Kohen D, Bird AC: Visual prognosis of disciform degeneration in myopia. *Ophthalmology* 1983, 90:923–926.

43.• Quaranta M, Arnold J, Coscas G, *et al.*: Indocyanine green angiographic features of pathologic myopia. *Am J Ophthalmol* 1996, 122:663–671.

ICG helps differentiate lacquer cracks from CNV.

44. Brancato R, Trabucchi G, Introini U, *et al.*: Indocyanine green angiography (ICGA) in pathological myopia. *Eur J Ophthalmol* 1996, 6:39–43.

45. Pece A, Brancato R, Avanza P, *et al.*: Laser photocoagulation of choroidal neovascularization in pathologic myopia: long-term results. *Int Ophthalmol* 1994–1995, 18:339–344.

46. Soubrane G, Pisan J: Myopie dégénerative: résultats de la photocoagulation des neovaisseaux sous-retiniens. In *Neovaisseaux Sous-Retiniens Maculaires Et Laser*. Edited by Coscas G, Soubrane G. Paris: Doin Editeurs; 1987:180–184.

47. Brancato R, Pece A, Avanza P, *et al.*: Photocoagulation scar expansion after laser therapy for choroidal neovascularization in degenerative myopia. *Retina* 1990, 10:239–243.

48. Deutman AF, Hendikse F, Hoyng C: Traitement des néovaisseaux sous-retiniens dans la myopie dégéenerative. *Ophtalmologie* 1989, 3:299–301.

49. Clark FM, Freeman WR, Goldbaum MH: Digital overlay of fluorescein angiograms and fundus images for treatment of subretinal neovascularization. *Retina* 1992, 12:118–126.

50. Singerman LJ, Kalski RS: Tunable dye laser for choroidal neovascularization complicating age-related macular degeneration. *Retina* 1989, 9:247–257.

51. Gass JDM, Clarkson JG: Angioid streaks and disciform macular detachment in Paget's disease (osteitis deformans). *Am J Ophthalmol* 1983, 75:576–586.

52. Green WR, Friedman-Kien A, Banfield WG: Angioid streaks in Ehlers-Danlos syndrome. *Arch Ophthalmol* 1966, 76:197–204.

53. Singerman LJ: Angioid streaks in thalassemia major [letter]. *Br J Ophthalmol* 1983, 67:558.

54. Singerman LJ, Hatem G: Laser treatment of choroidal neovascular membranes in angioid streaks. *Retina* 1981, 1:75–83.

55. Clarkson JG, Altman RD: Angioid streaks. *Surv Ophthalmol* 1982, 26:235–246.

56. Lebwohl M, Phelps RG, Yannuzzi L, *et al.*: Diagnosis of pseudoxanthoma elasticum by scar biopsy in patients without characteristic skin lesions. *N Engl J Med* 1987, 317:347–350.

57.• Quaranta M, Cohen SY, Krott R, *et al.*: Indocyanine green videoangiography of angioid streaks. *Am J Ophthalmol* 1995, 119:136–142.

ICG videoangiography may allow more precise localization of CNV than fluorescein angiography in patients with angoid streaks.

58. Singerman LJ, Rice TA, Novak MA, *et al.*: Red krypton and/or green and/or blue-green argon laser photocoagulation in treatment of angioid streaks. *Invest Ophthalmol Vis Sci* 1984, 25(Suppl):89.

59. Singerman LJ: Stries angioides: traitment par le laser à argon et le laser à krypton. In *Neovaisseaux Sous-Retiniens Maculaires et Laser*. Edited by Coscas G, Soubrane G. Paris: Doin Editeurs; 1987:221–223.

60. Pece A, Avanza P, Galli L, *et al.*: Laser photocoagulation of choroidal neovascularization in angioid streaks. *Retina* 1997, 17:12–16.

61. Gelisken O, Hendrikse F, Deutman AF: A long-term follow-up study of laser coagulation of neovascular membrane in angioid streaks. *Am J Ophthalmol* 1988, 105:299–303.

62. Nozik RA, Dorsch W: A new chorioretinopathy associated with anterior uveitis. *Am J Ophthalmol* 1973, 76:758–762.

63. Dreyer RF, Gass JDM: Multifocal choroiditis and panuveitis: a syndrome that mimics ocular histoplasmosis. *Arch Ophthalmol* 1984, 12:1776–1784.

64. Watzke RC, Packer AJ, Folk JC, *et al.*: Punctate inner choroidopathy. *Am J Ophthalmol* 1984, 98:572–584.

65. Palestine AG, Nussenblatt RB, Parver LM, *et al.*: Progressive subretinal fibrosis and uveitis syndrome. *Br J Ophthalmol* 1984, 68:667–673.

66. Morgan CM, Schatz H: Recurrent multifocal choroiditis. *Ophthalmology* 1986, 93:1138–1143.

67. Yannuzzi LA, Sorenson J, Shakin J, *et al.*: Acute disseminated chorioretinal spots: the New York experience. Presented at the Eighth Annual Meeting of the Macula Society, Marathon, Florida, 1985.

68. Singerman LJ: In discussion, Morgan CM, Schatz H: Recurrent multifocal choroiditis. *Ophthalmology* 1986, 93:1143–1147.

69. Callanan D, Gass JDM: Multifocal choroiditis and choroidal neovascularization associated with the multiple evanescent white dot and acute idiopathic blind spot enlargement syndrome. *Ophthalmology* 1992, 99:1678–1685.

70. Brown J Jr, Folk JC, Reddy CV, *et al.*: Visual prognosis of multifocal choroiditis, punctate inner choroidopathy, and the diffuse subretinal fibrosis syndrome. *Ophthalmology* 1996, 103:1100–1105.

71. Coscas G, Soubrane G, Delayre T, *et al.*: Treatment of subretinal neovessels in idiopathic recurrent multifocal choroiditis. *Bull Soc Ophtalmol Fr* 1989, 89:1275–1279.

72. Laatikainen L, Erkkila H: A follow-up study on serpiginous choroiditis. *Acta Ophthalmol (Copenh)* 1981, 59:707–718.

73. Mansour AM, Jampol LM, Packo KH, *et al.*: Macular serpiginous choroiditis. *Retina* 1988, 8:125–131.

74. Hardy RA, Schatz H: Macular geographic helicoid choroidopathy. *Arch Ophthalmol* 1987, 105:1237–1242.

75. Masi RJ, O'Connor GR, Kimura SJ: Anterior uveitis in geographic or serpiginous choroiditis. *Am J Ophthalmol* 1978, 86:228–232.

76. Chisholm IH, Gass JDM, Hutton WL: The late stage of serpiginous (geographic) choroiditis. *Am J Ophthalmol* 1976, 82:343–351.

77. Friberg TR: Serpiginous choroiditis with branch vein occlusion and bilateral periphlebitis. *Arch Ophthalmol* 1988, 106:585–586.

78. Wojno T, Meredith TA: Unusual findings in serpiginous choroiditis. *Am J Ophthalmol* 1982, 94:650–655.

79. Blumenkranz MS, Gass JD, Clarkson JG: Atypical serpiginous choroiditis. *Arch Ophthalmol* 1982, 100:1773–1775.

80. Wu JS, Lewis H, Fine SL, *et al.*: Clinicopathologic findings in a patient with serpiginous choroiditis and treated choroidal neovascularization. *Retina* 1989, 9:292–301.

81. Jampol LM, Orth D, Daily MJ, *et al.*: Subretinal neovascularization with geographic (serpiginous) choroiditis. *Am J Ophthalmol* 1979, 88:683–689.

82. Hooper PL, Kaplan HJ: Triple agent immunosuppression in serpiginous choroiditis. *Ophthalmology* 1991, 98:944–951.

83. Eagling EM: Ocular damage after blunt trauma to the eye. *Br J Ophthalmol* 1974, 58:126–140.

84. Fuller B, Gitter KA: Traumatic choroidal rupture with late serous detachment of the macula: report of successful argon laser treatment. *Arch Ophthalmol* 1973, 89:354–355.

85. Smith RE, Kelley JS: Late macular complications of choroidal ruptures. *Am J Ophthalmol* 1974, 77:650–658.

86. Gross JG, King LP, de Juan E Jr, *et al.*: Subfoveal neovascular membrane removal in patients with traumatic choroidal rupture. *Ophthalmology* 1996, 103:579–585.

87. Gass JDM, Guerry RK, Jack RL, *et al.*: Choroidal osteoma. *Arch Ophthalmol* 1978, 96:428–435.

88. Grand MG, Burgess DB, Singerman LJ, *et al.*: Choroidal osteoma: treatment of associated subretinal neovascular membranes. *Retina* 1984, 4:84–89.

89. Shields CL, Shields JA, Augsburger JJ: Choroidal osteoma. *Surv Ophthalmol* 1988, 33:17–27.

90. Teich SA, Walsh JB: Choroidal osteoma. *Ophthalmology* 1981, 88:696–698.

91. Rose SJ, Burke JF, Brockhurst RJ: Argon laser photoablation of a choroidal osteoma. *Retina* 1991, 11:224–228.

92. Grand G, Burgess D, Singerman LJ, Ramsey J:. Choroidal osteoma: treatment of associated subretinal neovascular membranes. *Retina* 1984, 4:84–89.

93. Morrison DL, Magargal LE, Ehrlich DR, *et al.*: Review of choroidal osteoma: successful krypton red laser photocoagulation of an associated subretinal neovascular membrane in involving the fovea. *Ophthalmic Surg* 1987, 18:299–303.

94. Munier F, Othenin-Girard P: Subretinal neovascularization secondary to choroidal septic metastasis from acute bacterial endocarditis. *Retina* 1992, 12:108–112.

95. Coll GE, Lewis H: Metastatic choroidal abscess and choroidal neovascular membrane associated with *Staphylococcus aureus* endocarditis in a heroin user. *Retina* 1994, 14:256–259.

96. Chung YM, Yeh TS, Sheu SJ, *et al.*: Macular subretinal neovascularization in choroidal tuberculosis. *Ann Ophthalmol* 1989, 21:225–229.

97. Deutman AF, Grizzard WS: Rubella retinopathy and subretinal neovascularization. *Am J Ophthalmol* 1987, 85:82–87.

98. Miller SA, Bresnick GH, Chandra SR: Choroidal neovascular membrane in Best's vitelliform macular dystrophy. *Am J Ophthalmol* 1976, 82:252–255.

99. Klein R, Lewis RA, Meyers SM, *et al.*: Subretinal neovascularization associated with fundus flavimaculatus. *Arch Ophthalmol* 1978, 96:2054–2057.

100. Robinson D, Tiedeman J: Choroideremia associated with a subretinal neovascular membrane: a case report. *Retina* 1987, 7:70–74.

101. Holz FG, Haimovici R, Wagner DG, *et al.*: Recurrent choroidal neovascularization after laser photocoagulation in Sorsby's fundus dystrophy. *Retina* 1994, 14:329–334.

102. Stern RM, Zakov ZN, Zegarra HZ, *et al.*: Multiple recurrent serosanguineous retinal pigment epithelial detachments in black women. *Am J Ophthalmol* 1985, 100:560–569.

103. Yannuzzi LA, Sorenson J, Spaide RF, *et al.*: Idiopathic polypoidal choroidal vasculopathy (IPCV). *Retina* 1990, 10:1–8.

104. Singerman LJ, Addiego R, Lamkin JC, *et al.*: Laser treatment of less common macular diseases. *Lasers In Ophthalmic Surgery*. Edited by Karlin DB. Cambridge, MA: Blackwell Science; 1995, 152–178.

105. Yannuzzi LA, Ciardella A, Spaide RF, *et al.*: The expanding clinical spectrum of idiopathic polypoidal choroidal vasculopathy. *Arch Ophthalmol* 1997, 115:478–485.

106. Gass JDM: Idiopathic juxtafoveal telangiectasia. *Arch Ophthalmol* 1982, 100:769–780.

107. Millay RH, Klein ML, Handelman IL, *et al.*: Abnormal glucose metabolism and parafoveal telangiectasia. *Am J Ophthalmol* 1986, 102:363–370.

108. Chew EY, Murphy RP, Newsome DA, *et al.*: Parafoveal telangiectasis and diabetic retinopathy. *Arch Ophthalmol* 1986, 104:71–75.

109. Geeraets WJ, Berry ER: Ocular and spectral characteristics as related to hazards from laser and other sources. *Am J Ophthalmol* 1968, 66:15–20.

110. Bischoff PM, Flower RW: Ten years' experience with choroidal angiography using indocyanine green dye: a new routine examination or an epilogue? *Doc Ophthalmol* 1985, 60:235–291.

111. Chang TS, Freund KB, de la Cruz Z, *et al.*: Clinicopathologic correlation of choroidal neovascularization demonstrated by indocyanine green angiography in a patient with retention of good visual acuity for almost four years. *Retina* 1994, 14:114–124.

112. Lim JI, Sternberg P Jr, Capone A, *et al.*: Selective use of indocyanine green angiography for occult choroidal neovascularization. *Am J Ophthalmol* 1995, 120:75–82.

113. Sorenson JA, Yannuzzi LA, Slakter JS, *et al.*: A pilot study of digital indocyanine green videoangiography for recurrent occult choroidal neovascularization in age-related macular degeneration. *Arch Ophthalmol* 1994, 112:473–479.

114. Avvad FK, Duker JS, Reichel E, *et al.*: The digital indocyanine green videoangiography characteristics of defined neovascularization. *Ophthalmology* 1995, 102:401–405.

115. Quaranta M, Cohen SY, Krott R, *et al.*: Indocyanine green videoangiography of angioid streaks. *Am J Ophthalmol* 1995, 119:136–142.

116. Vander J, Morgan C, Schatz H: Growth rate of subretinal neovascularization in age-related macular degeneration. *Ophthalmology* 1989, 96:1422–1426.

117. Singerman LJ, Hionis R: In discussion, Vander J, Morgan C, Schatz H: Growth rate of subretinal neovascularization in age-related macular degeneration. *Ophthalmology* 1989, 96:1426–1469.

118. Moorfields Macular Study Group: Treatment of senile disciform macular degeneration: a single-blind randomised trial by argon laser photocoagulation. *Br J Ophthalmol* 1982, 66:745–753.

119. Singerman LJ: Fluorescein angiography: practical role in the office management of macular diseases. *Ophthalmology* 1986, 93:1209–1215.

120. Macular Photocoagulation Study Group: Evaluation of argon green vs. krypton red laser for photocoagulation of subfoveal choroidal neovascularization in the Macular Photocoagulation Study. *Arch Ophthalmol* 1994, 112:1176–1184.

121. The Canadian Ophthalmology Study Group: Argon green vs. krypton red laser photocoagulation for extrafoveal choroidal neovascularization: one-year results in ocular histoplasmosis. *Arch Ophthalmol* 1994, 112:1166–1173.

122. Bloom SM: Thermal papillitis after dye red photocoagulation of a peripapillary choroidal neovascular membrane. *Retina* 1990, 10:261–264.

123. Turcotte P, Maguire MG, Fine SL: Visual results after laser treatment for peripapillary choroidal neovascular membranes. *Retina* 1991, 11:295–300.

124. Macular Photocoagulation Study Group: Laser photocoagulation for neovascular lesions nasal to the fovea: results from clinical trials for lesions secondary to ocular histoplasmosis or idiopathic causes. *Arch Ophthalmol* 1995, 113:56–61.

125. Macular Photocoagulation Study Group: The influence of treatment extent on the visual acuity of eyes treated with krypton laser for juxtafoveal choroidal neovascularization. *Arch Ophthalmol* 1995, 113:190–194.

126. Singerman LJ: Red krypton laser therapy of macular and retinal diseases. *Retina* 1982, 2:15–28.

127. Chamberlain JA, Bressler NM, Bressler SB, *et al.*: The use of fundus photographs and fluorescein angiograms in the identification and treatment of choroidal neovascularization in the Macular Photocoagulation Study. *Ophthalmology* 1989, 96:1526–1534.

128. Monahan PM, Gitter KA, Eichler JD, *et al.*: Evaluation of persistence of subretinal membranes using digitized angiographic analysis. *Retina* 1993, 13:196–201.

129. Rice TA, Murphy RP, Fine SL, *et al.*: Stability of argon laser photocoagulation scars in ocular histoplasmosis. In *Management of Retinal, Vascular, and Macular Disorders.* Edited by Fine SL, Owens SL. Baltimore: Williams and Wilkins; 1983:187–190.

130. Lewis H: Intraoperative fibrinolysis of submacular hemorrhage with tissue plasminogen activator and surgical drainage. *Am J Ophthalmol* 1994, 118:559–568.

131. Pharmacological Therapy for Macular Degeneration Study Group: Interferon α-2a is ineffective for patients with choroidal neovascularization secondary to age-related macular degeneration: results of a prospective randomized placebo-controlled clinical trial. *Arch Ophthalmol* 1997, 115:865–872.

132. Bergink GJ, Deutman AF, van den Broek JF *et al.*: Radiation therapy for subfoveal choroidal neovascular membranes in age-related macular degeneration: a pilot study. *Graefes Arch Clin Exp Ophthalmol* 1994, 232:591–598.

133. Hart PM, Archer DB, Chakravarty U: Asymmetry of disciform scarring in bilateral disease when one eye is treated with radiotherapy. *Br J Ophthalmol* 1995, 79:562–568.

134. Kliman GH, Puliafito CA, Stern SD, *et al.*: Phthalocyanine photodynamic therapy: new strategy for closure of choroidal neovascularization. *Lasers Surg Med* 1994, 15:2–10.

135. Miller JW, Walsh AW, Kramer M, *et al.*: Photodynamic therapy of experimental choroidal neovascularization using lipoprotein-delivered benzoporphyrin. *Arch Ophthalmol* 1995, 113:810–818.

136. Algvere PV, Berglin L, Gouras P, *et al.*: Transplantation of fetal retinal pigment epithelium in age-related macular degeneration with subfoveal neovascularization. *Graefes Arch Clin Exp Ophthalmol* 1994, 232:707–716.

CHAPTER 9

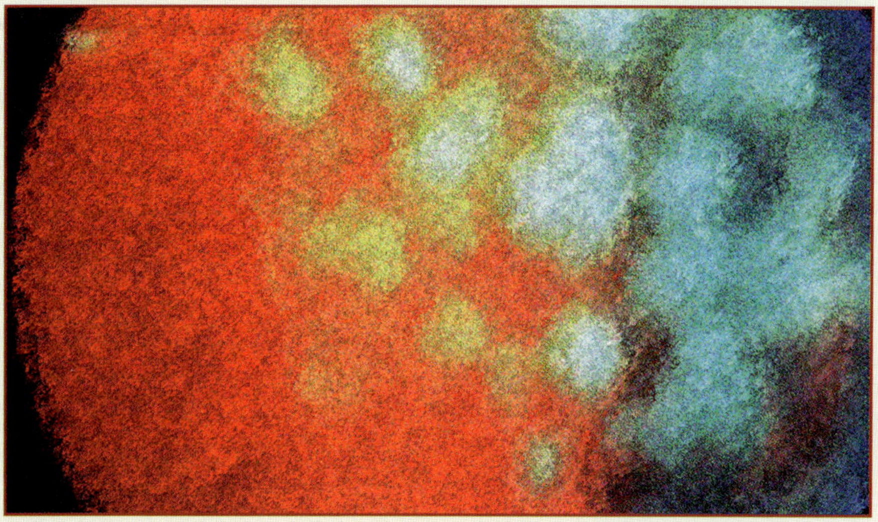

Laser Treatment of Less Common Macular Diseases

JOHN H. NIFFENEGGER
LAWRENCE J. SINGERMAN
HERNANDO ZEGARRA
SCOTT D. PENDERGAST

The less common macular diseases constitute a significant proportion of the conditions encountered by a laser surgeon. This chapter reviews idiopathic central serous chorioretinopathy, juxtafoveal telangiectasis, retinal arterial macroaneurysms, Coats disease, capillary hemangiomas, cavernous hemangiomas of the retina, arteriovenous communications of the retina, radiation retinopathy, nonarterial macroaneurysms, and cystoid macular edema.

IDIOPATHIC CENTRAL SEROUS CHOROIDOPATHY

Overview

Central serous choroidopathy (CSC) is classically described as a unilateral serous retinal detachment typically involving the fovea. It is associated with retinal pigment epithelial (RPE) disturbance, and occurs mostly in men in the third, fourth, or fifth decades [1]. Important variants include CSC in older patients or pregnant patients, chronic CSC, and bilateral CSC. Patients commonly complain of decreased vision, metamorphopsia, micropsia, and eccentric scotoma [1]. CSC is usually self-limited and may be recurrent. Visual recovery and resolution of subretinal fluid may be hastened by photocoagulation.

Pathology and pathogenesis

The etiology of CSC remains controversial. A primary disturbance of the RPE has been hypothesized [2,3]. A precipitating insult to the RPE may lead to its poor adherence to Bruch's membrane or to impairment of RPE-mediated ionic flow. A localized delay in arterial filling followed by choroidal hyperperfusion and venous hyperemia in the area of the damaged RPE has been noted to correspond with areas of pigment epithelial detachment (PED) or focal leakage on indocyanine green (ICG) videoangiography studies [4].

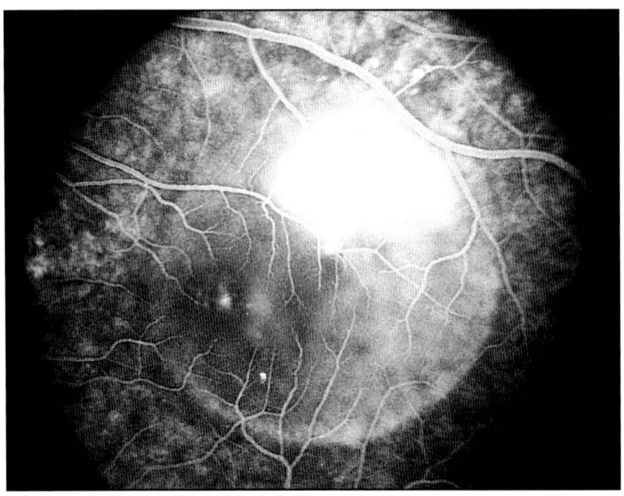

FIGURE 9-1. Fluorescein angiogram of central serous choroidopathy. Venous phase demonstrates smokestack leakage from a small pigment epithelial detachment (PED), superonasal to the fovea, which fills a large, round, sensory detachment. Note the small PEDs located just nasal to the fovea and inferior to the fovea.

Psychological stress and certain personality profiles ("type A") may be predisposing factors [1,5]. Pregnancy and systemic corticosteroids have also been associated with CSC [6,7]. Paraproteinemias have also been associated with CSC, although this is rare [8].

Clinical features

The classic finding in CSC is focal disturbance in the RPE with overlying serous retinal detachment (Fig. 9-1)[2]. Typically, the fovea is involved. The RPE disturbances are usually central pinpoint areas of leakage, but the area of disturbance may be larger than one half of a disc diameter [3]. Multiple foci of RPE leakage and disruption may also be present [9,10].

Pigment epithelial detachments, usually central, are the source of leakage in a minority of cases [1,11]. They may arise outside of or in the absence of associated serous retinal detachment [1,11,12]. A variant of CSC featuring bullous exudative retinal detachment (usually inferior and bilateral) has been reported and often features multiple or large PEDs underlying the detachment [13]. Another variant of CSC is characterized by atrophic RPE tracts descending from the macula and connecting a macular RPE leak to a dependent exudative detachment [10].

Pigment changes indistinguishable from age-related macular degeneration occur more frequently in eyes with CSC compared with noninvolved fellow eyes [14•]. RPE alterations are particularly noticeable in chronic or recurring cases [15,16]. Severe vision loss has been found in eyes with subretinal fibrin that later evolved into subretinal scarring, choroidal neovascularization (CNV), or RPE tear [17]. ICG angiography is helpful to differentiate CSC from CNV. Hyperfluorescence in CSC is first visible in the midphase of the ICG angiogram. Later dispersion of the hyperfluorescence and a distinctive silhouetting of the larger choroidal vessels are evident in CSC [18•].

Fine intraretinal lipid deposition has been reported, but hemorrhage is distinctly uncommon and should prompt a thorough search for CNV [10,19,20]. In chronic CSC, other retinal changes such as CME, cystic degeneration, parafoveal telangiectasis with leakage, choroidal folds, and atrophy of the chorioretinal capillaries have also been reported [10]. Progressive RPE decompensation, often bilateral, has been reported as a distinct, chronic form of CSC, although not all such cases have clearly followed earlier attacks of classic CSC [2,21]. Significant and progressive visual decline is associated with this variant despite that involved areas may appear normal or only mildly affected.

Fluorescein angiography

Most angiograms reveal isolated leaks, but multifocal leakage is not uncommon (Fig. 9-1) [3]. Most leaks arise in the macula [3,11]. The most common pattern is a pinpoint leak that slowly enlarges ("ink blot"). The classic "smokestack" pattern is seen in a minority of patients. A PED may exist under a pinpoint leak, with an overlying serous retinal detachment. Leakage from the RPE disturbance manifests as early hyperfluorescence, with later diffusion of dye into the serous retinal detachment [2,11]. Window defects resulting from focal or diffuse RPE atrophy also frequently cause early hyperfluorescence, which may be seen within tracts connecting macular leaks to inferior detachments.

Prognosis

The course of CSC is variable, but visual prognosis in typical forms of the condition is usually good [2]. Most cases spontaneously resolve within 3 to 6 months, with retention of normal or near-normal visual acuity, although some have subtle visual disturbances or significant abnormalities on visual function tests [22]. A small percentage of patients may suffer significant, permanent reduction in vision following a single severe attack.

A few patients develop chronic disease, or more severe or atypical forms, with large exudative detachments, multifocal leakage, or extensive RPE atrophy [10]. CSC in older patients (*eg*, those over 60 years of age) may have a poorer prognosis as well [23]. In all cases, recurrences are common and may be more so at or near a previously affected site. Like initial attacks, recurrences tend to resolve spontaneously. Multiple recurrences, indicative of widespread RPE changes, also indicate a poor prognosis.

Treatment

Laser treatment decreases the duration of subretinal fluid accumulation and speeds visual recovery but may not improve final visual acuity [9,14•,24,25]. No medical treatment (*eg*, antibiotics, corticosteroids, tranquilizers) has been found to be effective. Whether the recurrence rate is affected by laser treatment is controversial [9,11,16,26,27]. Two studies suggest a statistically significant reduction in recurrence rate with mean follow-up periods of 4.8 years and longer than 10 years, respectively [28].

Photocoagulation is reserved only for certain cases of CSC. Generally, observation for at least 4 months is advisable, because typical attacks often resolve spontaneously [11,12,19,26,27]. Treatment may be considered after multiple recurrences, if the attack has significant visual impact, or for more severe cases (multiple leaks or severe visual loss). Patients over 50 years of age or with lesions close to the fovea should be observed for as long as possible.

Argon green and krypton red lasers have been used, generally at settings of 200 µm and 0.1 to 0.2 seconds, creating light burns [9,11,16,19]. Treatment should be directed at the site of the leakage, because indirect treatment has not been found to be effective [24,27]. Treatment close to the fovea or within the papillomacular bundle should be avoided if possible. If either is necessary, the lightest possible treatment should be applied using a krypton red source.

In most cases, one treatment session is sufficient to induce resolution of the serous retinal detachment within several weeks. For PED with associated exudative bullous retinal detachment, treatment of the entire PED is recommended unless it is large or central. For CSC associated with atrophic RPE tracts and inferior retinal detachments, treatment may be directed to the focal areas of leakage, usually seen in or near the macula. Argon green laser treatments to produce a gray burn at the level of the RPE (50 to 100 µm, 0.2 to 0.3 seconds, and 50 to 150 mW) have been used [29].

CNV is a rare complication of photocoagulation. In a series of 1824 CSC-affected eyes treated with photocoagulation, 11 developed CNV at the site of photocoagulation in an area known to be free of CNV prior to treatment [30]. In patients over 55 years of age with findings consistent with CSC, exudative age-related macular degeneration should be ruled out with careful pretreatment contact lens examination and angiography [1,31].

JUXTAFOVEAL TELANGIECTASIS

Overview

Several subgroups of idiopathic juxtafoveal telangiectasis (IJT) have been described [32]. Gass and Blodi [33] categorized retinal IJT into three groups. Other diseases with retinal involvement, such as diabetes, venous occlusive disease, radiation retinopathy, sickle cell anemia–related hemoglobinopathies, Coats disease, and ocular ischemia, have findings similar to those of IJT [34]. Most patients with IJT experience slow visual loss beginning in adulthood.

Clinical features

Group 1 is nonfamilial and probably of developmental origin. Easily visible telangiectasis and intraretinal exudation resemble Coats syndrome. Most patients are male, and 94% have unilateral disease. Group 2 occurs during middle age and is bilateral in 98% of patients. Careful contact biomicroscopy reveals occult juxtafoveolar telangiectasis, minimal exudation, superficial retinal crystalline deposits, and right angle venules [35,36]. Late in the course of group 2 disease, foveolar atrophy, intraretinal pigment plaques, and CNV may develop. Group 3, less common than group 1 or 2, has bilateral, easily visible telangiectasis; minimal exudation; and capillary occlusion.

Pathology and pathogenesis

Pathogenesis of this condition is unknown, and only one familial case has been reported [32]. In group 1, the telangiectasis appears to be caused primarily by retinal capillary leakage and may be considered as a type of Coats disease that only affects the macula. In group 2, the findings may be caused by capillary diffusion abnormalities, possibly as a result of chronic, low-grade congestion related to the pattern of venules draining the affected area. Capillary occlusion appears to be the predominant process in group 3. Others have suggested that the retinal vascular changes in the bilateral forms are secondary to a primary disorder of the RPE. Histopathologic examination of one patient with typical bilateral disease revealed thickened capillary walls and luminal narrowing secondary to multilayered basement membrane proliferation [37]. The apparent telangiectasis observed on fluorescein angiography was thought to result from rapid diffusion of dye into thickened vessel walls.

Fluorescein angiography

Clinical findings in IJT may be subtle. Mild edema observed with contact lens biomicroscopy may be the only visible change on examination. Fluorescein angiography in IJT shows fine, fusiform, tortuous, variably sized capillaries and vessel tortuosity affecting the superficial and deep capillary plexus. Microaneurysms are common in the unilateral subtype (group 1). The affected vessels fill completely and promptly, and leakage of dye is seen in late phases (Fig. 9-2). Typical cystoid macular edema may develop. Hypofluorescence results from RPE hyperplasia or hemorrhage (in the setting of CNV). Besides capillary leakage, RPE window defects also account for hyperfluorescence, especially in bilateral disease.

Prognosis

The course and visual prognosis of IJT is somewhat variable. In all groups, typically a mild to moderate decline in vision is associated with metamorphopsia. There may be a slow progression with time, but patients generally maintain good vision in at least one eye for many years. Visual decline in unilateral IJT is caused by intraretinal edema and exudate and is usually minimal. CNV is more common in patients in group 2. Capillary occlusion contributes to visual loss in patients in group 3. Cystic retinal changes and lamellar macular holes can occur in all groups.

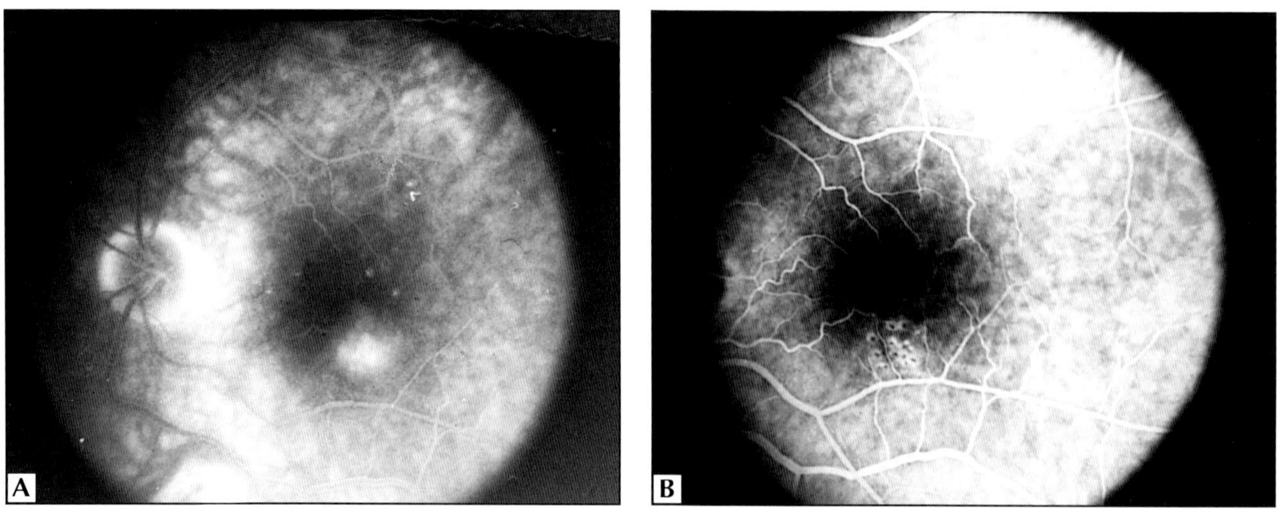

FIGURE 9-2. A, Diffuse ooze of fluorescein is seen in the late phase of the angiogram in a patient with group 2 idiopathic juxtafoveal telangiectasis associated with intraretinal crystals and slight intraretinal exudate (visual acuity 20/40). **B,** Same eye as in *panel A*. Midphase angiogram, 3 months after grid laser treatment to area of telangiectasis. Intraretinal exudates and edema are improved (visual acuity 20/30).

Photocoagulation

Photocoagulation of IJT has had variable success, depending in part on which group is treated [33]. Photocoagulation is probably beneficial in group 1 and frequently induces resolution of edema and exudate. However, because the natural history of this form is often self-limited, observation is probably warranted. In group 2, treatment can reduce exudation (Fig. 9-2) but is less commonly needed before the development of CNV. Group 3 is predominantly associated with capillary closure and usually is not amenable to laser treatment.

In cases of persistent or progressive visual loss due to increasing macular edema with or without exudate, treatment with argon green or dye yellow laser can be considered. Light to moderate intensity burns of 100 to 500 μm and a duration of 0.05 to 0.1 seconds should be applied in a grid pattern to areas of leakage outside the foveal avascular zone. Multiple treatment sessions are preferable to a heavier single treatment. Not all abnormal vessels need to be destroyed or treated directly. Treatment should be performed sparingly to reduce occurrence of bothersome pericentral scotomas. CNV complicating IJT should also be considered for laser treatment (Fig. 9-3).

RETINAL ARTERIAL MACROANEURYSMS

Overview

Acquired dilatations of the retinal arterial system are termed *retinal arterial macroaneurysms* [38,39]. The incidence clearly increases with age, peaking in the seventh and eighth decades. Women are more commonly affected than men by a ratio of approximately 4 to 1. Approximately 75% of patients with retinal macroaneurysms have hypertension [40–43]. Atherosclerotic heart disease, dyslipidemias, and polycythemia are less strongly associated [42,44]. Affected patients also seem to be at a higher risk for stroke [45]. Because of these associations with systemic disease, patients with retinal arterial macroaneurysms should be considered for thorough medical evaluation.

Coexistent findings may include generalized arterial narrowing, vascular tortuosity, caliber irregularity, sheathings, and exudate, as well as intra-arterial plaques and emboli (Fig. 9-4). Vein or artery occlusion (in the same or fellow eye) may also be seen, as may occlusion of the affected artery distal to the macroaneurysm. Arterial changes similar to macroaneurysms have also been seen with arteriovenous malformations of the retina [46].

Pathology and pathogenesis

Histopathologically, the affected arterial wall is thickened by hyalin, fibrin, lipid, and foamy macrophages [43]. It is hypothesized that arterial macroaneurysms result from focal vascular decompensation following injury by systemic hypertension or local vaso-occlusion (thromboembolic disease) [38,43,45].

Clinical features

Retinal arterial macroaneurysms tend to be unilateral and may arise multiply, even along the same vessel, although most lesions are solitary [38,39]. Macroaneurysms are most commonly located along a temporal arcade. Although they may be silent, many retinal arterial macroaneurysms present with visual loss, either acute (secondary to hemorrhage or rupture) or chronic (secondary to macular edema, exudate, and detachment).

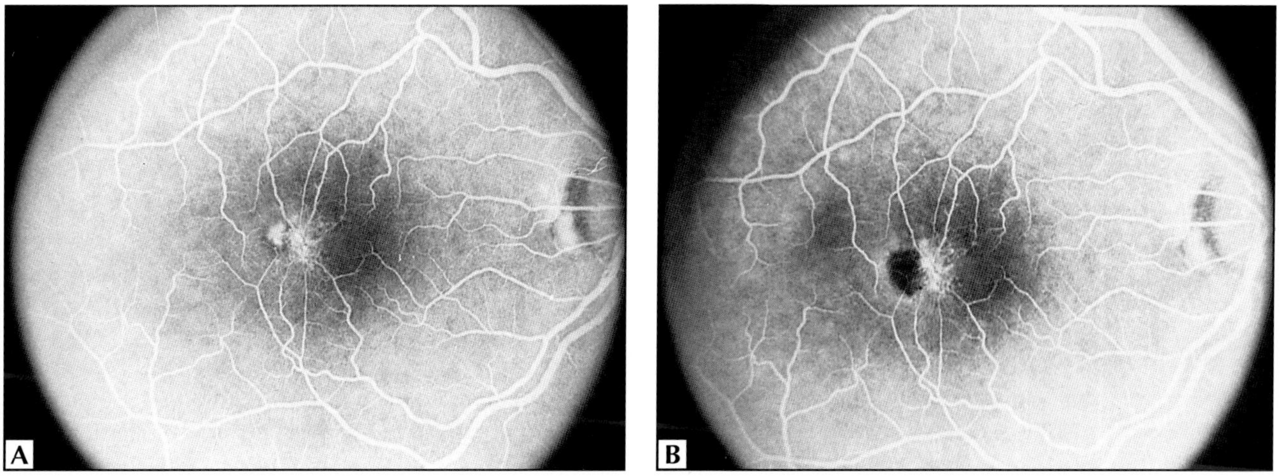

FIGURE 9-3. **A,** Choroidal neovascularization (CNV) complicating group 2 idiopathic juxtafoveal telangiectasis. Well-defined hyperfluorescence temporal to the fovea and telangiectasis (visual acuity 20/40). **B,** Same eye, 3 weeks after treatment. The CNV has been obliterated by laser photocoagulation.

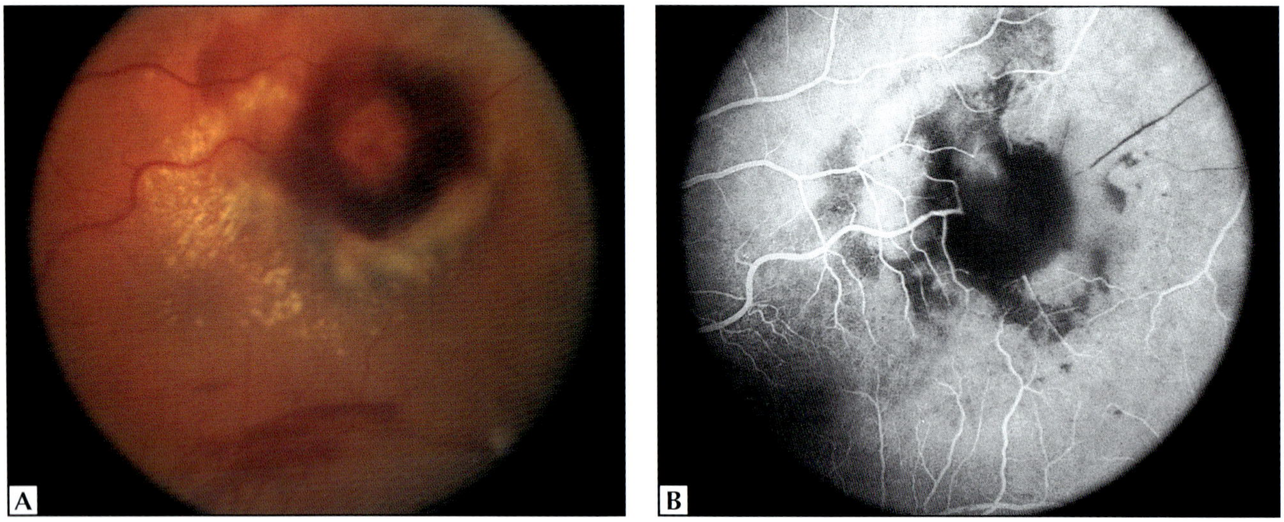

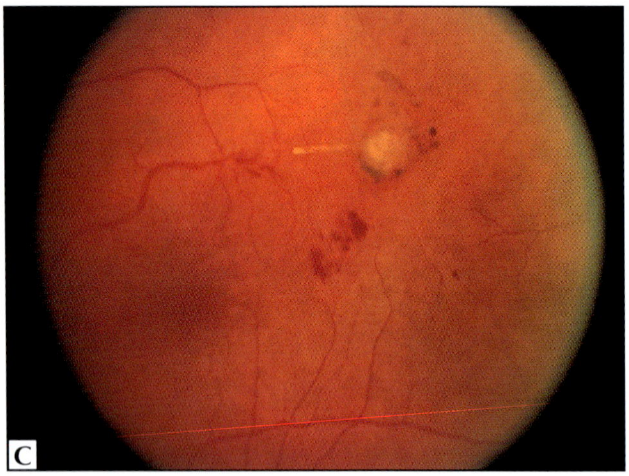

FIGURE 9-4. **A,** Intraretinal, subretinal, and preretinal hemorrhage surrounds a retinal arterial macroaneurysm located in the temporal arcade. Hard exudate extends into the fovea (visual acuity 20/200). **B,** Same eye 1 month after laser photocoagulation. Hemorrhage and exudate block leakage from the macroaneurysm. A filling defect of the distal artery segment indicates that branch retinal artery occlusion is present. **C,** One year after argon green laser photocoagulation of the lesion, visual acuity has improved to 20/25. Note the resolution of hemorrhage and exudate.

Retinal macroaneurysms appear as a focal, red, saccular or fusiform dilations of the arterial wall. The saccular type may be more prone to hemorrhage [44]. The exudate often surrounds the macroaneurysm in a circinate pattern but may migrate into the macula, regardless of aneurysm location (Fig. 9-4). Macroaneurysms located closer to the optic nerve seem more likely to bleed or rupture. Distal macroaneurysms are usually exudative and less prone to hemorrhage, as are macroaneurysms associated with vein occlusions. Involuted macroaneurysms appear as translucent, vascular outpouchings or shrunken, round, gray-white lesions along an artery.

Fluorescein angiography

Typically, the macroaneurysm fills early in the arterial phase [38,39,45]. Filling may be delayed, incomplete, or irregular as a result of intraluminal thrombus, endothelial cell proliferation, or involution. Hemorrhage, exudate, or arterial hyalinization may block the typical hyperfluorescence (Fig. 9-4). Late staining and leakage are common at the wall of the macroaneurysm, as well as along the proximal arterial segment. Macular capillary leakage and edema may also be demonstrated.

Prognosis

Many patients are asymptomatic as long as the aneurysm does not affect the macula [44]. Often a macroaneurysm closes spontaneously, without causing visual loss. Rupture or hemorrhage of a macroaneurysm is typically followed directly by involution. Less commonly, recurrent hemorrhage or reactivation of a quiescent or involuted macroaneurysm occurs [39].

Symptomatic macroaneurysms often lead to visual loss. Permanent, significantly decreased vision may be seen in the setting of long-standing and severe macular edema, exudate, and hemorrhage (particularly of a subfoveal type) [45]. Prognosis with macroaneurysms associated with acute preretinal or vitreous hemorrhage seems better than that with macroaneurysms associated with exudate affecting the macula. Simple intraretinal hemorrhage often clears without sequelae [39].

Treatment

Visual recovery may be expedited by laser photocoagulation [38,39,45]. Treatment should be considered in patients in whom the macroaneurysm shows significant or increasing leakage affecting or threatening the fovea, especially in the presence of a persistent loss of vision after 1 to 3 months of observation. Unless persistent dense vitreous hemorrhage prompts vitrectomy, a hemorrhagic or ruptured macroaneurysm without active leakage usually does not require treatment because spontaneous involution usually follows.

Elimination of leakage is the goal of laser therapy [47]. Extra care should be taken in the setting of vitreous hemorrhage and overtreatment should be avoided, because this finding increases the likelihood of distal arteriolar occlusion or perforation [46]. Retinal macroaneurysms are best treated with argon green or dye yellow wavelengths because of the enhanced absorption of these wavelengths by hemoglobin [38,39,47,48]. Photocoagulation treatment strategies can be direct, indirect, or a combination. Both techniques use low- to moderate-energy 200- to 500-µm burns with a duration of 0.2 to 0.5 seconds. With the direct method, treatment generally begins near the edge, overlapping onto adjacent retina. The center of the macroaneurysm is then partially or fully treated with larger, lighter burns, proceeding proximally to distally and avoiding feeder vessels. The larger and lighter burns may decrease the risk of hemorrhage and artery occlusions. With the indirect strategy, laser is applied in a pattern of one to three rows of nearly confluent laser burns around and adjacent to the macroaneurysm, again beginning proximally.

Closure of the macroaneurysm is usually accelerated by the photocoagulation, leading to a gradual improvement over several months [39]. Fluorescein angiographic evidence of persistent leakage may indicate that repeat treatment is necessary. With resolution of a macroaneurysm, visual acuity often improves, except in the setting of significant foveal exudate, edema, or hemorrhage [38,39,47]. Complications of laser treatment include branch retinal artery occlusion (Fig. 9-4), hemorrhage, choroidal rupture, and subretinal neovascularization [38,39,41,49].

COATS DISEASE

Overview

Coats disease is a primary disorder of the retinal vasculature featuring prominent irregular, incompetent telangiectases of large and small retinal vessels. The disorder is most likely developmental, with no evident genetic basis [50,51].

Coats disease primarily affects men (approximately 80% of cases) and is usually unilateral (at least 90% of cases). When bilateral, it is usually asymmetric [52,53]. Findings diagnostically indistinguishable from Coats disease are seen in 3% to 5% of patients with retinitis pigmentosa and have been reported in association with several other inherited disorders, including facioscapulohumeral muscular dystrophy [54].

Pathology and pathogenesis

Findings are consistent with a noninflammatory exudative vasculopathy [55,56]. Apparent loss of the blood–retina barrier leads to telangiectasis and leakage, with secondary changes in the retina, especially the inner retina. Vessels are thickened and hyalinized, leading to aneurysmal dilation with or without obliteration, exudation, hemorrhage, diffuse glial proliferation, RPE hyperplasia, and destruction of the retinal architecture.

Clinical features

Peak incidence of Coats disease is at the end of the first decade, with the vast majority of affected patients presenting by age 30 [50,52,53]. It has been diagnosed in infants. Children younger than 4 years of age may present with leukocoria and are often referred to specialists to rule out retinoblastoma. Some adults also present with minimal visual loss. Other presentations include neovascular glaucoma and severe exudative retinal detachment with profound visual loss.

Various clinical findings are possible. The temporal fundus, particularly the superotemporal quadrant, is most commonly affected. Capillary telangiectasis is the most common sign (Fig. 9-5) [57]. Mild disease is associated with minimal leakage. Tortuosity, kinking, and telangiectasis increase, with involvement of venules and arterioles as well as capillaries seen in more severe disease [50]. The major vessels develop "grape cluster" or "light bulb" configurations, beading, aneurysmal changes, and other irregularities [50,52,55,56,58,59]. Associated changes include vascular obstruction, sheathed and sclerotic vessels, microaneurysms, small vessel and capillary dropout, and abnormal arteriovenous shunting.

Inherent vascular incompetence leads to retinal thickening, edema, hemorrhage, and exudate (*ie*, subretinal, intraretinal, and preretinal). Serous detachment of the sensory retina, sometimes total, may develop. Subretinal refractile crystals and pigmentary changes frequently follow exudative detachment. Retinal and iris neovascularization, with neovascular glaucoma, iridocyclitis, cataracts, and disc edema, is a man-

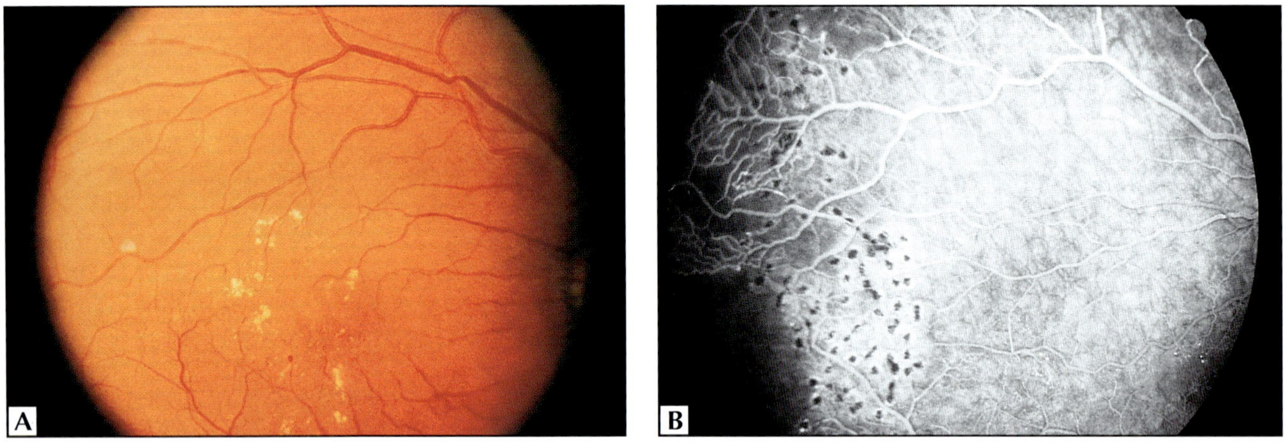

FIGURE 9-5. **A,** Telangiectasis and intraretinal exudates are visible in the temporal macula of this patient with Coats disease. **B,** Fluorescein angiogram demonstrates telangiectasis of the macular vessels. The temporal vessels have beading, capillary dropout, and abnormal arteriovenous shunting. Note the photocoagulation in the area of abnormal vessels.

ifestation of severe posterior disease. Traction retinal detachment results from vitreous condensations, veils, and bands.

Vision loss most often results from leakage and exudation. CME, circinate maculopathy, and exudative macular detachment can develop with either macular or peripheral retinal vasculopathy. In severe cases, a disciform mass may form centrally. Capillary nonperfusion of the macula may further contribute to visual loss.

Fluorescein angiography

Typical vascular changes and their extent are well imaged by fluorescein angiography. Angiography may demonstrate changes not readily seen on examination and highlight the irregular telangiectasis of capillary beds and associated venules and arterioles [50,53]. Capillary nonperfusion, microaneurysms, vascular beading, and abnormal vascular communications ("shunting" through dilated capillaries) are common (Fig. 9-5). Intraretinal neovascular channels may occur. Intraretinal and subretinal leakage of fluorescein begins early in the venous phase and persists [51]. Characteristic CME may develop, and subretinal pooling may be seen locally or in dependent areas remote from the abnormal vessels.

Prognosis

Coats disease has a variable course and rarely may go into remission [50,52,59]. Limited disease may fluctuate, with little or no progression. Patients with limited paramacular telangiectasis, mild edema, and exudate may be observed without treatment. Regardless of initial severity, progression involving all quadrants can lead to total exudative retinal detachment, secondary glaucoma, or other complications. Progression may be gradual or rapid, progressing from limited disease to total exudative retinal detachment within a year. Significant progression is more likely with more extensive vascular involvement. Prognosis seems to be worse if three or more quadrants of the retina are involved. Coats disease tends to be more severe in young children (*ie,* younger than 4 years of age); patients who are younger at presentation are more likely to have widespread disease and extensive sequelae [50,52].

Treatment

Treatment is effective in stabilizing (and occasionally improving) vision in most patients, as well as in preserving the eye [50,52,53,56]. Early treatment seems to be more effective, especially when the retina is attached. Older, more reliable patients with good visual acuity and limited disease that spares the macula may simply be observed. Extramacular lesions with subretinal exudate should be treated before frank retinal detachment or macular exudate develops. Patients with recent loss of vision and exudate from focal paramacular telangiectasis may be among the best candidates for treatment. Extra care should be used in treating disease near the fovea, especially in the papillomacular bundle.

Treatment in children should be prompt and aggressive. In severe cases, all peripheral lesions should be treated, even when the prognosis for central vision is guarded, to prevent large exudative retinal detachments. Treatment type depends on extent, duration, and location of the vascular abnormalities and exudate and may include photocoagulation, cryotherapy, diathermy, scleral buckling, external drainage of subretinal fluid, and even pars plana vitrectomy for significant traction detachment.

Clinical examination and fluorescein angiography should be used to ensure that all affected areas are treated with photocoagulation. Laser photocoagulation is performed with the argon green or dye yellow laser, using a spot size of 100 to 500 μm for a duration of 0.2 to 0.5 seconds. Burns are applied directly to the anomalous vessels to cause spasm or whitening. The therapeutic endpoint is obliteration of the telangiectatic vessels. Therapy can also be directed to adjacent retina and abnormal capillary beds. Extra care is necessary when treating the macula. Cryotherapy is needed in lesions that are peripheral or accompanied by large exudative retinal detachments; such cases may require prior drainage of subretinal fluid. Diathermy and scleral buckling, along with drainage of subretinal fluid, have also been used.

Multiple sessions are often needed, especially in young patients. Resolution of the disease is gradual, usually beginning 4 to 6 weeks after therapy. Complete resolution of exudate may take over 1 year. Epiretinal membrane formation, pigmentary changes, hemorrhage, inflammation, and scotoma have also developed after laser treatment or cryotherapy [51,60].

Even with successful treatment, the disease can recur in areas of previously normal vessels, even many years after initial therapy. Long-term follow-up, at least biannually, is recommended.

CAPILLARY HEMANGIOMAS

Overview

Capillary hemangiomas are benign vascular hamartomas of the retina and, occasionally, of the optic nerve [61,62]. These lesions may be isolated or part of a familial syndrome, such as von Hippel-Lindau disease [63–69]. Capillary hemangiomalike lesions have also been reported rarely in association with retinitis pigmentosa and neurofibromatosis [70,71]. These lesions are uncommon, but the incidence in men and women is similar [64,67,68,72]. New lesions have been discovered in patients of all ages but most often present in the second and third decades and are rarely seen after the fourth. Younger patients often have a family history positive for the presence of the condition.

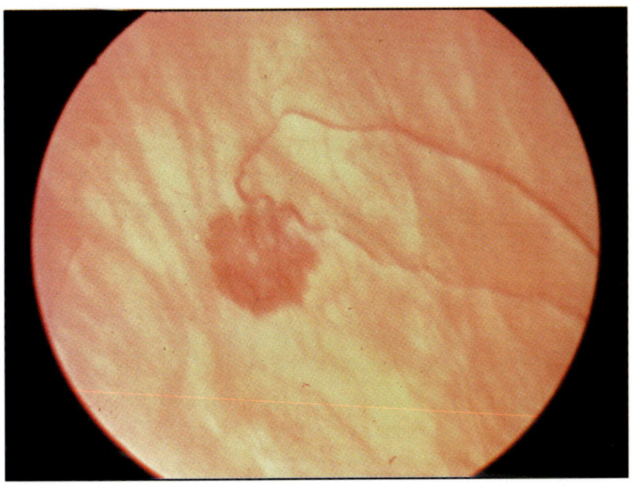

FIGURE 9-6. This capillary hemangioma was found in a patient in whom von Hippel-Lindau disease was later diagnosed. Note the multiple large, irregular, tortuous, branching, interconnected capillary proliferations and the feeder vessels.

Von Hippel-Lindau disease is inherited as an autosomal dominant trait with high penetrance and variable expressivity [64]. It is unusual for an affected patient to have all manifestations of the syndrome. Family history is not always positive, however, because of the late and silent manifestations of von Hippel-Lindau disease. It remains unclear what percentage of retinal angiomas is truly familial, but it may be higher than the accepted 20% [62,72,73]. Retinal capillary hemangiomas are present in two thirds or more of patients with von Hippel-Lindau disease and are the most common manifestation, causing the presenting symptoms in most patients [64,67]. The most common causes of death are cerebellar hemangioblastoma and renal cell carcinoma [64,67]. Other associated abnormalities include pheochromocytoma and, less frequently, polycythemia; medullary and spinal hemangioblastomas; angiomas of the skin; and cysts of the liver, kidney, pancreas, epididymis, adrenal glands, ovaries, lung, bone, omentum, and thyroid [64,67,74]. Bladder hemangiomas and islet cell tumors of the pancreas have also been reported [64].

Pathology and pathogenesis

Capillary hemangiomas are composed of multiple large, irregular, tortuous, branching, interconnected capillary proliferations of variable caliber (Fig. 9-6) [65,74]. The remainder of the retinal vasculature appears normal. Smaller hemangiomas may contain fairly normal capillaries and arterioles. Large tumors may breach the internal limiting membrane and lead to preretinal neovascularization and overlying vitreous condensations. Regressed lesions develop a hyperplastic RPE response, fibroglial scarring, and retinal thinning.

Clinical features

Capillary hemangiomas most frequently affect the midperiphery and periphery. They can present in single or multiple manifestations [63,64,74,75]. Incidence of bilaterality is variable but may be as high as 50% [62,74].

Typical endophytic capillary hemangiomas seem to arise from the inner retina and initially appear similar to microaneurysms. Larger lesions form fleshy, well-defined, elevated, oval to round, solitary orange-red nodules [62,64,66,75,76]. These are found in all locations, including at the optic nerve, and may enlarge to many disc diameters in size. Initially, feeder vessels may not be markedly abnormal, particularly if the lesion is smaller than 1 disc diameter (Fig. 9-6). In larger lesions, they develop tortuosity and dilatation, along with arterialization of the draining vein. The afferent and efferent vessels assume a similar color as a result of admixture of the arterial and venous circulations.

Sessile and exophytic lesions involve the deeper or outer retina, extend into the subretinal space and arise frequently around the optic nerve. These lesions often do not develop obvious feeder vessels. Examination may reveal only whitening of the overlying retina and a few dilated retinal capillaries extending posteriorly into the tumor. Surface hemorrhage may be another sign. Hemangiomas may cause macular edema (sometimes CME), retinal exudate (intraretinal or subretinal), retinal hemorrhage (preretinal, intraretinal, or subretinal), and exudative retinal detachment [77,78]. Vitreous reaction and preretinal fibrosis, macular pucker, and preretinal neovascularization are not uncommon and can lead to traction retinal detachment [79–82]. Rhegmatogenous retinal detachment may occur following breaks caused by surface traction, especially at the posterior base of the lesion between the afferent and efferent vessels.

Many lesions, perhaps up to 50%, are clinically silent [64]. In symptomatic patients, the spectrum of findings on presentation includes painless blurred vision, floaters, visual field loss, scotoma, metamorphopsia, micropsia, or even a blind, painful eye. Decreased vision is the most common symptom, usually resulting from chronic macular edema. Leukocoria may be the presenting sign in young patients if exudate is extensive.

Von Hippel-Lindau disease should be ruled out in patients presenting with retinal capillary hemangiomas. [64]. Work-up should include a careful family history (which may be falsely negative) and neurologic and physical examinations, including measurement of standing and supine blood pressures. Annual testing includes complete blood counts, urine catecholamines and metanephrines, and renal ultrasound. Tests to be performed at presentation and biannually thereafter include head and abdominal computer tomography (CT) scans. Examination of family members, particularly children and young adults, should be considered. Retinal examinations, including fluorescein angiography, should be performed at least annually in patients with suspected von Hippel-Lindau disease. Lifetime surveillance for new or recurrent lesions, with examinations at least every 6 months, is recommended for patients with retinal capillary hemangiomas.

Fluorescein angiography

Early perfusion and rapid dye transit of the tumor are typically seen on fluorescein angiography [61,78]. Perfusion of the angioma is retinal in origin. Transit of dye is rapid. Fluorescein leakage and staining may be confined within the tumor or may extend intraretinally, intravitreally, or into the subretinal space. Small or encapsulated lesions may not leak and may be difficult to demonstrate [77]. Usually no macular leakage is found, even with significant exudate. Fluorescein angiography of deeper tumors, particularly juxtapapillary and optic nerve tumors, demonstrates fine vascular networks, also filling early [61,66]. Afferent and efferent vessels are rarely evident with these exophytic tumors.

Prognosis

Progression to severe visual loss or other end-stage complications occurs in approximately 50% of patients, even with treatment. Progression is generally slow [73]. Some lesions, particularly smaller ones, are static or progress very slowly. Other lesions may grow rapidly, with worsening exudate leading to exudative or tractional retinal detachment, neovascular glaucoma, blindness, and phthisis. Progression can be rapid and aggressive, but spontaneous regression has also been reported [74]. Although their maximal growth occurs before puberty, capillary hemangiomas can grow in the third and fourth decades and sometimes later. New lesions may arise anywhere, including near areas of previous treatment. Development of new lesions may occur more often in eyes with multiple lesions.

Treatment

Prompt treatment is important because retinal capillary hemangiomas often cause visual loss, and treatment is significantly easier and more effective for smaller lesions with less exudate [68,72]. The exception to this rule is an optic nerve tumor [61,66], in which treatment itself can significantly diminish vision. Observation is warranted at least until associated exudate is significant.

Smaller lesions can be treated with laser photocoagulation. Reasonable clinical responses have occurred in lesions smaller than 2.5 disc diameters. Argon green or dye yellow laser has been used to treat retinal capillary hemangiomas directly with confluent burns of 100 to 1000 μm (depending on lesion size) and long duration (0.2 to 0.5 seconds). The endpoint is a significant whitening or blanching over the entire angioma. Small spot size and high intensity are avoided to minimize the risk of hemorrhage. The goal of treatment should be complete obliteration of the tumor with visible shrinkage, whitening, and nonperfusion on fluorescein angiography. Response to treatment can be delayed, especially with larger lesions, and multiple sessions are often necessary (and may also be safer). Treatment sessions should be separated by approximately 1 to 2 weeks. Regular follow-up, including fluorescein angiography, should be performed every 6 months, with re-treatment if reperfusion occurs. New lesions should be sought and treated. Laser photocoagulation of feeder vessels is not a widely accepted practice as a result of the higher risk of significant scotoma from vascular occlusion or full-thickness retinal damage.

Optic nerve and juxtapapillary lesions must be managed carefully because treatment may significantly reduce vision. Low to moderate surface photocoagulation may be repeated over several months. Treatment of "selected portions" of the tumors may also be beneficial, but overall prognosis is still poor. High-intensity treatment to larger areas contributes to visual loss, scotoma, and epiretinal membrane formation.

Smaller retinal capillary hemangiomas often respond to laser therapy, but recurrences and treatment failures do occur, with progression to rubeosis, neovascular glaucoma, exudative retinal detachment, and phthisis. Complications of photocoagulation include epiretinal membrane, scotoma, and hemorrhage. Worsened subretinal fluid or exudate is common but is usually mild and transient and may be worse following cryotherapy. Exact incidence of these complications is uncertain and difficult to distinguish from the natural history of the disorder itself.

Cryotherapy is preferred for large anterior lesions or in eyes with hazy media. The double-freeze thaw technique is recommended, with no more than 12 cycles per session to avoid an increased risk of proliferative vitreoretinopathy (PVR). Multiple sessions may be necessary, repeated at intervals of approximately 6 to 8 weeks. Complications of cryotherapy are similar to those of laser treatment or untreated capillary hemangiomas. Excessively vigorous cryotherapy may be associated with higher rates of PVR.

Combinations of pars plana vitrectomy, scleral buckling, drainage of subretinal fluid, and cryotherapy may be needed for large, unresponsive, or complicated capillary hemangiomas. Transscleral diathermy has also been used, as well as surgical eyewall resection. Epiretinal membranes should be managed by treating the associated tumor and waiting at least 6 months, because successful treatment of the hemangioma may induce spontaneous regression of the epiretinal membrane.

Visual outcome following treatment is better when the lesion is smaller than 2.5 disc diameters. Even with successful treatment of the tumor, permanent visual deficit, resulting from sequelae such as subfoveal hemorrhage, subfoveal lipid epiretinal membrane, and traction retinal detachment, is not uncommon.

CAVERNOUS HEMANGIOMAS OF THE RETINA

Overview

Cavernous hemangiomas, like capillary hemangiomas, are benign vascular hamartomas that affect the retina and, occasionally, the optic nerve [83–86]. They are equally rare in men and women and usually present in early adulthood. Typically, they are isolated congenital malformations; they have also been seen in association with similar neurological or cutaneous lesions, suggestive of a phakomatosis [87–89]. Individuals affected by such a syndrome may develop angiomas anywhere in the central nervous system, heralded by seizure, cranial nerve palsy, paresthesias, or focal neurologic deficits. Cutaneous angiomas have also been reported but are an inconsistent manifestation of this syndrome, which is transmitted in an autosomal dominant pattern.

Pathology and pathogenesis

Cavernous hemangiomas arise within the inner half of the retina, but large lesions may involve outer retina as well [85,90]. These tumors consist of numerous dilated, interconnected, thin-walled vessels. The luminal caliber is greater than that seen in the capillary variety. Normal endothelial cells and pericytes account for the characteristic absence of leakage, exudate, and edema.

Clinical features

These lesions are almost always monocular and solitary [85,87]. Often located posterior to the equator but outside the temporal arcades, they appear as sessile, thin-walled, grape-like clusters of saccular aneurysms. The individual saccules can vary in size from small microaneurysms up to as large as 1 disc diameter, and the overall lesion size can be several disc diameters, projecting into the vitreous. The saccules themselves are usually filled with dark venous blood and may appear only partially filled—sluggish flow leads to separation of clear plasma above from erythrocytes below.

The remaining retina and major vessels generally appear uninvolved, although twin vessels have been associated. Fibrous epiretinal membrane often partially covers the tumor. Occasionally, small superficial hemorrhages, adjacent pigmentary clumping, or hypopigmentation develops. Vitreous hemorrhage complicates up to 10% of cases and is the most common cause of visual loss. Subretinal and intraretinal hemorrhages also occur but are usually mild [62,84,85].

Patients with newly developed cavernous hemangioma of the retina should undergo a careful family history, a thorough physical evaluation with attention to the skin and neurologic systems, and CT or magnetic resonance imaging (MRI) scan of the brain. Family members should also be examined, particularly in the setting of a positive family history or systemic findings consistent with a hereditary syndrome.

Fluorescein angiography

Delayed perfusion is evident on fluorescein angiography, suggesting that the lesions are relatively isolated from the retinal circulation [83–85]. Hypofluorescence is present in the arterial phase, with slow filling occurring in the mid- to late venous phase. Plasma-erythrocyte layering is particularly prominent on fluorescein angiography, with hyperfluorescent caps in the saccules, particularly in the late phases. Usually no leakage of dye is found, although mild late diffusion into the overlying vitreous may be found; moreover, no arteriovenous shunts, significant feeder vessels, or involvement of the remainder of the retinal circulation are commonly seen.

Prognosis

The course of cavernous hemangiomas is usually nonprogressive [84,85]. Some lesions show progressive thickening and hyalinization. Exudation is rare, but surface fibroglial tissue may increase over time. Visual prognosis is excellent in most cases, and the lesions usually may be followed without treatment.

Treatment

In cases of significant recurrent hemorrhage, ablation with photocoagulation or cryotherapy may be considered [84,85,87]. Laser photocoagulation, if required, should be applied confluently to the surface of the tumor and possibly the adjacent retina, avoiding major vessels. Ablation may prove to be incomplete, and retreatment may be necessary. Optic nerve lesions should rarely, if ever, be treated, due to the potential for optic nerve injury with visual field loss or decreased vision. Other potential complications of laser treatment include growth of the lesion, vitreous hemorrhage, and epiretinal membrane formation, with subsequent macular distortion.

ARTERIOVENOUS COMMUNICATIONS OF THE RETINA

Overview

Arteriovenous communications of the retina are rare, congenital, direct communications between the arterial and venous circulations without an intervening normal capillary bed [91–94]. These shunts may appear as sporadic, isolated findings or as part of the systemic Wyburn-Mason syndrome. They affect men and women equally and are most often diagnosed in young adults (*ie*, typically younger than 30 years of age).

In general, arteriovenous communications do not demonstrate a well-defined inheritance pattern, even when part of the Wyburn-Mason syndrome [91,92]. This rare phakomatosis is characterized by monocular retinal shunts associated with similar arteriovenous malformations of the ipsilateral central nervous system, including the midbrain, cerebral hemispheres, and, often, the visual pathways [92–95]. Incidence of central nervous system lesions in patients with retinal shunts is hard to quantify precisely, and estimates range from 17% to 81% [93]. Other sites for potential malformations include the orbit, ipsilateral face and paranasal structures, eyelids, skin, lung, and spine [92]. Neurologic symptoms are variable [93,94]. Cutaneous findings are infrequent but include nevus flammeus and ipsilateral facial vessel dilation [92,96]. Because of its prominent systemic findings and relatively larger ocular lesions, the Wyburn-Mason syndrome is usually diagnosed earlier in life than isolated arteriovenous malformations.

Pathology and pathogenesis

Histopathologically, large arteriovenous communications occupy the full thickness of the retina [94,95]. Involved arteries and veins are difficult to distinguish. Each vessel has a fibromuscular medial coat of variable thickness and a wide, almost acellular fibrohyaline adventitial coat. Adjacent retinal changes include loss of ganglion cells and nerve fibers, as well as attenuation and cystic degeneration. Outside the lesion, the retina and its vasculature appear normal. An arteriovenous malformation of the optic nerve can replace much of the nerve's normal structure.

Clinical features

Arteriovenous communications of the retina are usually unilateral and may be single or multiple in an affected eye. The temporal quadrants and the papillomacular bundle are more commonly affected (Fig. 9-7). Arteriovenous communications vary in appearance from obscure, barely visible anastomoses to a "bag of worms" or mass of dilated vessels with indistinct arterial and venous components [93]. No pulsation is present. Small foci of retinal degeneration and pigmentation may be found; however, usually no optic atrophy is seen.

Arteriovenous malformations have been divided into three grades [91,92]. Grade 1 lesions are communications between a small arteriole and a small venule; grade 2 lesions are communications between a branch artery and a branch vein; and grade 3 ("diffuse type") communications demonstrate widespread, marked dilation of most of or all the vascular system. The Wyburn-Mason syndrome is usually is associated with grades 2 and 3 lesions.

Visual acuity typically correlates inversely with the clinical grade [91,92]. Patients with grade 3 lesions often have visual acuity insufficient for more than finger counting. This severe visual loss often leads to earlier diagnosis. Location is also important, as vascular malformations directly involving the macula or disc produce more visual compromise. At the other end of the spectrum are smaller peripheral lesions that are clinically silent.

Complications of arteriovenous communications of the retina are infrequent but include intraretinal hemorrhage, vitreous or preretinal hemorrhage, vascular occlusion, optic atrophy, choroidal and retinal ischemia, and neovascular glaucoma [91,92,97]. These lesions have been associated with other vascular anomalies such as retinal macrovessels (with grade 1 lesions), leaking macroaneurysms, and twin vessels, but they are usually seen without other retinal vascular anomalies [98].

Fluorescein angiography

Malformations typically fill rapidly in the arterial phase, with a greatly reduced transit time and venous filling immediately after arterial filling [91,92]. As a result, axial rather than peripheral filling of the involved veins may be found ("arterial laminar flow"), especially in larger lesions. Late staining of affected veins is possible, and slight leakage may be present in some larger, decompensating malformations. Accompanying capillary changes include leakage inside the area affected by the malformation, adjacent dropout, microaneurysms, and microvascular dilations. Choroidal and retinal ischemia may also be seen.

Prognosis

Many arteriovenous communications of the retina, especially group 1 lesions, are asymptomatic and stationary, although some increased tortuosity, sclerosis, and remodeling may occur [91,92,97]. Spontaneous regression can occur [99]. Visual loss may occur due to macular edema, macular hemorrhage, direct macular involvement, visual field loss secondary to optic pathway lesions, and optic atrophy of the fellow eye if there has been chiasmal involvement. Amblyopia may significantly limit the response to treatment [91,92,96].

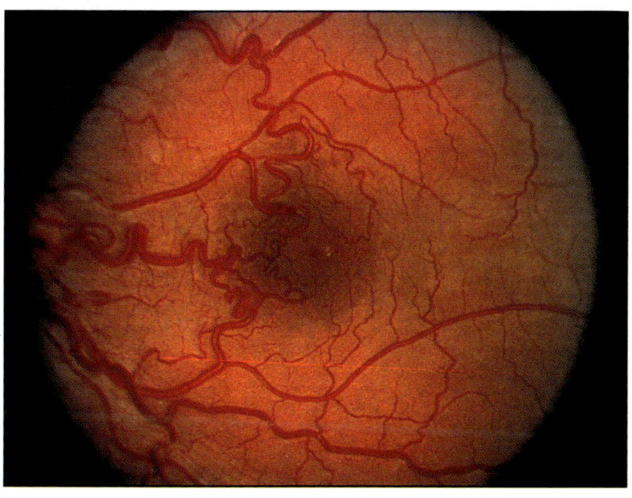

FIGURE 9-7. Grade 2 arteriovenous malformations in a patient with the Wyburn-Mason syndrome are tortuous and dilated.

Treatment

Treatment is usually not indicated unless the lesions are complicated by vein occlusion or neovascular glaucoma [97]. Panretinal photocoagulation or peripheral cryotherapy are better options than is direct photocoagulation, which may be complicated by bleeding, secondary ischemia, and failure to close the malformation.

RADIATION RETINOPATHY

Overview

Radiation retinopathy is an occlusive microangiopathy that has been reported following local or external radiation therapies for many conditions of the eye, orbit, sinuses, and central nervous system [100–110]. External beam doses of less than 30 Gy, in daily fractions of no more than 2 Gy, are believed to be significantly less likely to lead to radiation retinopathy, but the condition has been reported following dosages of 15 to 20 Gy [100,101]. Significantly higher doses of local radiation modalities (plaques, implants) may be needed to produce equivalent disease.

Radiation retinopathy usually presents 6 months to 3 years after treatment but may occur several weeks to decades later [111,112]. Latency may be shorter with therapy for plaque. Retinopathy is usually slowly progressive. The condition is often more severe in patients receiving chemotherapy and those with diabetes [105]. Hypertension and collagen vascular disease have also been postulated as risk factors for the development or exacerbation of radiation retinopathy [106,108]. Some patients with hereditary retinoblastoma may have an unusually severe response to radiation therapy.

Pathology and pathogenesis

Primary vascular insult, with occlusion and decompensation, occurs in radiation retinopathy [102,103,105]. Other retinal vascular changes include degenerative changes of the media and adventitia, loss of endothelial cells and pericytes, multifocal inner retinal ischemic atrophy, RPE changes, and cystic intraretinal changes and exudates. Ischemic optic nerve changes also occur (radiation neuropathy).

Clinical features

Patients often present with symptoms of blurred vision, either mild or severe, or floaters. The most common signs on examination include intraretinal hard exudates and hemorrhage, telangiectasis of retinal capillaries, microaneurysms, and cotton wool spots. Other changes include intraretinal and macular edema, RPE hyperplasia with or without atrophy, vascular sheathing, arterial attenuation and occlusion, and segmental vascular dilatation (Fig. 9-8). Proliferative retinopathy of the disc or elsewhere, with sequelae including vitreous hemorrhage and traction retinal detachment, may be seen. CNV has been reported [110].

Fluorescein angiography

Capillary nonperfusion can be extensive (Fig. 9-8), and, if severe, occlusion of larger arterioles may be seen [102,107]. Irregular, telangiectatic capillaries and microaneurysms often leak, and further leakage may be noted at the disc or from areas of neovascularization. Hyperfluorescence or hypofluorescence caused by pigmentary alterations and defects are common in chronic and severe cases.

Prognosis and treatment

Complications of radiation retinopathy can be treated with laser photocoagulation [100,104,106,107,110]. Indications and techniques similar to those developed for diabetic macular edema can be used to direct treatment. Argon green laser applications at settings of 50 to 100 μm and 0.05 to 0.1 seconds are applied to focal microaneurysms and other sites of leakage [100]. Alternatively, a grid pattern using argon green or krypton red with spacing of approximately one burn width is used for areas of diffuse leakage and capillary nonperfusion associated with macular edema (50 to 100 μm, 0.05 seconds in a grid pattern to the RPE in the area of the vascular changes) [104]. Additional light treatments may be necessary. For proliferative retinopathy, panretinal photocoagulation has been found to be effective in inducing regression [100,111]. Early treatment of radiation retinopathy has been suggested for macular edema or CNV, because prognosis is generally poor without treatment [104,110]. Cases most likely to benefit from treatment include those with mild to moderate edema without cystoid changes, severe nonperfusion, or severe visual loss. Significant macular ischemia is a contraindication to laser treatment. As there is some variability in the amount of radiation exposure necessary to produce radiation retinopathy, repeated evaluation of patients receiving as little as 20 Gy should be performed for at least three years after radiation treatment [101,110,112].

NONARTERIAL MACROANEURYSMS

Macroaneurysms may develop from retinal veins, capillaries, or collateral vessels following venous occlusion [113,114]. These macroaneurysms tend to be saccular and may arise multiply in a given eye. They are similar in size to arterial macroaneurysms and have been graded as small (100 to 149 μm), medium (150 to 249 μm), or large (250 μm or larger) [114]. Most are medium size.

On fluorescein angiography, venous macroaneurysms are usually associated with major branch veins or venules and are well-circumscribed saccular lesions that hyperfluoresce in the mid- to late phases of the angiogram. Capillary macroaneurysms appear to be on the venous side and fill from adjacent capillary beds. Filling is delayed, and late staining of the walls as well as adjacent capillary bed irregularity may be found. Macroaneurysms of collateral vessels are usually obvious.

Nonarterial macroaneurysms have been associated with surrounding retinal edema, serous macular detach-

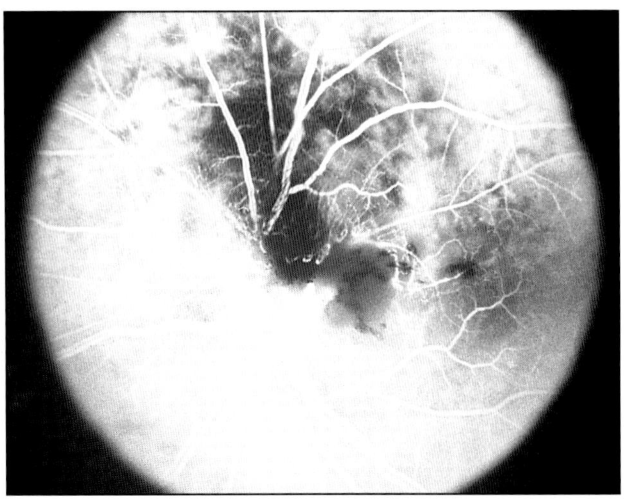

FIGURE 9-8. Fluorescein angiogram of an eye with severe radiation retinopathy demonstrates extensive capillary nonperfusion, occlusion of larger arterioles, telangiectatic capillaries, microaneurysms, and leakage from neovascularization.

ment, intraretinal hemorrhage, and exudates. Argon laser treatment has been used to obliterate capillary macroaneurysms and to treat venous aneurysms indirectly, with some visual benefit. Before treatment, the visual impact of the macroaneurysm must be carefully weighed against other potential coincident causes of visual loss (*eg*, CME, ischemia, neovascularization, and vitreous hemorrhage, among others).

CYSTOID MACULAR EDEMA

In aphakic or pseudophakic CME associated with vitreous strand incarceration in the surgical wound, several investigators have used yttrium-aluminum-garnet (YAG) vitreolysis, with variable success in improving vision [115–117]. Most clinical studies to date, however, have been small, nonrandomized, and poorly controlled. Therefore, efficacy of this technique is not well established [116]. No clear correlation exists between CME and anterior anatomic derangement, and some investigators believe that response to YAG vitreolysis is the exception rather than the rule [116]. However, in certain clinical situations, this technique may be useful, and significant complications are rare [115]. Prophylactic vitreolysis is probably not warranted, and chronic CME is probably less likely to respond [115].

Vitreolysis is usually performed with a contact lens to enhance magnification, focus, and energy delivery [115]. Treatment near the corneal scleral wound, where the vitreous strands are narrower and more easily visualized, is probably more effective. Disruption of the thinnest accessible distal portion of the strand is recommended [115]. Single pulses of low energy (1.0 to 1.5 mJ) are usually sufficient. Several attempts over multiple sessions are often necessary to lyse the vitreous adhesions completely. Transient corneal stromal white opacities or small iris hemorrhages may occur, but these resolve spontaneously. Rare complications, including retinal detachment and elevated intraocular pressure, have also been reported. Prophylactic topical anti-inflammatory and antiglaucoma agents are often used. Direct retinal photocoagulation of aphakic CME has been performed but has not been widely adopted [116, 119].

Photocoagulation of CME associated with retinitis pigmentosa has also been attempted, with initially encouraging results [118]. Additional clinical trials of this approach are required to define its efficacy fully. Available information remains insufficient to warrant widespread recommendations, and it is probably premature to use laser photocoagulation to treat macular edema in retinitis pigmentosa [119].

REFERENCES AND RECOMMENDED READING

Recently published papers of particular interest have been highlighted as:

- • Of special interest
- •• Of outstanding interest

1. Gass JDM: Pathogenesis of disciform detachment of the neuroepithelium. II. Idiopathic central serous retinopathy. *Am J Ophthalmol* 1967, 63 (Suppl):1–39.

2. Levine R, Brucker AJ, Robinson F: Long-term follow-up of idiopathic central serous chorioretinopathy by fluorescein angiography. *Ophthalmology* 1989, 96:854–859.

3. Spitznas M, Huke J.: Number, shape, and topography of leakage points in acute type 1 central serous retinopathy. *Graefes Arch Clin Exp Ophthalmol* 1987, 225:437–440.

4. Prunte C, Flammer J: Choroidal capillary and venous congestion in central serous chorioretinopathy. *Am J Ophthalmol* 1996, 121:26–34.

5. Yannuzzi LA: Type-A behavior and central serous chorioretinopathy. *Retina* 1987, 7:111–130.

6. Fastenberg DM, Ober RR: Central serous choroidopathy in pregnancy. *Arch Ophthalmol* 1983, 101:1055–1058.

7. Harada T, Harada K: Six cases of central serous choroidopathy induced by systemic corticosteroid therapy. *Doc Ophthalmologica* 1985, 60:37–44.

8. Cohen SM, Kokame GT, Gass JD: Paraproteinemias associated with serous detachments of the retinal pigment epithelium and neurosensory retina. *Retina* 1996, 16:467–473.

9. Gass JDM: Photocoagulation treatment of idiopathic central serous choroidopathy. *Trans Am Acad Ophthalmol Otolaryngol* 1977, 83:456–467.

10. Yannuzzi LA, Shakin JL, Fisher YL, Altomonte MA: Peripheral retinal detachments and retinal pigment epithelial atrophic tracts secondary to central serous pigment epitheliopathy. *Ophthalmology* 1984, 91:1554–1572.

11. Novak MA, Singerman LJ, Rice TA: Krypton and argon laser photocoagulation for central serous chorioretinopathy. *Retina* 1987, 7:162–169.

12. Schatz H, Madeira D, Johnson RN, McDonald HR: Central serous chorioretinopathy occurring in patients 60 years of age and older. *Ophthalmology* 1992, 99:63–67.

13. Mazzuca DE, Benson WE: Central serous retinopathy: variants. *Surv Ophthalmol* 1986, 31:170–174.

14.• Yap EY, Robertson DM: The long-term outcome of central serous chorioretinopathy. *Arch Ophthalmol* 1996, 114:689–692.

The decreased rate of CSC recurrence reported after direct laser photocoagulation was sustained for follow-up beyond 10 years.

15. Roseman RL, Olk RJ: Grid laser photocoagulation for atypical central serous chorioretinopathy. *Ophthalmic Surg* 1988, 19:786–791.

16. Annesley WH, Augsburger JJ, Shakin JL: Ten year follow-up of photocoagulated central serous chorioretinopathy. *Trans Am Ophthalmol Soc* 1981, 79:355–346.

17. Schatz H, McDonald HR, Johnson RN, *et al.*: Subretinal fibrosis in central serous chorioretinopathy. *Ophthalmology* 1995, 102:1077–1088.

18.• Spaide RF, Hall L, Hass A, *et al.*: Indocyanine green videoangiography of older patients with central serous chorioretinopathy. *Retina* 1996, 16:203–213.

ICG angiography is helpful to differentiate CSC from CNV.

19. Robertson DM: Argon laser photocoagulation treatment in central serous retinopathy. *Ophthalmology* 1986, 93:972–974.

20. Gomolin JES: Choroidal neovascularization and central serous chorioretinopathy. *Can J Ophthalmol* 1989, 24:20–23.

21. Gilbert M, Owens SL, Smoth PD, Fine SL: Long-term follow-up of central serous chorioretinopathy. *Br J Ophthalmol* 1984, 68:815–820.

22. Folk JC, Thompson HS, Han DP, Brown CK: Visual function abnormalities in central serous retinopathy. *Arch Ophthalmol* 1984,102:1299–1302.

23. Spaide RF, Campeas L, Haas A, *et al.*: Central serous chorioretinopathy in younger and older adults. *Ophthalmology* 1996, 103:2070–2079.

24. Watzke RC, Burton TC, Woolson RF: Direct and indirect laser photocoagulation of central serous choroidopathy. *Am J Ophthalmol* 1979, 88:914–918.

25. Weinberger D, Kremer I, Sira IB: The treatment of foveal central serous choroidopathy by krypton red laser. *Ann Ophthalmol* 1990, 22:35–38.

26. Slusher MM: Krypton red laser photocoagulation in selected cases of central serous chorioretinopathy. *Retina* 1986, 6:81–84.

27. Robertson DM, Ilstrup D: Direct, indirect, and sham laser photocoagulation in the management of central serous retinopathy. *Am J Ophthalmol* 1983, 95:457–466.

28. Burumcek E, Mudun A, Karacorlu S, Arslan MO: Laser photocoagulation for persistent central serous retinopathy: results of long-term follow-up. *Ophthalmology* 1997, 104:616–622

29. Jalkh AE, Jabbour N, Avila MP, *et al.*: Retinal pigment epithelium decompensation. II. Laser treatment. *Ophthalmology* 1984, 91:1549–1553.

30. Matsunaga H, Nangoh K, Uyama M, *et al.*: Occurrence of choroidal neovascularization following photocoagulation treatment for central serous retinopathy [In Japanese]. *Nippon-Ganka-Gakkai-Zasshi* 1995, 99:460–468.

31. Robertson DM: Argon laser photocoagulation treatment in central serous retinopathy. *Ophthalmology* 1986, 93:972–974.

32. Hutton WL, Snyder WB, Fuller D, Vaiser A: Focal parafoveal retinal telangiectasis. *Arch Ophthalmol* 1978, 96:1362–1367.

33. Gass JD, Blodi BA: Idiopathic juxtafoveolar retinal telangiectasis. Update of classification and follow-up study. *Ophthalmology* 1993, 100:1536–1546.

34. Chew EY, Murphy RP, Newsome DA, Fine SL: Parafoveal telangiectasis and diabetic retinopathy. *Arch Ophthalmol* 1986, 104:71–75.

35. Gass JDM: Idiopathic juxtafoveal retinal telangiectasia. *Arch Ophthalmol* 1982, 100:769–780

36. Moisseiev J, Lewis H, Bartov E, *et al.*: Superficial retinal refractile deposits in juxtafoveal telangiectasis. *Am J Ophthalmol* 1990, 109:604–605.

37. Green WR, Quigley HA, de la Cruz Z, Cohen B: Parafoveal retinal telangiectasis. Light and electron microscopy studies. *Trans Ophthalmol Soc UK* 1980, 100:162–170.

38. Rabb MF, Gagliano DA, Teske MP: Retinal arterial macroaneurysm. *Surv Ophthalmol* 1988, 33:73–96.

39. Lavin ML, Marsh RJ, Peart S, Rehman A: Retinal arterial macroaneurysms: a retrospective study of 40 patients. *Br J Ophthalmol* 1987, 71:817–825

40. Asdourian GK, Goldberg MF, Jampol L, Rabb M: Retinal macroaneurysms. *Arch Ophthalmol* 1977, 95:624–628.

41. Panton RW, Goldberg MF, Farber MD: Retinal arterial macroaneurysms: risk factors and natural history. *Br J Ophthalmol* 1990, 74:595–600.

42. Nadel AJ, Gupta KK: Macroaneurysms of the retinal arteries. *Arch Ophthalmol* 1976, 94:1092–1096.

43. Fichte C, Streeten BW, Friedman AH: A histopathologic study of retinal artery aneurysms. *Am J Ophthalmol* 1978, 85:509–518.

44. Abdel-Khalek MN, Richardson J: Retinal macroaneurysm: natural history and guidelines for treatment. *Br J Ophthalmol* 1986, 70:2–11.

45. Lewis RA, Norton EW, Gass JDM: Acquired arterial macroaneurysms of the retina. *Br J Ophthalmol* 1987, 60:21–30.

46. Tilanus MD, Hoyng C, Deutman AF, *et al.*: Congenital arteriovenous communications and the development of two types of leaking retinal macroaneurysms. *Am J Ophthalmol* 1991, 112:31–33.

47. Mainster MA, Whitacre MM: Dye yellow photocoagulation of retinal arterial macroaneurysms. *Am J Ophthalmol* 1988, 105:97–98.

48. Joondeph BC, Joondeph HC, Blair NP: Retinal macroaneurysms treated with the yellow dye laser. *Retina* 1989, 9:187–192.

49. Russell SR, Folk JC: Branch retinal artery occlusion after dye yellow photocoagulation of an arterial macroaneurysm. *Am J Ophthalmol* 1987, 104:186–187.

50. Gass JDM: A fluorescein angiographic study of macular dysfunction secondary to retinal vascular disease. V. Retinal telangiectasis. *Arch Ophthalmol* 1968, 80:592–605.

51. McGrand JC: Photocoagulation in Coats' disease. *Trans Ophthalmol Soc UK* 1970, 90:47–56.

52. Ridley ME, Shields JA, Brown GC, Tasman W: Coats' disease. Evaluation of management. *Ophthalmology* 1982, 89:1381–1387.

53. Harris GS: Coats' disease, diagnosis and treatment. *Can J Ophthalmol* 1970, 5:311–320.

54. Gurwin EB, Fitzsimons RB, Sehmi KS, Bird AC: Retinal telangiectasis in facioscapulohumeral muscular dystrophy. *Arch Ophthalmol* 1985, 103:1695–1700.

55. Tripathi K, Ashton N: Electron microscopical study of Coats' disease. *Br J Ophthalmol* 1971, 55:289–301.

56. Green WR: Bilateral Coats' disease. Massive gliosis of the retina. *Arch Ophthalmol* 1967, 77:378–383.

57. Pe'er J: Calcifications in Coats' disease. *Am J Ophthalmol* 1988, 106:742–743.

58. Farkas TG, Potts AM, Boone C: Some pathological and biochemical aspects of Coats' disease. *Am J Ophthalmol* 1973, 75:289–301.

59. Deutsch TA, Rabb MF, Jampol LM: Spontaneous regression of retinal lesions in Coats' disease. *Can J Ophthalmol* 1982, 17:169–172

60. Arrig PG, Lahav M, Hutchins RK, Weiter JJ: Pigmentary retinal degeneration and Coats' disease: a case study. *Ophthalmic Surg* 1988, 19:432–436.

61. Yimoyines DJ, Topilow HW, Abedin S, McMeel J: Bilateral peripapillary exophytic retinal hemangioblastoma. *Ophthalmology* 1982, 89:1388–1392.

62. Gass JDM: Treatment of retinal vascular anomalies. *Trans Am Acad Ophthalmol Otolaryngol* 1977, 83:432–445.

63. Apple DJ, Goldberg MF, Wyhinny GJ: Argon laser treatment of von Hippel-Lindau retinal angiomas. II. Histopathology of treated lesions. *Arch Ophthalmol* 1974, 92:126–130.

64. Hardwig P, Robertson DM: von Hippel-Lindau disease: a familial, often lethal, multisystem phakomatosis. *Ophthalmology* 1984, 91:263–270.

65. Mottow-Lippa L, Tso MOM, Peyman GA, Chejfec G: von Hippel angiomatosis. A light, electron microscopic, and immunoperoxidase characterization. *Ophthalmology* 1983, 90:848–855.

66. Gass JDM, Braunstein R: Sessile and exophytic capillary angiomas of the juxtapapillary region and optic nerve head. *Arch Ophthalmol* 1980, 98:1790–1797.

67. Melmon KL, Rosen SW: Lindau's disease. Review of the literature and study of a large kindred. *Am J Med* 1964, 36:595–617.

68. Blodi CF, Russell SR, Pulido JS, Folk JC: Direct and feeder vessel photocoagulation of retinal angiomas with dye yellow laser. *Ophthalmology* 1990, 97:791–797.

69. DeJong PTVM, Verkaart RJF, van de Vooren MJ, *et al.*: Twin vessels in von Hippel-Lindau disease. *Am J Ophthalmol* 1988, 105:165–169.

70. Kollaritis CR, Mehelas TJ, Shealy TR, Zahn JR: Von Hippel tumors in siblings with retinitis pigmentosa. *Ann Ophthalmol* 1982, 14:256–259.

71. Dobyns WB, Michels VV, Groover RV, *et al.*: Familial cavernous malformation of the central nervous system and retina. *Ann Neurol* 1987, 21:579–583.

72. Annesley WH, Leonard BC, Shields JA, Tasman WS: Fifteen year review of treated cases of retinal angiomatosis. *Trans Am Acad Ophthalmol Otolarnyngol* 1977, 83:446–453.

73. Usher CH: On a few hereditary eye affections. *Trans Ophthalmol Soc U K* 1935, 55:164–193.

74. Whitson JT, Welch RB, Green WR: von Hippel-Lindau disease: case report of a patient with spontaneous regression of a retinal angioma. *Retina* 1986, 6:253–259.

75. Sellors PJ, Archer D: The management of retinal angiomatosis. *Trans Ophthalmol Soc U K* 1970, 89:529–543.

76. Lowden BA, Harris GS: Pheochromocytoma and von Hippel-Lindau's disease. *Can J Ophthalmol* 1976, 11:282–288.

77. Goldberg MF, Koenig S: Argon laser treatment of von Hippel-Lindau retinal angiomas. *Arch Ophthalmol* 1974, 92:121–124.

78. Kremer I, Gilad E, Ben-Sira I: Juxtapapillary exophytic retinal capillary hemangioma treated by yellow krypton (568 nm) laser photocoagulation. *Ophthalmic Surg* 1988, 19:743–747.

79. Nicholson DH, Anderson LS, Blodi C: Rhegmatogenous retinal detachment in angiomatosis retinae. *Am J Ophthalmol* 1986, 101:187–189.

80. Laatikainen L, Immonen I, Summanen P: Peripheral retinal angiomalike lesion and macular pucker. *Am J Ophthalmol* 1989, 108:563–566.

81. Schwartz PL, Trubowitsi G, Fastenberg DM, Stein M: Macular pucker and retinal angioma. *Ophthalmic Surg* 1987, 18:677–679.

82. Schwartz PL, Fastenberg DM, Shakin JL: Management of macular puckers associated with retinal angiomas. *Ophthalmic Surg* 1990, 21:550–556.

83. Drummond JW, Hall D, Steen WH, Lusk JE: Cavernous hemangioma of the optic disc. *Ann Ophthalmol* 1980, 12:1017–1018.

84. Klein M, Goldberg MF, Cotlier E: Cavernous hemangioma of the retina: report of four cases. *Ann Ophthalmol* 1975, 7:1214–1221.

85. Gass JDM: Cavernous hemangioma of the retina. A neuro-oculo-cutaneous syndrome. *Am J Ophthalmol* 1971, 71:799–814.

86. Moffat KP, Lee MS, Ghosh M: Retinal cavernous hemangioma. *Can J Ophthalmol* 1988, 23:133–135.

87. Pancurak G, Goldberg MF, Frenkel M, Crowell RM: Cavernous hemangiomas of the retina: genetic and central nervous system involvement. *Retina* 1985, 5:215–220.

88. Schwartz AC, Weaver RG, Bloomfield R, Tyler M: Cavernous hemangioma of the retina, cutaneous angiomas, and intracranial vascular lesion by computed tomography and nuclear magnetic resonance imaging. *Am J Ophthalmol* 1984, 98:483–487.

89. Goldberg RE, Pheasant TR, Shields JA: Cavernous hemangiomas of the retina. A four-generation pedigree with neurocutaneous manifestations and an example of bilateral retinal involvement. *Arch Ophthalmol* 1979, 97:2321–2324.

90. Messmer E, Font RL, Laqua H, *et al.*: Cavernous hemangioma of the retina. Immunohistochemical and ultrastructural observations. *Arch Ophthalmol* 1984, 102:413–418.

91. Archer DB, Deutman A, Ernests JT, Krill AE: Arteriovenous communications of the retina. *Am J Ophthalmol* 1973, 75:225–241.

92. Mansour AM, Walsh JB, Henkind P: Arteriovenous anastomoses of the retina. *Ophthalmology* 1987, 94:35–40.

93. Cameron ME: Congenital arterio-venous aneurysm of the retina. *Br J Ophthalmol* 1958, 42:655.

94. Wyburn-Mason R: Arteriovenous aneurysm of midbrain and retina, facial naevi and mental changes. *Brain* 1943, 66:164–203.

95. Cameron ME, Greer CH: Congenital arterio-venous aneurysm of the retina. A postmortem report. *Br J Ophthalmol* 1968, 52:768–772.

96. Brodsky MC, Hoyt WF, Higashida RT, *et al.*: Bonnet-Dechaume-Blanc Syndrome with large facial angioma. *Arch Ophthalmol* 1987, 105:844–845.

97. Mansour AM, Wells CG, Jampol LM, Kalina RE: Ocular complications of arteriovenous communications of the retina. *Arch Ophthalmol* 1989, 107:232–236.

98. Brown GC, Donoso LA, Magargal LE, *et al.*: Congenital retinal macrovessels. *Arch Ophthalmol* 1982, 100:1430–1436.

99. Varma R, Goldberg RE, Spaeth GL: Applications of digital image analysis: the topography of an optic disc coloboma and alterations in the retinal vessels in an arteriovenous malformation. *Trans Pa Acad Ophthalmol Otolaryngol* 1987, 39:588–591.

100. Kinyoun JL, Chittum ME, Wells CG: Photocoagulation treatment of radiation retinopathy. *Am J Ophthalmol* 1988, 105:470–478.

101. Miller ML, Goldberg SH, Bullock JD: Radiation retinopathy after standard radiotherapy for thyroid-related ophthalmopathy [letter]. *Am J Ophthalmol* 1991, 112:600–601.

102. Hayreh SS: Post-radiation retinopathy. A fluorescence fundus angiographic study. *Br J Ophthalmol* 1970, 54:705–714.

103. Egbert PR, Fajardo LF, Donaldson SS, Moazed K: Posterior ocular abnormalities after irradiation for retinoblastoma: a histopathological study. *Br J Ophthalmol* 1980, 64:660–665.

104. Axer-Siegel R, Kremer I, Ben-Sira I, Weiss J: Radiation retinopathy treated with red krypton laser. *Ann Ophthalmol* 1989, 21:272–276.

105. Viebahn M, Barricks ME, Osterloh MD: Synergism between diabetic and radiation retinopathy: case report and review. *Br J Ophthalmol* 1991, 75:629–632.

106. Chee PH: Radiation retinopathy. *Am J Ophthalmol* 1968, 66:860–865.

107. Gass JDM: A fluorescein angiographic study of macular dysfunction secondary to retinal vascular disease. VI. X-ray irradiation, carotid artery occlusion, collagen vascular disease, and vitritis. *Arch Ophthalmol* 1968, 80:606–617.

108. Wara WM, Irvine AR, Neger RE, *et al.*: Radiation retinopathy. *Int J Radiat Oncol Biol Phys* 1979, 5:81–83.

109. Midena E, Segato T, Piermarrocchi S, *et al.*: Retinopathy following radiation therapy of paranasal sinus and nasopharyngeal carcinoma. *Retina* 1987, 7:142–147.

110. Amoaku WMK, Archer DB: Fluorescein angiographic features, natural course, and treatment of radiation retinopathy. *Eye* 1990, 4:657–667.

111. Chaudhuri PR, Austin DJ, Rosenthal AR: Treatment of radiation retinopathy. *Br J Ophthalmol* 1981, 65:623–625.

112. Amoaku WMK, Archer DB: Cephalic radiation and retinal vasculopathy. *Eye* 1990, 4:195–203.

113. Schulman J, Jampol LM, Goldberg MF: Large capillary aneurysms secondary to retinal venous obstruction. *Br J Ophthalmol* 1981, 65:36–41.

114. Cousins SW, Flynn HW, Clarkson JG: Macroaneurysms associated with retinal branch vein occlusion *Am J Ophthalmol* 1990, 109:567–570.

115. Katzen LE, Fleischman JA: YAG laser treatment of cystoid macular edema. *Am J Ophthalmol* 1983, 95:589–592.

116. Yannuzzi LA: A perspective on the treatment of aphakic cystoid macular edema. *Surv Ophthalmol* 1984, 28(suppl):540–543.

117. Steinert RF, Wasson PJ: Neodymium:YAG laser anterior vitreolysis for Irvine-Gass cystoid macular edema. *J Cataract Refract Surg* 1989, 15:304–307.

118. Weingeist TA: YAG laser treatment of cystoid macular edema [letter]. *Am J Ophthalmol* 1983, 96:407–409.

119. Jampol LM, Sanders DR, Kraff MC: Prophylaxis and therapy of aphakic cystoid macular edema. *Surv Ophthalmol* 1984, 28(Suppl):535–539.

120. Newsome DA, Blacharski PA: Grid photocoagulation for macular edema in patients with retinitis pigmentosa. *Am J Ophthalmol* 1987, 103:161–166.

121. Heckenlively JR: Grid photocoagulation for macular edema in patients with retinitis pigmentosa [letter]. *Am J Ophthalmol* 1987, 104:94.

CHAPTER **10**

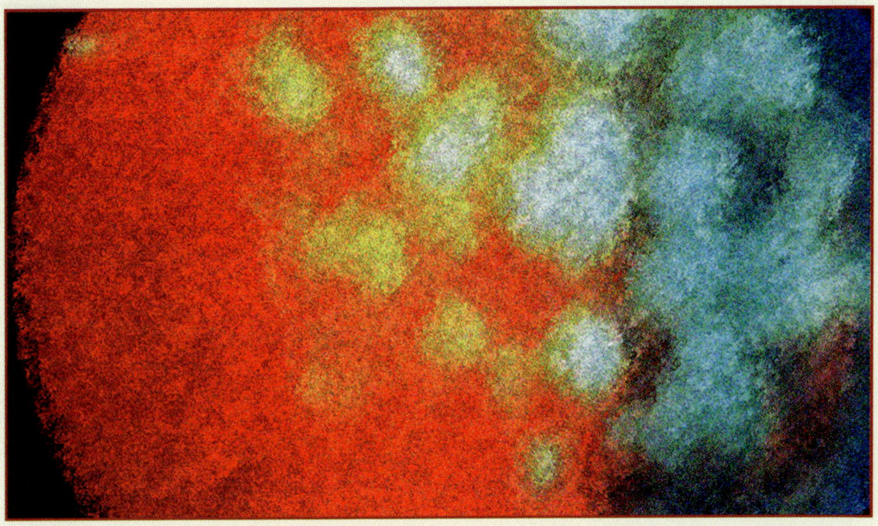

Photodynamic Therapy for Ocular Tumors and Neovascularization

JOAN W. MILLER
EVANGELOS S. GRAGOUDAS

Photodynamic therapy (PDT) combines the application of low-intensity, nonthermal light with a photosensitizing agent to produce effects on tissue. Early investigations in animal models and early pilot studies of human ocular tumors yielded mixed results with earlier-generation photosensitizers. More recently, PDT with newer photosensitizing agents has shown encouraging results in the treatment of tumors and neovascularization. These newer photosensitizing agents have increased absorption at longer wavelengths and produce less skin photosensitivity. The improved efficacy of PDT demonstrated in recent experimental and clinical studies suggests that PDT shows promise as a primary treatment modality for ocular neovascularization and tumors.

The foundation of modern PDT consists of a large body of observations and investigations into the nature of photodynamic reactions, research that has spanned most of this century [1,2]. The modern era of clinical PDT (then termed *photoradiation therapy*) began in the 1970s when reports of long-term cures after light radiation treatment of animal tumors 24 to 48 hours after intravenous hematoporphyrin administration were published [3,4]. Subsequently, numerous clinical studies have used PDT to treat malignancies at various sites, including the bladder, lung, head and neck, brain, blood, uterus, and gastrointestinal tract. Most reports concluded that superficial and minimally invasive disease responds best to PDT. The treatment of large tumors generally required higher light or photosensitizer doses to produce a complete response and were associated with an increased rate of complications. These earlier studies often lacked standardized inclusion criteria, treatment protocols and endpoints, definition of response rates, and lengths of follow-up, making interpretation of the results difficult. Improved photosensitizers, advances in photosensitizer delivery and light dosimetry, and the adoption of increasingly rigorous study designs should allow clinicians and regulatory agencies to evaluate the efficacy of PDT in comparison with other, more established forms of therapy.

MECHANISM OF ACTION

Photodynamic therapy requires the administration of a photosensitizing dye, usually intravenously, which localizes to the target tissues. Light irradiation of these tissues at an absorption maximum of the dye elevates the photosensitizer from its electronic ground state to a higher level (excited) triplet state. The excited photosensitizer quickly returns to the ground state, and, in the process, transfers energy to other molecules. When this energy is transferred to molecular oxygen (type II mechanism), singlet oxygen is formed, which then reacts with proteins, nucleic acids, and lipid membranes [5]. When the excited photosensitizer transfers energy to other compounds (type I mechanism), superoxide, hydroxyl, and other free radicals may be formed [6]. Cellular injury mediated by singlet oxygen in the type II mechanism is the predominant pathway of tissue injury secondary to PDT and requires adequate levels of oxygen in the target tissues. Photodynamic tissue effects are not dependent on increasing the temperature of the target tissues and thus differ from conventional thermal photocoagulation or dye-enhanced thermal photocoagulation.

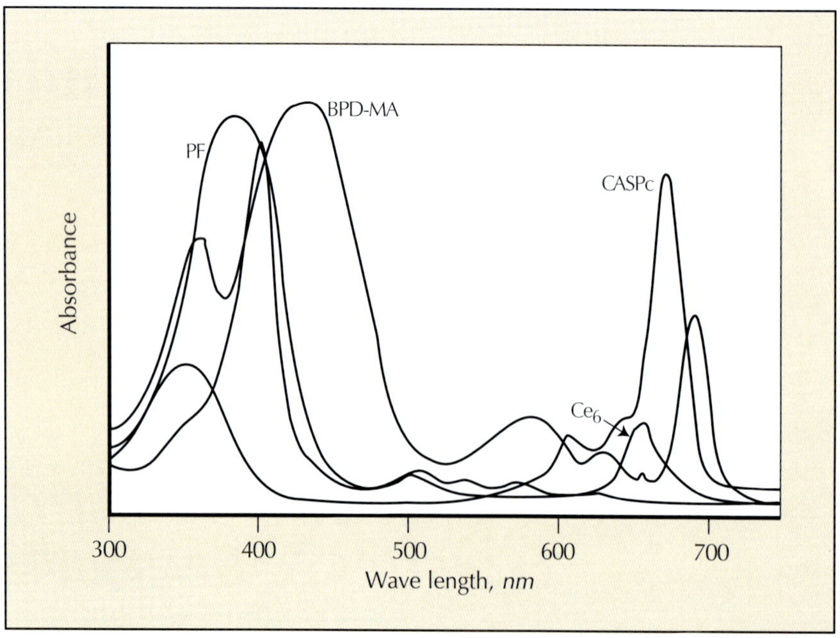

FIGURE 10-1. Absorption spectra of selected photosensitizers that have been used in photodynamic therapy. BPD-MA—benzoporphyrin derivative monoacid ring A; CASPc—chloroaluminum sulfonated phthalocyanine; Ce6—chlorin e6; PF—Photofrin. (*From* Liu and Anderson [1]; with permission.)

The multiple factors governing the effectiveness of a given photosensitizer depend in part on its photophysical and physicochemical properties. The absorption spectrum of the photosensitizer dictates the wavelengths of the radiation beam that may be suitable for PDT. Generally, the wavelength(s) selected coincide with an absorption maximum of the photosensitizer. The absorption spectrum of several photosensitizers that have been used in ophthalmology are superimposed in Figure 10-1. Other important considerations include the metabolism, pH, and route of administration of the photosensitizer. A key consideration in PDT is the ability of the photosensitizer to localize preferentially in target tissues, which damages the target tissue and minimizes collateral damage to surrounding tissues [7]. One strategy to increase selectivity is to use lipoproteins. When porphyrin photosensitizers are preincorporated into liposomes or precomplexed with lipoproteins, their delivery to neoplastic tissues is increased [8,9]. This increase may result from the fact that cells with high mitotic activity, such as tumor cells and neovascular endothelial cells, were found to have a high-expression low-density lipoprotein (LDL) receptor (such as the apo B/E receptor) [10], which might lead to more efficient uptake of LDL-bound molecules by receptor-mediated endocytosis [11]. Photosensitizers may be retained in tumors because of a larger interstitial space and poor lymphatic network [12]. Another strategy to increase selectivity is to bind the photosensitizer to an antibody directed at the target tissue [13].

The subcellular target may also vary among photosensitizers [14]. Some photosensitizers primarily damage the plasma membrane and mitochondria, whereas others cause nuclear or lysosomal damage. Despite evidence for direct damage to tumor cells under some circumstances, most data suggest that occlusion of tumor vasculature is an important mechanism leading to tumor cell death. PDT-induced damage to endothelial cells results in platelet adhesion and degranulation, leading to stasis and aggregation of blood cells and vascular occlusion. Tumor cell necrosis results from the subsequent tissue ischemia [15].

Many light sources can be used for PDT, including broad-band light from incandescent or arc lamps, or monochromatic light from tunable argon-pumped dye lasers or diode lasers. Broad light bands may enhance the photodynamic effect if they excite secondary absorption peaks of the photosensitizer. Slit lamp delivery of laser light allows for spatial confinement and is particularly suited to intraocular applications [16,17,18••]. PDT is typically performed with low irradiances such as 150 to 200 mW/cm^2, which limits any tissue-warming and thermal effects. However, these low irradiances are impractical for ophthalmic applications because they require long treatment times (*eg,* 16 minutes and 36 seconds for 150 J/cm^2), making it difficult for the user to maintain alignment of the treatment beam, using a contact lens and viewing the fundus with slit lamp biomicroscopy under dim illumination. Research in our laboratory indicated that irradiances up to 1800 mW/cm^2 did not produce significant thermal effect as evidenced by collagen denaturation [19]. Ocular applications using 600 mW/cm^2 have been adopted in preclinical and clinical studies [20,21,22•]. The mild hyperthermia that may be produced with higher irradiances may act synergistically with PDT to potentiate cell killing [23].

TABLE 10-1 THERAPEUTIC PHOTOSENSITIZERS USED FOR TREATMENT OF OCULAR TUMORS AND NEOVASCULARIZATION

- Xanthene derivatives
  - Rose bengal
- Tetrapyrrole derivatives
  - Hematoporphyrin derivative
  - Photofrin (porfimer sodium/dihematoporphyrin ether)
  - Benzoporphyrin derivative
  - Tin etiopurpurin
- Chlorins and bacteriochlorins
  - Chlorin e6
  - Bacteriochlorin a
- Phthalocyanines
  - Chloroaluminum sulfonated phthalocyanine

PHOTOSENSITIZERS IN OPHTHALMOLOGY

Several major classes of photosensitizers have been used in vitro and in vivo in animal models for the study of mechanisms of photodynamic injury and to develop an optimal agent for PDT for human malignancies (Table 10-1). Among these agents, the tetrapyrroles, phthalocyanines, benzophenoxazines, and xanthenes have been used for ocular applications. Porphyrin derivatives such as hematoporphyrin derivative (HPD) and porfimer sodium (Photofrin) are the most widely studied photodynamic agents. HPD is a complex mixture of porphyrins that is synthesized from hematoporphyrin [24]. PDT with HPD is generally performed with a 630-nm wavelength light to increase tissue penetration and decrease absorption by other tissue chromophores. Drawbacks of this agent are its small absorption peak at longer wavelengths (Fig. 10-1) and the prolonged skin photosensitivity lasting 1 month or more after therapy. Porfimer sodium is a partially purified component of HPD that is more potent and produces reduced skin toxicity than does HPD [25]. Porfimer sodium has been approved for human use in Canada for the treatment of superficial bladder cancer. In Japan, early cancers of the lung, esophagus, stomach, and cervix have been treated [26]. Phase III clinical trials in North America and Europe have shown some beneficial effect for the palliative treatment of lung and esophageal cancers and for prophylactic treatment for papillary bladder cancer [27].

The chlorins, bacteriochlorins, and benzoporphyrin derivatives are newer porphyrin derivatives with favorable properties and have recently been used for PDT (Table 10-1). Chlorin derivatives such as monoaspartyl chlorin e6 are effective photosensitizers in animal tumor models [28]. Bacteriochlorin a is a chlorin derivative that has an absorption maximum at 760 nm and a higher molar absorption coefficient compared with HPD [29]. Benzoporphyrin derivative (BPD) is another modified porphyrin that has an absorption maximum of about 690 nm and is phototoxic in vivo. BPD is rapidly inactivated or cleared from the body with no significant phototoxicity after 24 hours [30]. It has been used to treat ocular neovascularization and tumors, and its safety and efficacy after intravenous administration are currently being evaluated in human clinical trials of macular degeneration and other diseases [22•,27]. Tin ethyl etiopurpurin ($SNET_2$), which absorbs at 637 nm, has been used to treat experimental choroidal neovascularization and is in early clinical trials [31]. Compared with HPD, these newer-generation photosensitizers share important characteristics, such as higher absorption peaks at longer wavelengths and diminished phototoxicity.

Phthalocyanines are another class of photosensitizers with a strong absorption band at 675 nm [32,33]. Central metals, such as zinc and aluminum, are incorporated into their structure to increase the triplet state and singlet oxygen yields. Their solubility and cellular localization are at least partially determined by the number and charge of their side chains. The phthalocyanines are cleared more rapidly and produce substantially less skin toxicity than do HPD, Photofrin, or dihematoporphyrin ether (DHE) [33]. Phthalocyanines have been investigated in experimental models of ocular neovascularization and ocular tumors, but their safety for use in humans has not yet been determined [34–36]. Texaphyrins are pure, synthetic, water-soluble macrocycles that are formulated with central metallic ions. Lutetium texaphyrin absorbs at 732 nm and is stable, pure, and water soluble and shows rapid skin clearance and no skin photosensitization [37]. Its efficacy has been demonstrated in the treatment of experimental tumors and atheromatous plaque, and it has been studied in Phase I studies of patients with metastatic cancer [38,39•]. Xanthene derivatives also have photosensitizing properties [40,41]. Rose bengal is a halogenated fluorescein derivative with increased singlet oxygen yields and photosensitizing ability and has been used to produce photochemically mediated vascular damage of ocular vessels [42–44].

OCULAR TUMORS

Accumulating knowledge regarding the mechanism of photochemically mediated injury suggests that it may offer improved selectivity compared with conventional thermal photocoagulation for selected ocular disorders. The initial distribution of photoactive dyes in vascular structures after intravenous administration and the high transmission of the ocular media (cornea, lens, and vitreous) may allow destruction of vascular structures in the eye, with reduced collateral damage to adjacent tissues. The enhanced binding to new vessels (including those associated with neoplastic tissues) exhibited by porphyrin photosensitizers may increase this selectivity. To investigate this possibility, various experimental and human studies have been performed using PDT for the treatment of ocular tumors and neovascularization.

Iris and ciliary body melanoma

Clinical studies

Several case reports describe PDT for treatment of human iris and ciliary body melanoma. In 1984, Tse *et al.* [45] treated two ciliary body melanomas and one iris melanoma with HPD and transcorneal red light (xenon arc lamp or argon-pumped dye laser at 630 nm), with low irradiances (18 to 200 mW/cm^2) and high fluences (1400 J/cm^2 and 2566 J/cm^2). Necrosis of both tumors was incomplete as shown by histopathologic examination, but the tumor treated with the higher fluence showed an increased depth of necrosis. The iris melanoma received 1080 J/cm^2 and showed complete clinical response. One year later, few residual tumor cells at the peripheral iris were seen histopathologically. Sery *et al.* [46] treated a patient with diffuse multinodular iris melanoma with HPD given at 2.5 mg/kg and 632-nm red light from an argon-pumped dye laser delivered by a fiberoptic probe and found no response.

A combined photodynamic and photothermal approach for the treatment of iris melanoma has also been reported. Chambers *et al.* [47] treated a patient with iris melanoma with DHE, 2.5 mg/kg, and both 647-nm and 676-nm red light (76 J/cm^2, 31,850 mW/cm^2). The tumor was subsequently re-treated with 544-nm green light and similar treatment parameters, with noticeable surface whitening. Transient iritis developed and the tumor regressed from 1 to 6 months after treatment, with no evidence of recurrence after 13 months. In 1992, Davidorf and Davidorf [25] treated four patients with iris melanoma with either HPD or DHE. Their first patient was treated with HPD, 2.5 mg/kg, and 630-nm red light at 106J/cm^2 and developed severe refractory iritis requiring enucleation. Histopathologic evaluation of the eye revealed subtotal tumor necrosis. The other three patients were given DHE and were treated with a combination of krypton red and argon green laser light delivered through a slit lamp until whitening of the tumor surface appeared. All three patients had complete clinical regression of the tumor.

Some complications noted with PDT for human iris and ciliary body melanomas, such as iris neovascularization and neovascular glaucoma, are also seen with other treatment modalities [45,48]. Severe uveitis is associated with high fluences and photosensitizer doses and may be the result of sudden and extensive necrosis of neoplastic tissues [25,35]. This complication might theoretically be minimized by the treatment of large tumors in multiple sessions.

Experimental studies

These pilot human studies have been inconclusive regarding the efficacy of PDT and indicate the need for improved understanding of light dosimetry and other factors limiting photodynamic injury. Accordingly, investigators at our institution and others have pursued PDT research using experimental models. The simplest tumor model is the Greene hamster melanoma model in which Greene hamster melanoma cells are grown in culture and are injected into the anterior chamber of rabbits [49–54]. Tumor nodules rapidly proliferate, filling the anterior chamber, and, if untreated, eventually lead to ocular perforation. The photosensitizer is injected intravenously through an ear vein; the anterior segment tumors are treated with laser light at the absorption maximum of the photosensitizer using an optical fiber or slit lamp delivery. The optimal time interval from injection of the photosensitizer to light irradiation may depend on the photosensitizer chosen and is a current area of investigation. Immediately after light irradiation, no change may be discernible in the appearance of the tumor. Conversely, surface hemorrhages, vascular occlusion or narrowing, and surface edema and exudate may be noted. Anterior chamber inflammation and a slight increase in the size of the tumors (caused by edema) may be seen in the days following treatment. Anterior segment fluorescein angiography as early as 20 minutes after treatment shows profound hypofluorescence, indicating occlusion of surface tumor vessels [52].

Studies using the Greene hamster model and HPD or DHE have, in most cases, shown only partial tumor necrosis by histopathologic examination—results similar to those reported in humans [49]. Complete necrosis has been reported in small tumors of up to 4 mm in height with HPD, 2.5 mg/kg, and a fluence of 102 J/cm^2 or greater (irradiance: 71 mW/cm^2) [51,53]. When using this model, high doses of HPD (7.5 to 10 mg/kg) or energy levels of more than 180 J/cm^2 caused unacceptable ocular toxicity, including corneal and conjunctival edema and intraocular hemorrhage and inflammation [51]. Histopathologic study of eyes after experimental anterior chamber melanoma with HPD phototherapy suggests that occlusion of tumor vessels is the predominant mechanism responsible for tumor necrosis [54]. Direct PDT effects on tumors have also been reported [54].

In our laboratory, this anterior chamber model has been used to study the feasibility of PDT with newer generation photosensitizers such as chloroaluminum sulfonated phthalocyanine (CASPc) or benzoporphyrin-derivative monoacid ring A (BPD-MA) (Schmidt *et al.*, unpublished data) [35]. Panagopoulos *et al.* [35] performed PDT 24 hours after the intravenous administration of CASPc, 5 mg/kg, using 675-nm red light at nonthermal power densities (63 to 216 mW/cm^2) (Fig. 10-2). Tumors treated with light or dye alone showed continued growth. Four eyes treated with 3 to 10 J/cm^2 (10 to 48 mW/cm^2) after intravenous CASPc administration experienced tumor regrowth after initial growth arrest. Eyes that received 20 J/cm^2 or greater had permanent growth arrest, which was confirmed histopathologically. Those that received the highest light doses (57 to 60 J/cm^2) or very high doses of CASPc (16 to 30 mg/kg) showed permanent growth arrest but developed corneal edema, hyphema, and severe anterior segment inflammation.

Others used the same model to perform PDT using BPD-MA precomplexed with LDL (Schmidt *et al.*, unpublished data). This mode of delivery has been shown in animal models to increase dye accumulation in experimental tumors [9]. After irradiation with 692-nm red light using energies of 100 J/cm^2 (150 mW/cm^2), necrosis of anterior chamber tumors was seen histopathologically. PDT using newer photosensitizers such as CASPc and BPD appears to be effective in the treatment of Greene hamster melanoma tumors [35] (Schmidt *et al.*, unpublished data). However, the Greene hamster melanoma models have several limitations. Physical damage to adjacent structures such as the cornea and lens, which has been observed with this model, may be related in part to the abnormal location of these tumors as well as to the effects of PDT. Tumor cells that are not visible at the time of PDT remain untreated and continue to grow and thus preclude long-term follow-up of affected eyes. The Greene ham-

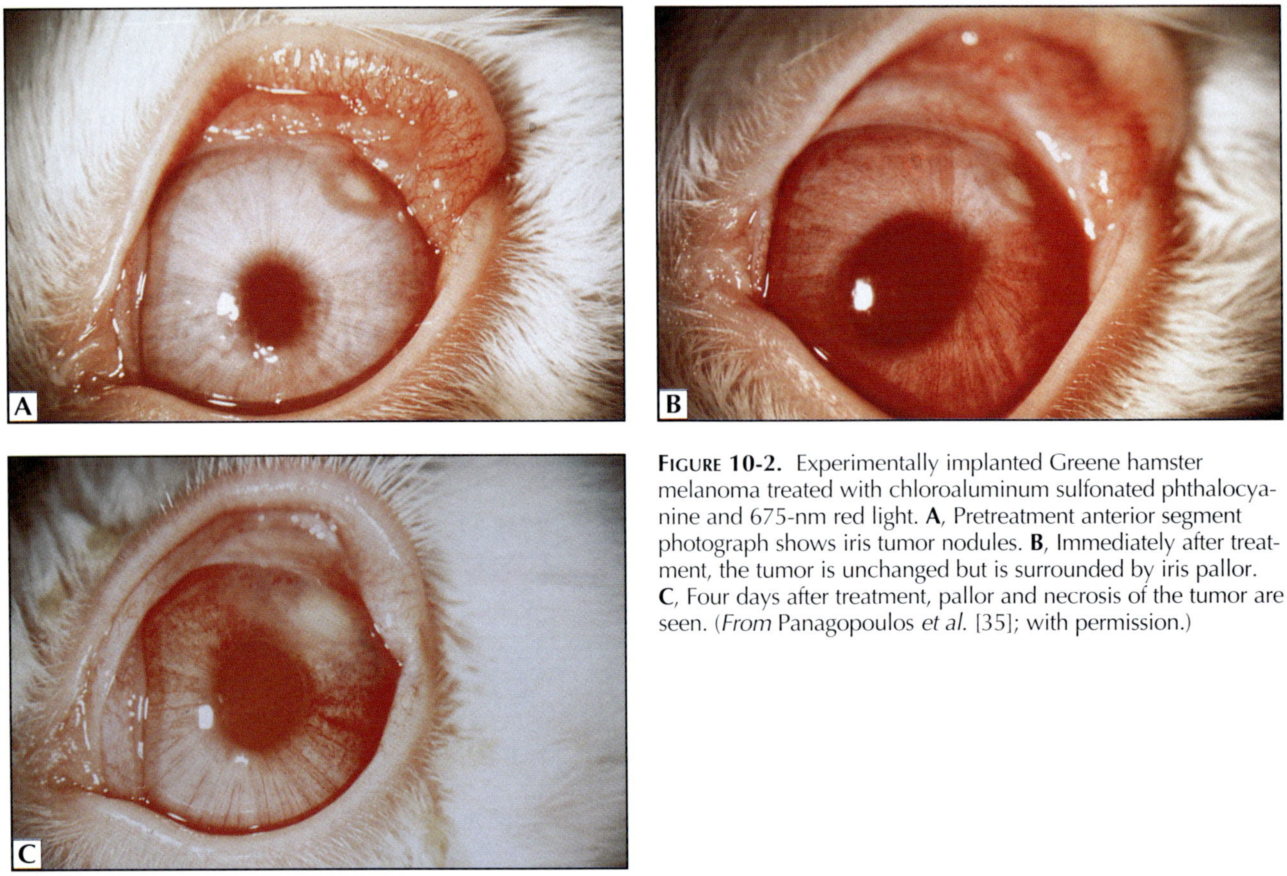

FIGURE 10-2. Experimentally implanted Greene hamster melanoma treated with chloroaluminum sulfonated phthalocyanine and 675-nm red light. **A**, Pretreatment anterior segment photograph shows iris tumor nodules. **B**, Immediately after treatment, the tumor is unchanged but is surrounded by iris pallor. **C**, Four days after treatment, pallor and necrosis of the tumor are seen. (*From* Panagopoulos *et al.* [35]; with permission.)

ster models have also been criticized as a melanoma model because their lack of pigmentation may make these tumors more susceptible to PDT-mediated injury. Newer models with pigmented melanoma cells may address this criticism.

Choroidal melanoma

Clinical studies

The treatment of choroidal melanoma with PDT has been described in a few clinical reports. Tse *et al.* [45] treated three patients with choroidal melanoma with HPD, 3 to 5 mg/kg, and transcorneal red light delivered through a xenon arc lamp or an argon-pumped dye laser (630 nm). Two patients treated with 64 or 850 J/cm^2 showed no histologic evidence of tumor necrosis. The third patient received a higher fluence (2160 J/cm^2) but tumor necrosis was limited to a depth of only 2 to 3 mm. Bruce [55,56] treated 24 patients with choroidal melanoma with HPD, 2.5 mg/kg, followed 72 hours later by transcorneal and transscleral exposure to 630-nm red light (200 to 6800 J/cm^2) from an argon pumped dye laser. Skin sensitivity, chemosis, iritis, and reduced visual acuity occurred in all 24 patients. Improvement in visual acuity occurred only in patients with tumors farther than 4 mm from the macula. Postoperative conjunctival chemosis and iritis were treated with topical steroids and cycloplegic drops, with resolution over 6 weeks. Less common complications were cataract, vitreitis, choroidal detachment, and exudative retinal detachment. Patients with small- and medium-sized tumors responded best, but no definitive statement was made regarding the number of patients cured [56]. An interim report by the same author had previously stated that complete regression was seen in eight of 11 patients with small tumors (<500 mm^3), whereas large tumors remained stable for 3 to 4 months, but all tumors regrew [55,56]. Histopathologic specimens from 10 eyes treated with PDT and subsequently enucleated for tumor recurrence or lack of initial response were reported to show extrascleral extension in three patients and viable and necrotic tumor, inflammation, and chorioretinal scarring in all 10 patients (Bruce RA, personal communication).

Murphree *et al.* [57] treated seven patients with choroidal melanoma using HPD, 2.5 mg/kg, and transcorneal and transscleral red light and reported only one complete response, in a patient with an amelanotic melanoma who was treated twice. More recently, Favilla *et al.* [58] treated 19 patients with choroidal melanoma using HPD, 5 to 7.5 mg/kg, and transpupillary (and transcleral in three patients) 620- to 630-nm red light (Fig. 10-3). All tumors were less than 10 mm in height and all but one were less than 7 mm in height. Complete response was recorded in six patients who had tumors of light or moderate pigmentation. No regression was seen in eight patients, five of whom had darkly pigmented tumors.

In general, these clinical studies indicate that small melanomas or those that are nonpigmented or lightly pigmented may respond favorably to PDT, whereas large melanomas are not responsive. Increased light absorption by chromophores, such as melanocytes or blood, may contribute to the incomplete eradication of large tumors [46]. Other possible factors include the choice of photosensitizer, low or nonhomogenous oxygen concentrations within the tumor, or inadequate distribution or quenching of the photosensitizer. The results of these studies indicate that PDT for choroidal melanomas has not yet been proved to be as effective as existing methods of treatment, such as charged-particle and plaque radiotherapy [59].

Experimental studies

Investigators in our laboratory and elsewhere have treated experimental choroidal melanoma with newer-generation photosensitizers [60–63,64•]. In these experiments, tumor cells such as the Greene hamster melanoma are injected into the suprachoroidal space, and growth is monitored by indirect ophthalmoscopy, fundus photography, and, in some cases, echography and color Doppler imaging [62]. Tumors are then treated with laser light delivered through the slit lamp. Schmidt-Erfurth *et al.* [60] treated experimental subchoroidal Greene hamster melanoma with BPD-MA, 2 mg/kg, precomplexed with lipoprotein and 692-nm red light. Complete necrosis of tumors was confirmed by histopathologic examination after treatment with 100 J/cm^2. Complications included transient vitreitis and a self-limited exudative retinal detachment in 50% of treated eyes, which largely resolved within 48 hours. As described previously, the Greene hamster melanoma model, whether in the anterior or posterior segment, may be easier to treat with PDT because of its lack of pigmentation.

To overcome the limitations of a nonpigmented melanoma model, Hu *et al.* [65] of our institution have established a pigmented choroidal melanoma model in the rabbit and have used it to evaluate the effect of PDT on the destruction of choroidal melanoma. Tumor-bearing rabbits were injected with CASPc, 5mg/kg, and 24 hours later tumors were irradiated with

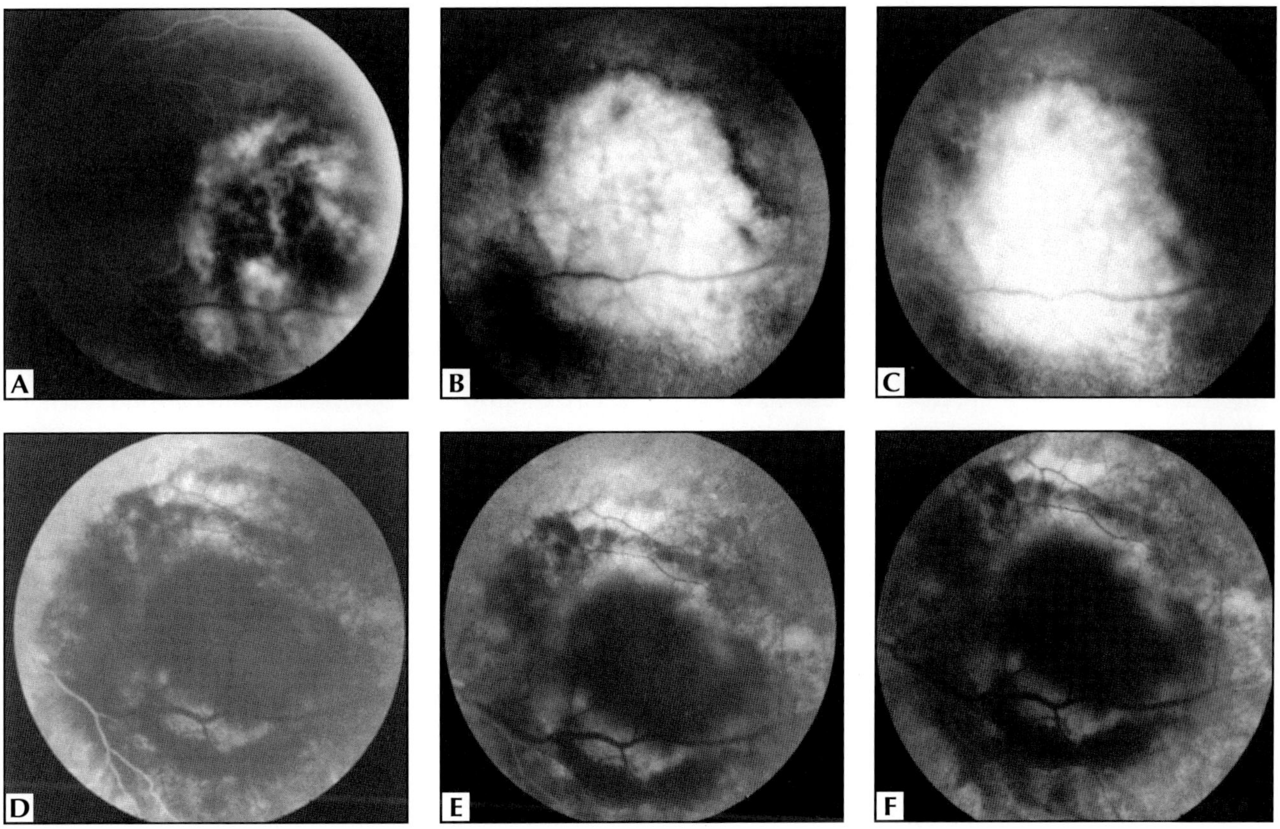

FIGURE 10-3. **A**, Early; **B**, Middle; **C**, Late frames of fluorescein angiography of choroidal melanoma. **D**, Early; **E**, Middle; **F**, Late frames after photodynamic therapy with hematoporphyrin derivative; decreased leakage of fluorescein from surface vessels is present. (*From* Favilla *et al.* [58]; with permission.)

675-nm red light from an argon-pumped dye laser. Complete tumor arrest was accomplished with light doses of 35 to 60 J/cm^2 [61••]. PDT using BPD was also effective in treating experimental pigmented choroidal melanoma [64•]. In 18 rabbit eyes treated with PDT using BPD, regression was seen in all tumors treated with 60 J/cm^2. Histologic examination showed acute vascular damage through the full thickness of the tumor (up to 4.6 mm) [66]. These experimental studies suggest that PDT with newer photosensitizing agents and modified treatment strategies holds promise for the treatment of human choroidal melanoma.

Retinoblastoma

Clinical studies

Few reports exist of patients with retinoblastoma who have been treated with PDT. Murphree *et al.* [57] treated six patients with recurrent retinoblastoma with HPD and subthermal threshold 630-nm red light. Despite initial regression, tumor growth resumed in all six patients. Ohnishi *et al.* [67] performed PDT with HPD, 2.5 and 5 mg/kg, and the argon laser (488 to 514.5 nm) in five children with retinoblastoma. Four of five eyes had had previous ionizing radiation treatment. In the case treated initially with PDT using HPD, 5 mg/kg (300 mW/cm^2, 270 J/cm^2), angionecrosis, thrombus formation, and tumor cell death were seen to a depth of about 6 mm. Choroidal hemorrhage developed in one patient during PDT; it was stopped by thermal photocoagulation. Tractional retinal detachment occurred in another child and was attributed to excessive ionizing radiation. Using an approach similar to that of Ohnishi, Murphree [68] successfully treated two patients with recurrent retinoblastoma with HPD followed by continuous-wave argon green laser photocoagulation. The lack of pigmentation in retinoblastoma should facilitate tissue penetration and increase the efficacy of PDT. However, this treatment approach is likely to be ineffective in eyes with vitreous seeding because the absence of tumor vasculature in these areas would preclude photosensitizer uptake [69]. It is difficult to draw any conclusions based on the limited treatment experience with this modality. In animal models, necrosis of experimental retinoblastoma-like tumors can be produced after PDT, but high photosensitizer doses may be associated with complications such as retinal edema, detachment, and choroidal hemorrhage [69–72]. Pending further reports, the treatment of human retinoblastoma with PDT remains investigational.

OCULAR NEOVASCULARIZATION

The rationale for using PDT to occlude pathologic neovascularization developed from observations first recognized in treating tumors. Porphyrin photosensitizing dyes preferentially localize to neovascular tissue in tumors and elsewhere, so that tumor damage from PDT occurs secondary to vascular occlusion. The mechanism of vascular thrombosis in the eye is similar to that previously described for ocular tumors, and its rate is also directly related to light intensity, photosensitizer doses, and oxygen concentration [42–44]. The potential for PDT to produce selective closure of ocular neovascularization with decreased collateral damage to other structures has been investigated in several experimental studies and is in clinical trial in macular degeneration.

Corneal neovascularization

PDT of experimental corneal neovascularization (induced by intrastromal injection of interleukin-2) was performed by Epstein *et al.* [73], using intravenous DHE and irradiation 72 hours later with light at 514 nm. Significant reduction in corneal neovascularization was observed, with side effects including blepharitis and iris injury. Pallikaris *et al.* [74] used phthalocyanine and 675-nm light to treat experimental corneal neovascularization induced by intrastromal silk sutures in rabbits. Neovascularization appeared thrombosed histologically in the first few days after PDT, although some larger vessels appeared patent by the 20th postoperative day. Some thrombosis of normal iris vessels was noted, although the iris appeared to have recovered by 1 month following PDT. We found no clinical reports of PDT for corneal neovascularization.

Iris neovascularization

Currently, PDT of iris neovascularization has been restricted to use in experimental models. Experimental iris neovascularization may be produced in primates by photothermal occlusion of major retinal veins [75]. Using this model, Packer *et al.* [76] treated iris neovascularization with HPD, 3 mg/kg, and 675-nm red light (200 mW/cm^2, 540 J/cm^2). Twenty-four hours after PDT, reduction in fluorescein staining was marked as seen on iris angiography, but a substantial inflammatory anterior chamber reaction was also manifest. Iris neovascularization later recurred in one eye, which was then re-treated. Using a similar model, Miller *et al.* [34] in this laboratory treated experimental iris neovascularization with intravenous CASPc, 0.5 to 1.0 mg/kg, and 675-nm red laser light (200 mW, 34 to 102 J/cm^2) and found thrombotic occlusion of iris neovascularization as early as 1 hour after treatment (Fig. 10-4). Leaky iris vessels reappeared by day 7 in one treated eye, without evidence for recanalization of PDT-treated vessels. Minimal anterior chamber reaction and a transient rise in intraocular pressure occurred after treatment. Experimental iris neovascularization has also been successfully treated in our laboratory with PDT using liposomal BPD and 689-nm light [77]. The treatment of clinical iris neovascularization with PDT may have a role as adjunctive therapy in combination with standard retinal ablation.

Choroidal neovascularization

Photodynamic therapy is a potentially selective treatment modality for choroidal neovascularization (CNV), in which it may occlude neovascularization and spare the overlying neurosensory retina. This offers the potential to avoid the sudden decrease in vision that is a complication of thermal photocoagulation of subfoveal choroidal neovascular membrane. Various groups have studied the efficacy of various photosensitizers for PDT of experimental CNV, and at least two photosensitizers are in clinical trial.

Experimental CNV can be induced in the monkey eye following high-intensity laser injury in the macula. CNV typically develop 2 to 4 weeks after the laser injury [78] and last 13 weeks on average, although the CNV does regress at variable rates [79,80]. Thomas and Langhofer [81] treated one eye of a cynomolgus monkey with experimental CNV with DHE, 8 mg/kg, and argon green laser light. A single 1.6-J/cm^2 burn (200 µm, 0.1 second, 100 mW) 12 hours after DHE led to histologic evidence of occlusion of the neovascular complex, but without attendant occlusion of the choriocapillaris. An identical lesion treated without DHE did not show occlusion of the neovascular membrane. The light parameters used in this study imply a thermal component to the damage, in that the irradiance was 318 W/cm^2. In another study using the same model, Miller and Miller [16] irradiated experimental CNV after the injection of rose bengal, 40 mg/kg, with 1.5 to 7.6 J/cm^2 (12.7 mW/cm^2) delivered from a slit lamp using a cut-off filter that transmitted light above 510 nm and another that absorbed all light above 750 nm. They identified an effective therapeutic window for PDT, with irradiation performed between 40 and 70 minutes after dye injection, which damaged the CNV without damage to retinal vessels. Although CNV damage occurred, it was incomplete. Using the same model, Kliman *et al.* [36] used intravenous CASPc, 0.5 mg/kg, followed 24 hours later by 675-nm red light (1 to 10 mW, 15 seconds to 2 minutes) to produce closure of CNV as seen on fluorescein angiography and histopathology. The selectivity of effect and the damage to retinal structures were not described.

Studies have been done with SNET$_2$ in experimental CNV [31]. Closure of experimental CNV was achieved with an intravenous dye dose of 1 mg/kg

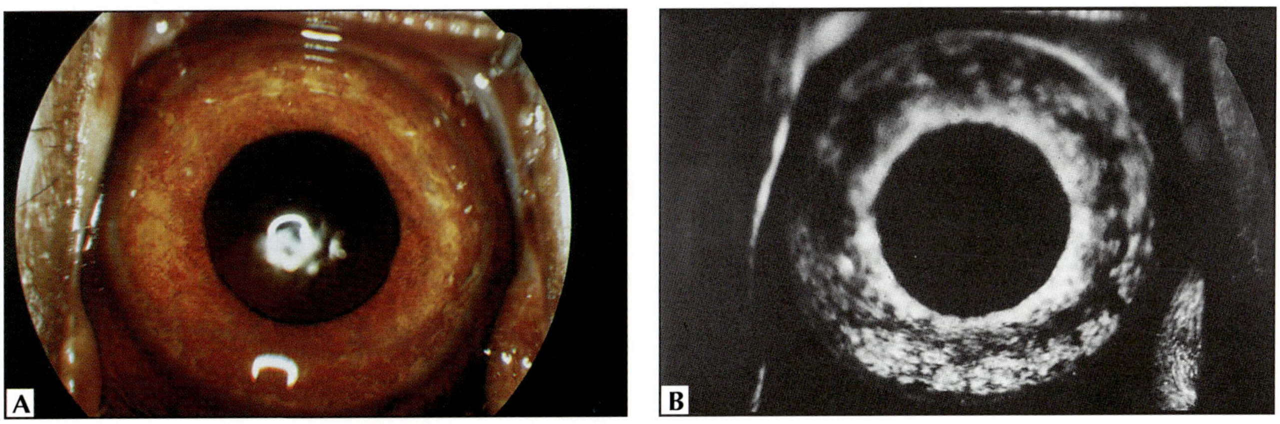

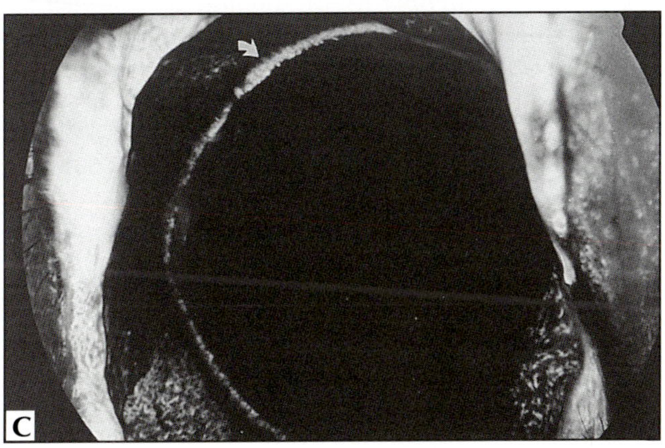

FIGURE 10-4. Photodynamic therapy for experimental iris neovascularization. **A**, Florid iris neovascularization is seen on iris photograph. **B**, New iris vessels leak on fluorescein angiogram. **C**, After treatment, marked hypoperfusion of iris vasculature is visualized on fluorescein angiography. (*From* Miller *et al.* [34]; with permission.)

using 665-nm red light with an irradiance of 600 mW/cm^2, fluence of 35 to 70 J/cm^2, and a spot size of 1200 μm, requiring light exposure between 60 and 120 seconds. Selectivity and the effects on normal retinal structures were not studied. Based on this preclinical work, a Phase I trial was initiated using PDT and $SNET_2$ to treat CNV. As of September 1997, 30 patients had been treated, with promising results (David Crean, personal communication, 1997).

Normal choroidal vasculature has been occluded using new photosensitizers, and it has been postulated that these dyes may prove useful in the treatment of CNV. Mori *et al.* [21] demonstrated occlusion of choroidal vessels in Japanese monkey eyes using 2 to 10 mg/kg of mono-l-aspartyl chlorin e6 (Npe6) and 664-nm light (0.4 to 7.5 J/cm^2). Obana *et al.* [82•] used ATX-S10, a new chlorin derivative, to occlude choriocapillaris and choroid in rabbits and rats using 2 to 12 mg/kg and 672-nm light at 3.5 J/cm^2.

In our laboratory, we have worked with a tetrapyrrol-derivative BPD-MA. This photosensitizer has a long absorption wavelength at 690 nm [30], allowing deeper tissue penetration and penetration through blood, fibrous tissue, and fluid—important components of CNV. When injected intravenously, BPD has a serum half-life of 30 minutes, and the highest tissue levels are reached in 3 hours, declining rapidly in the first 24 hours and reducing the risk of skin photosensitivity [83]. It was first used in clinical trials in patients with malignant skin tumors [84].

Initial studies of experimental CNV used a lipoprotein-associated preparation of BPD at doses of 1 to 2 mg/kg and 692-nm light, with a 1250-μm spot size. Closure of CNV was seen when irradiation was performed 1 to 80 minutes after dye injection, with a fluence of 50 to 150 J/cm^2 and irradiance of 150 to 600 mW/cm^2 [17]. No thermal damage, as assessed by electron microscopic examination of collagen fibrils, was seen at irradiances as high as 1800 mW/cm^2 [19]. By using higher irradiances, one could perform the irradiation much more quickly (166 seconds versus 666 seconds for 100 J/cm^2), making treatment of CNV much more practical.

Dosimetry of PDT for CNV was refined using the liposomal preparation of BPD, with fundus photography, fluorescein angiography, and light and electron microscopic examination [18]. The liposomal preparation provided a solubilized formulation of BPD for reliable administration that could be used clinically. BPD fundus angiography, using a fundus camera and digital imaging system with filters altered to optimize detection of BPD fluorescence, demonstrated accumulation of liposomal BPD in experimental CNV [85]. Dye doses of 0.25 to 1.0 mg/kg of liposomal BPD were studied, and a minimal dose of 0.375 mg/kg caused effective and reproducible closure of CNV using a 1250-μm spot size of 692-nm light with an irradiance of 600 mW/cm^2 and a fluence of 150 J/cm^2 [18]. Irradiation was performed 5 to 120 minutes after dye injection, but irradiation at 5 minutes after dye injection caused occlusion of choroidal vessels in the normal eye, whereas irradiation after 50 minutes caused occlusion in only 41% of the CNV.

Because the CNV in this model arose from a laser injury, it was difficult to assess the selectivity of PDT effect. Therefore, experiments were carried out in normal retina and choroid to determine the effects on normal retina and choroid using the same PDT parameters. A grading scheme for assessing the damage to retina and choroid was devised. Damage to the retinal pigment epithelium (RPE) and choriocapillaris was seen in all irradiated eyes. The grading scheme was based on the damage to the neurosensory retina, retinal vessels, and medium to large choroidal vessels. Grade I damage described occasional pyknosis in the outer nuclear layer (ONL), grade II described less than 20% pyknosis in ONL, grade III described less than 50% pyknosis in the ONL, grade IV described more than 50% pyknosis in the ONL, and grade V described more than 50% pyknosis in the ONL and damage to large choroidal vessels, alone or also to retinal vessels. Some damage to the photoreceptors was seen in all grades, typically mild vacuolization and disorientation of the inner and outer segments of the photoreceptors. PDT with 1 mg/kg liposomal BPD led to grade V damage to the retina and choroid. When PDT was performed with liposomal BPD doses of 0.25, 0.375, or 0.5 mg/kg at 20 to 50 minutes after dye injection, the retinal structure was well preserved. The optimal dosimetry, based on the effects on experimental CNV and normal retina and choroid, was thought to be a dye dose of 0.375 mg/kg (approximately 6 mg/m^2), 600 mW/cm^2, 150 J/cm^2 with irradiation performed 20 to 50 minutes after the bolus intravenous dye injection.

Dosimetry experiments in the monkey model of experimental CNV were done using a bolus intravenous injection of liposomal BPD and showed no toxicity. Liposomal drugs, however, are typically administered as an intravenous infusion, and it was believed that clinical application of this therapy should not use a bolus injection. Further studies were undertaken to evaluate efficacy of PDT using BPD administered as an intravenous infusion [20]. Slow infusion of BPD (over 45 minutes) showed effective closure of experimental CNV when PDT was performed within 30 to 45 minutes of the start of dye infusion, similar to the bolus injection but providing a smaller time window for selective treatment. A faster infusion (10 minutes) was tested and showed effective closure when irradiation was performed 20 to 30 minutes from the start of infusion using a spot size of 1250 to 3000 μm of 689-nm light, at 600 mW/cm^2 and 150 J/cm^2. Closure of CNV was demonstrated angiographically (Fig. 10-5), and light microscopy demonstrated occluded vessels in the area of CNV, closure of the associated choriocapillaris, and sparing of the overlying retina. Using the same PDT parameters, treatment of normal retina and choroid produced a grade II lesion.

Studies were performed to examine longer-term effects of PDT using BPD on the treated CNV, normal retina, and choroid [86]. Persistent closure (as long as 4 weeks) of CNV was observed in eyes that had been treated with the optimal parameters. Histopathology demonstrated a fibrous scar covered by proliferating RPE, with few open capillaries. In normal eyes treated with PDT, the choriocapillaris had reperfused by 4 weeks and the RPE appeared to be repopulated with variable pigmentation. Pigmented macrophages were noted overlying the RPE, along with mild disorganization of the photoreceptor outer segments. It appeared that the noted damage to the RPE and choriocapillaris had recovered after 4 to 7 weeks.

Because early clinical studies suggested that PDT might need to be repeated, studies were undertaken to assess recovery of multiple PDT treatments of normal eyes [87•]. Three sequential PDT treatments were performed in the same area of normal retina and choroid. Three doses of liposomal BPD were used (6, 12, and 18 mg/m^2), with the light doses kept constant (689 nm, 600 mW/cm^2, 100 J/cm^2). Treatments were separated by 2 weeks, and histopathologic examination was performed at 2 and 6 weeks after the third treatment. Minimal damage was seen in the group treated at 6 mg/m^2, with recovery comparable to the single treatment at 0.375 mg/kg (approximately 6 mg/m^2). Higher dye doses, however, led to significant cumulative damage to the normal retina, choroid, and optic nerve.

Based on these preclinical studies, a Phase I/II trial was initiated in March 1995 to study PDT of CNV using liposomal BPD [22]. The trial, designed primarily as a safety trial, was sponsored by QLT Phototherapeutics (Vancouver, British Columbia) and CIBAVision Ophthalmics (Bulach, Switzerland). Patients with subfoveal CNV secondary to age-related macular degeneration and other etiologies were enrolled and treated after

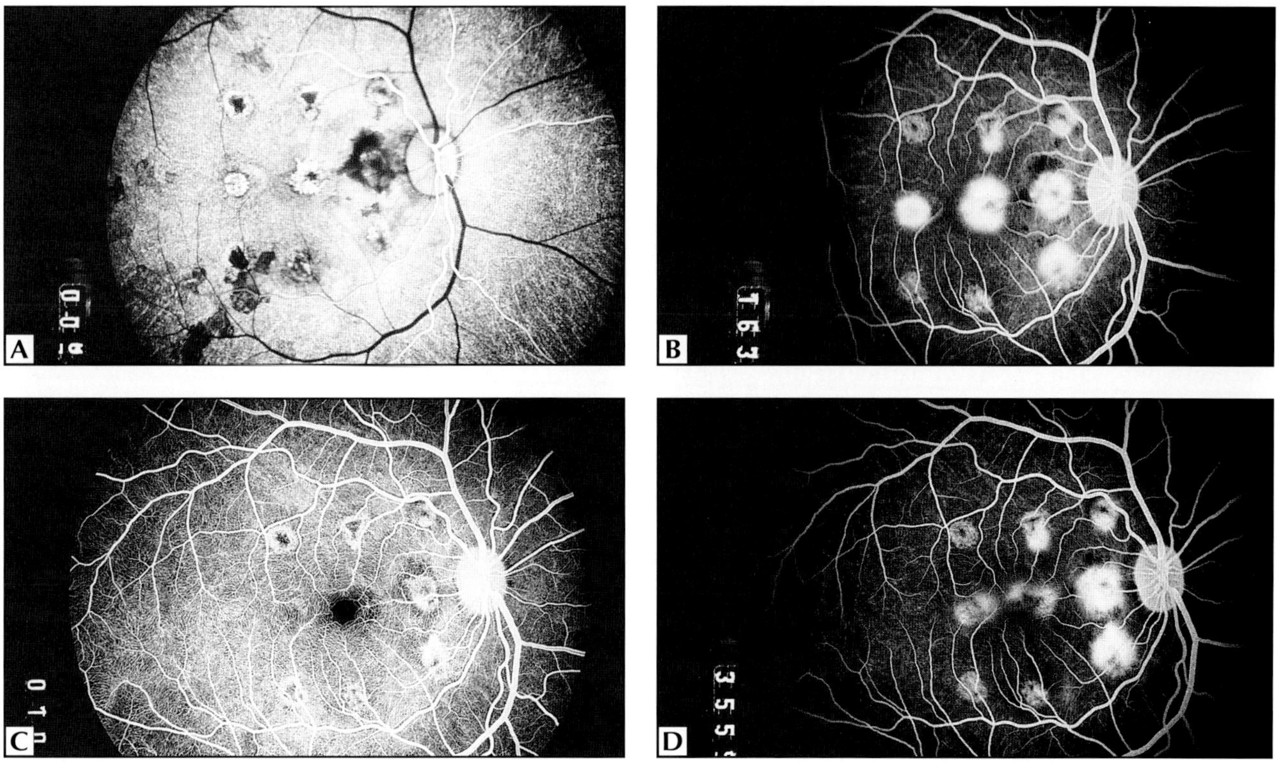

FIGURE 10-5. Photodynamic therapy (PDT) of experimental choroidal neovascularization (CNV) using liposomal benzoporphyrin derivative (BPD). **A**, Early-phase fluorescein angiogram of CNV prior to PDT showing typical lacy pattern of hyperfluorescence in areas of CNV; **B**, Leakage is evident in the late-phase angiogram. **C**, Twenty-four hours after PDT to the lesion in the central macula, a second lesion, temporal the first, shows perfusion of retinal vessels in the early-phase angiogram with no perfusion of the CNV. **D**, The late-phase angiogram, shows some staining at the edges of the PDT-treated areas. The CNV not treated with PDT, in the nasal and inferonasal macula, continue to leak fluorescein. (*From* Husain *et al.* [20]; with permission.)

informed consent. The treating centers were the Massachusetts Eye and Ear Infirmary in Boston, University Eye Hospital in Lubeck, Jules Gonin Hospital in Lausanne, and University Hospital in Geneva; the angiograms were interpreted by the Wilmer Reading Center in Baltimore. In total, 61 patients were enrolled in dose-escalating regimens, using a dye dose of 6 or 12 mg/m^2 of liposomal BPD and a light dose of 50 to 150 J/cm^2 administered 20 or 30 minutes after the start of dye infusion. Patients were observed in follow-up for 12 weeks with refracted visual acuity using Bailey-Lovey charts, ophthalmic examinations, and standardized fluorescein angiography.

Most cases showed absence of leakage from CNV in the early phase of the angiogram at 1 week's follow-up, which is consistent with occlusion of the CNV. By 4 weeks' follow-up, most patients showed leakage from a part of the original area of classic CNV. At 12 weeks' follow-up, recurrences or extension of CNV beyond the original border were seen in some cases. Adverse ocular events, including retinal vessel closure, were seen at the highest light dose and defined the acceptable upper limit of the light dose. Vision was stable in most cases during the 3 months of follow-up. No significant difference was noted between regimens. Multiple treatments were also assessed and did not show any improvement in the persistence of CNV closure, although multiple treatments were tolerated without any short-term loss of vision resulting from treatment.

A Phase III randomized, double-masked, placebo-controlled trial was initiated in December 1996 for patients with subfoveal CNV, either new or recurrent, with a classic component defined as fluorescein angiography, resulting from age-related macular degeneration. By October 1997, 609 patients had been enrolled by the 22 participating centers in North America and Europe. Patients are assessed at 3-month intervals with refracted visual acuity, ophthalmic examination, and standardized fluorescein angiography; they are re-treated if leakage is demonstrated angiographically. The study is designed to determine whether PDT using BPD can reduce the risk of visual loss from subfoveal CNV in age-related macular degeneration.

Conclusions

Photodynamic therapy has been used to treat ocular tumors and neovascularization in both clinical and experimental settings. Clinical investigations in the 1970s using these techniques showed mixed or disappointing results. Renewed interest in this form of therapy is related to the development of newer-generation photosensitizers and increasing scientific knowledge regarding basic mechanisms governing successful PDT. These newer photosensitizers show increased efficacy and markedly diminished cutaneous photosensitivity and are currently under investigation in the preclinical and clinical arenas. Further refinements in the tissue localization of photosensitizers and treatment protocols for PDT suggest that this therapeutic modality may one day become a standard form of therapy for many ocular disorders, including intraocular tumors and neovascularization.

References and Recommended Reading

Recently published papers of particular interest have been highlighted as:
- • Of interest
- •• Of outstanding interest

1. Liu H, Anderson R: Photodynamic therapy in dermatology: recent developments. *Dermatol Clin* 1993, 11:1–13.
2. Daniell M, Hill J: A history of photodynamic therapy. *Aust N Z J Surg* 1991, 61:340–348.
3. Diamond I, McDonagh A, Wilson C, *et al.*: Photodynamic therapy of malignant tumors. *Lancet* 1972, 2:1175–1177.
4. Dougherty T, Grindley G, Fiel R, *et al.*: Photoradiation therapy II: cure of animal tumors with hematoporphyrin derivative and light. *JNCI* 1975, 55:115–121.
5. Weishaupt K, Gomer C, Dougherty T: Identification of singlet oxygen as the cytotoxic agent in photo-inactivation of murine tumor. *Cancer Res* 1976, 36:2326–2329.
6. Buettner G, Oberly L: The apparent production of superoxide and hydroxyl radicals by hematoporphyrin and light as seen by spin-trapping. *FEBS Lett* 1980, 121:161–164.
7. Figge F, Weiland G, Manganiello L, *et al.*: Cancer detection and therapy: affinity of neoplastic, embryonic and traumatized tissues for porphyrins and metalloporphyrins. *J Proc Soc Exp Biol Med* 1948, 68:640–641.
8. Jori G, Tomio L, Reddi E, *et al.*: Preferential delivery of liposome-incorporated porphyrin to neoplastic cells in tumour-bearing rats. *Br J Cancer* 1983, 48:307–309.
9. Allison BA, Waterfield E, Richter AM, *et al.*: The effects of plasma lipoproteins on in vitro tumor cell killing and in vivo tumor photosensitization with benzoporphyrin derivative. *Photochem Photobiol* 1991, 54:709–715.
10. Jori G: Low density lipoprotein-liposome delivery system for tumor photosensitizers in vivo. In *Photodynamic Therapy, Basic Principles and Clinical Applications*. Edited by Henderson B, Dougherty T. New York: Dekker; 1992:173–186.

11. Kessel D: Porphyrin-lipoprotein association as a factor in porphyrin localization. *Can Let* 1986, 33:183–188.

12. Henderson B, Dougherty T: How does photodynamic therapy work? *Photochem Photobiol* 1992, 55:931–948.

13. Jiang F, Allison B, Liu D, *et al.*: Enhanced photodynamic killing of target cells by either monoclonal antibody or low density lipoprotein mediated delivery systems. *J Controlled Release* 1992, 19:41–58.

14. Nelson J, Liaw L-H, Orenstein A, *et al.*: Mechanism of tumor destruction following photodynamic therapy with hematoporphyrin derivative, chlorin, and phthalocyanine. *JNCI J* 1988, 80:1599–1605.

15. Castellani A, Pace G, Concioli M: Photodynamic effect of hematoporphyrin on blood microcirculation. *J Pathol Bacteriol* 1963, 86:99–102.

16. Miller H, Miller B: Photodynamic therapy of subretinal neovascularization in the monkey eye. *Arch Ophthalmol* 1993, 111:855–860.

17. Miller JW, Walsh AW, Kramer M, *et al.*: Photodynamic therapy of experimental choroidal neovascularization using lipoprotein-delivered benzoporphyrin. *Arch Ophthalmol* 1995, 113:810–818.

18.•• Kramer M, Miller J, Michaud N, *et al.*: Liposomal BPD verteporfin photodynamic therapy: selective treatment of choroidal neovascularization in monkeys. *Ophthalmology* 1996, 103:427–438.

Study in which dosimetry was established for the treatment of experimental CNV with PDT using liposomal BPD.

19. Moulton RS, Walsh AW, Miller JW, *et al.*: Response of retinal and choroidal vessels to photodynamic therapy using benzoporphyrin derivative monoacid [abstract]. *Invest Ophthalmol Vis Sci* 1993, 34:1169.

20. Husain D, Miller J, Michaud N, *et al.*: Intravenous infusion using liposomal benzoporphyrin derivative verteporfin for photodynamic therapy of experimental choroidal neovascularization. *Arch Ophthalmol* 1996, 114:978–985.

21.• Mori K, Ohta M, Katagiri T: Photodynamic therapy (PDT) with a combination of a new photosensitizer: NPe6 and a diode laser emitting at 664 nm. *Invest Ophthalmol Vis Sci* 1996, 37:S3177.

Photodynamic therapy of experimental CNV using a new photosensitizer, Npe6.

22.• Gragoudas E, Schmidt-Erfurth U, Sickenberg M, *et al.*: Results and preliminary dosimetry of photodynamic therapy for choroidal neovascularization in age-related macular degeneration in a Phase I/II trial. *Invest Ophthalmol Vis Sci* 1997, 38:S17.

Preliminary results of the first Phase I and II trial of verteporfin BPD-MA in PDT for CNV.

23. Waldow S, Dougherty T: Interaction of hyperthermia and photoradiation therapy. *Radiat Res* 1984, 97:380–385.

24. Bonnet R, Ridge R, Scourides P, *et al.*: On the nature of hematoporphyrin derivative. *J Chem Soc Perkins Trans* 1981, 1:3135–3140.

25. Davidorf J, Davidorf F: Treatment of iris melanoma with photodynamic therapy. *Ophthalm Surg* 1992, 23:522–527.

26. Kato H, Horai T, Furuse K, *et al.*: Photodynamic therapy of cancers: a clinical trial of porfimer sodium in Japan. *Jpn J Cancer Res* 1993, 84:1209–1214.

27. Levy J: Photosensitizers in photodynamic therapy. *Semin Oncol* 1994, 21(Suppl 15):4–10.

28. Nelson J, Roberts W, Berns MW: In vivo studies on the utilization of mono-l-aspartyl chlorin (NPe6) for photodynamic therapy. *Cancer Res* 1987, 47:4681–4685.

29. Schuitmaker J, van Best J, van Delft J, *et al.*: Bacteriochlorin a, a new photosensitizer in photodynamic therapy. *Invest Ophthalmol Vis Sci* 1990, 31:1444–1450.

30. Richter AM, Waterfield E, Jain AK, *et al.*: Photosensitising potency of structural analogues of benzoporphyrin derivative (BPD) in a mouse tumour model. *Br J Cancer* 1991, 63:87–93.

31.• Baumal C, Puliafito C, Pieroth L, *et al.*: Photodynamic therapy (PDT) of experimental choroidal neovascularization with tin ethyl etiopurpurin. *Invest Ophthalmol Vis Sci* 1996, 37:S122.

Photodynamic therapy of experimental CNV using a second-generation photosensitizer, tin ethyl etiopurpurin. This photosensitizer is now in clinical trial for CNV.

32. Kreimer-Birnbaum M: Modified porphyrins, chlorins, phthalocyanines, and purpurins: second-generation photosensitizers for photodynamic therapy. *Semin Hematol* 1989, 26:157–173.

33. Morgan A, Skalkos D: Second generation sensitizers: where are we and where should we be going? In *Proceedings of Society of Photo-optical Instrumentation Engineers* 1990, 6:87–106.

34. Miller JW, Stinson WG, Gregory WA, *et al.*: Phthalocyanine photodynamic therapy of experimental iris neovascularization. *Ophthalmology* 1991, 98:1711–1719.

35. Panagopoulos JA, Svitra PP, Puliafito CA, *et al.*: Photodynamic therapy for experimental intraocular melanoma using chloraluminum sulfonated phthalocyanine. *Arch Ophthalmol* 1989, 107:886–890.

36. Kliman CH, Stern D, Gregory WA, *et al.*: Angiography and photodynamic therapy of experimental choroidal neovascularization using phthalocyanine dye [abstract]. *Invest Ophthalmol Vis Sci* 1989, 30:371.

37. Young S, Woodburn K, Wright M, *et al.*: Lutetium texaphyrin (PCI-0123): a near-infrared, water-soluble photosensitizer. *Photochem Photobiol* 1996, 63:892–897.

38. Woodburn K, Fan Q, Kessel D, *et al.*: Phototherapy of cancer and atheromatous plaque with texaphyrins. *J Clin Laser Med Surg* 1996, 14:343–348.

39.• Woodburn K, Fan Q, Miles D, *et al.*: Localization and efficacy analysis of the phototherapeutic lutetium texaphyrin (PCI-0123) in the murine EMT6 sarcoma model. *Photochem Photobiol* 1997, 65:410–415.

Description of a new photosensitizer, lutetium texaphyrin, which has potential application in treatment of ocular neovascularization.

40. Yoshikawa K, Kurata H, Iwahara S, *et al.*: Photodynamic action of fluorescein dyes in DNA-damage and in vitro inactivation of transforming DNA in bacteria. *Mutation Res* 1978, 56:359–362.

41. Gandin E, Lion Y, Van De Vorst A, *et al.*: Quantum yield of singlet oxygen production by xanthene derivatives. *Photochem Photobiol* 1983, 37:271–278.

42. Wilson C, Hatchell D: Photodynamic retinal vascular thrombosis. *Invest Ophthalmol Vis Sci* 1991, 32: 2357–2365.

43. Royster A, Nanda S, Hatchell D, *et al.*: Photochemical initiation of thrombosis. *Arch Ophthalmol* 1988, 106:1608–1614.

44. Nanda S, Hatchell D, Tiedeman J, *et al.*: A new method of vascular occlusion. *Arch Ophthalmol* 1987, 105:1121–1124.

45. Tse D, Dutton J, Weingeist T, *et al.*: Hematoporphyrin photoradiation therapy for intraocular and orbital malignant melanoma. *Arch Ophthalmol* 1984, 102:833–838.

46. Sery T, Shields J, Augsburger J, *et al.*: Photodynamic therapy of human ocular cancer. *Ophthalmic Surg* 1987, 18:413–418.

47. Chambers R, Arnson D, Davidorf F, *et al.*: Treatment of iris melanoma with dihematoporphyrin ether and an ophthalmic laser delivery system. *Contemp Ophthalm Forum* 1986, 4:70–84.

48. Lewis R, Tse D, Phelphs C, *et al.*: Neovascular glaucoma after photoradiation therapy for uveal melanoma. *Arch Ophthalmol* 1984, 102:839–842.

49. Liu H, Chuo N: Hematoporphyrin phototherapy for experimental intraocular malignant melanoma. *Arch Ophthalmol* 1983, 101:901–903.

50. Gomer C, Jester J, Razum N, *et al.*: Photodynamic therapy of intraocular tumors, examination of hematoporphyrin derivative distribution and long-term damage in rabbit ocular tissue. *Cancer Res* 1985, 45:3718–3725.

51. Sery T, Dougherty T: Photoradiation of rabbit ocular malignant melanoma sensitized with hematoporphyrin derivative. *Curr Eye Res* 1984, 3:519–528.

52. Franken K, van Delft J, Dubelman T, *et al.*: Hematoporphyrin derivative photoradiation treatment of experimental malignant melanoma in the anterior chamber of the rabbit. *Curr Eye Res* 1985, 4:641–654.

53. Gomer C, Murphree A, Doiron D, *et al.*: Preclinical evaluation of ocular photoradiation therapy. In *Proceedings of the International Symposium on Porphyrins in Tumor Phototherapy*. Edited by Andreoni A, Cubeddu R. New York: Plenum Press; 1984.

54. Franken N, Vrensen G, van Delft J, *et al.*: Early morphological changes induced by photodynamic therapy in amelanotic Greene melanoma implanted in the anterior eye chamber of rabbits. *Lasers Surg Med* 1988, 3:27–34.

55. Bruce RJ: Evaluation of hematoporphyrin photoradiation therapy to treat choroidal melanoma. *Lasers Surg Med* 1984, 4:59–64.

56. Bruce RJ: Photoradiation therapy for choroidal malignant melanoma. In *A Clinical Manual: Photodynamic Therapy of Malignancies*. Edited by McCaughan JJ. Austin, TX: RG Landes; 1993.

57. Murphree A, Cote M, Gomer C: The evolution of photodynamic therapy techniques in the treatment of intraocular tumors. *Photochem Photobiol* 1987, 46:919–923.

58. Favilla I, Barry W, Gosbell A, *et al.*: Phototherapy of posterior uveal melanomas. *Br J Ophthalmol* 1991, 75:718–721.

59. Lingua R, Parel J: Photodynamic therapy for ocular tumors. *J Photochem Photobiol* 1991, 119–122.

60. Schmidt-Erfurth U, Bauman W, Gragoudas E, *et al.*: Photodynamic therapy of experimental choroidal melanoma using lipoprotein-delivered benzoporphyrin. *Ophthalmology* 1994, 101:89–99.

61.•• Gonzalez V, Hu L, Theodossiadis P, *et al.*: Photodynamic therapy of pigmented choroidal melanomas. *Invest Ophthalmol Vis Sci* 1995, 36:871–878.

Photodynamic therapy of experimental pigmented choroidal melanoma with CASPc.

62. Phillips A, Browne B, Allan D: Haematoporphyrin photosensitisation treatment of experimental choroidal melanoma. *Eye* 1987, 1:680–685.

63. Ozler S, Nelson S, Liggett P, *et al.*: Photodynamic therapy of experimental subchoroidal melanoma using chloraluminum sulfonated phthalocyanine. *Arch Ophthalmol* 1992, 110:555–561.

64.• Young L, Howard M, Hu L, *et al.*: Photodynamic therapy of pigmented choroidal melanomas using a liposomal preparation of benzoporphyrin derivative. *Arch Ophthalmol* 1996, 114:186–192.

Recent studies of PDT for experimental melanoma demonstrating increased efficacy using second-generation photosensitizing agents.

65. Hu L, Huh K, Gragoudas E, *et al.*: Establishment of pigmented choroidal melanomas in a rabbit model. *Retina* 1994, 14:264–269.

66. Kim R, Hu L, Foster S, *et al.*: Photodynamic therapy of pigmented choroidal melanomas of greater than 3 mm thickness. *Ophthalmology* 1996, 103:2029–2036.

67. Ohnishi Y, Yamana Y, Minei M: Photoradiation therapy using argon laser and a hematoporphyrin derivative for retinoblastoma: a preliminary report. *Jpn J Ophthalmol* 1986, 30:409–419.

68. Murphree A: Retinoblastoma. In *Retina*, vol 1. Edited by Ryan S, Ogden T. St. Louis: CV Mosby; 1989:544.

69. White L, Gomer C, Doiron D, *et al.*: Ineffective photodynamic therapy (PDT) in a poorly vascularized xenograft model. *Br J Cancer* 1988, 57:455–458.

70. Winther J, Ehlers N: Histopathological changes in an intraocular-like tumour following photodynamic therapy. *Acta Ophthalmol* 1988, 66:69–78.

71. Winther J, Overgaard J: Photodynamic therapy of experimental intraocular retinoblastomas: dose-response relationships to light energy and photofrin II. *Acta Ophthalmol* 1989, 67:44–50.

72. Winther J: Porphyrin photodynamic therapy in an experimental retinoblastoma model. *Ophthalmic Paediat Genet* 1987, 8:49–52.

73. Epstein R, Hendricks R, Harris D: Photodynamic therapy of corneal neovascularization. *Cornea* 1991, 10:424–432.

74. Pallikaris I, Miltiades M, Iliaki O, *et al.*: Effectiveness of corneal neovascularization photothrombosis using phthalocyanine and a diode laser (675 nm). *Lasers Surg Med* 1993, 13:197–203.

75. Virdi PS, Hayreh SS: Ocular neovascularization with retinal vascular occlusion. I. Association with experimental retinal vein occlusion. *Arch Ophthalmol* 1982, 100:331–341.

76. Packer AJ, Tse DT, Gu X-Q, *et al.*: Hematoporphyrin photoradiation therapy for iris neovascularization. A preliminary report. *Arch Ophthalmol* 1984, 102:1193–1197.

77. Husain D, Miller J, Kenney A, *et al.*: Photodynamic therapy and digital angiography of experimental iris neovascularization using liposomal benzoporphyrin derivative. *Ophthalmology* 1997, 104:1242–1250.

78. Ohkuma H, Ryan SJ: Experimental subretinal neovascularization in the monkey. *Arch Ophthalmol* 1983, 101:1102–1110.

79. Ryan SJ: Subretinal neovascularization: natural history of an experimental model. *Arch Ophthalmol* 1982, 100:1804–1809.

80. Miller H, Miller B, Ryan S: The role of retinal pigment epithelium in the involution of subretinal neovascularization. *Invest Ophthalmol Vis Sci* 1986, 27:1644–1652.

81. Thomas EL, Langhofer M: Closure of experimental subretinal neovascular vessels with dihematoporphyrin ether augmented argon green laser photocoagulation. *Photochem Photobiol* 1987, 46:881–886.

82.• Obana A, Gohto Y, Miki T, *et al.*: Photodynamic therapy of choroidal vessels using a newly developed chlorin derivative (ATX-S10). *Invest Ophthalmol Vis Sci* 1996, 37:S549.

Photodynamic therapy closure of normal choroidal vessels in the rabbit, using a new chlorin derivative.

83. Richter AM, Cerruti-Sola S, Sternberg ED, *et al.*: Biodistribution of tritiated benzoporphyrin derivative (3H-BPD-MA), a new potent photosensitizer, in normal and tumor-bearing mice. *J Photochem Photobiol* 1990, 5:231–244.

84. Lui J, Hruza L, Kollias N, *et al.*: Photodynamic therapy of malignant skin tumors with benzoporphyrin derivative-monoacid ring A (BPD-MA): Preliminary investigations. In *Proceedings of Lasers in Otolaryngology, Dermatology, and Tissue Welding*. Society of Photo-Optical Instrumentation Engineers. Bellingham, Washington, 1993; 1876:147–151.

85. Kramer M, Miller J, Delori F, *et al.*: Imaging of experimental choroidal neovascularization by liposomal BPD-MA angiography [abstract]. *Invest Ophthalmol Vis Sci* 1995, 36:S236.

86. Husain D, Miller J, Michaud N, *et al.*: Long term effect of photodynamic therapy (PDT) using liposomal benzoporphyrin derivative (BPD) on experimental choroidal neovascularization (CNV) and normal retina and choroid. *Invest Ophthalmol Vis Sci* 1996, 37:S223.

87.• Reinke M, Canakis C, Husain D, *et al.*: Photodynamic therapy (PDT) retreatment of normal retina and choroid in the primate. *Invest Ophthal Vis Sci* 1997, 38:S17.

An experimental study of the recovery of normal retina and choroid after multiple PDT treatments. Since the current clinical trials of PDT for CNV use multiple PDT treatments, the recovery of normal tissues from repeated treatments is an important issue.

SELECTED BIBLIOGRAPHY

Ciba Foundation: *Photosensitizing Compounds: Their Chemistry, Biology and Clinical Use*. New York: John Wiley & Sons; 1989.

Henderson BW, Dougherty TJ, eds: *Photodynamic Therapy*. New York: Marcel Dekker; 1992.

Husain D, Miller JW: Photodynamic therapy for macular degeneration. *Semin Ophthalmol* 1997, 12:14–25.

Kessel D: *Photodynamic Therapy of Neoplastic Disease*, vol 1. Boca Raton: CRC Press; 1990.

McCaughan JS Jr: *A Clinical Manual: Photodynamic Therapy of Malignancies*. Austin, TX: RG Landes; 1993.

CHAPTER 11

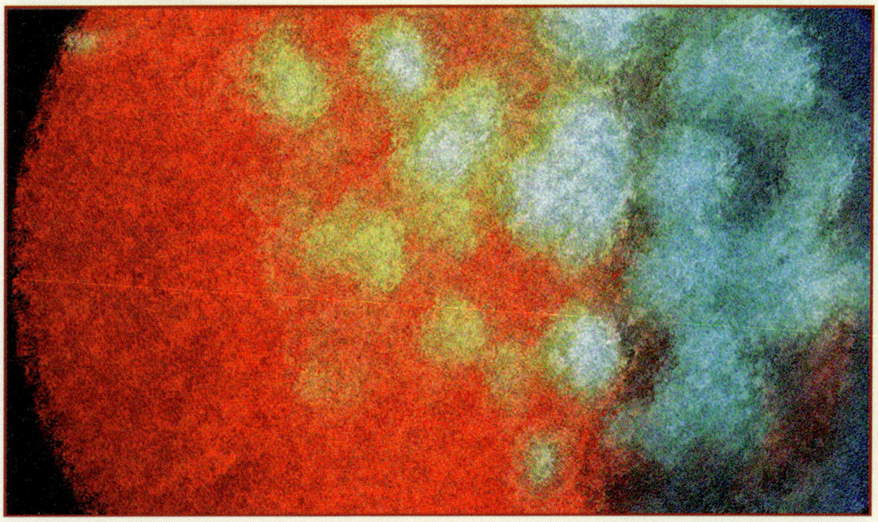

Photocoagulation Treatment of Pigmented Intraocular Tumors

LEONIDAS ZOGRAFOS
EVANGELOS S. GRAGOUDAS

At present, laser photocoagulation is often used in the conservative treatment of pigmented choroidal tumors. Photocoagulation is, however, rarely the sole or primary therapeutic modality. More often, photocoagulation is applied to treat the side effects of irradiation following conservative management of intraocular tumors. The use of new infrared lasers and laser lights in photodynamic therapy provides new alternatives for the conservative treatment of uveal melanoma.

One of the first applications of xenon photocoagulation, described in 1952 by Meyer-Schwickerath and Bornfeld [1], was the treatment of choroidal melanomas. This application was soon followed by photocoagulation for treatment of retinoblastomas, choroidal hemangiomas, and vascular tumors of the retina. Soon after its introduction, laser photocoagulation supplanted xenon photocoagulation for most ophthalmic applications. Nevertheless, laser photocoagulation's implementation in ocular oncology was slower, and xenon photocoagulation continues to be used today for certain indications.

Although photocoagulation is widely used, few reports in the ophthalmic literature discuss photocoagulation treatment of intraocular tumors, and even fewer reports have been published of large series of patients with sufficiently long follow-up to allow sound evaluation of the results.

PHOTOCOAGULATION TREATMENT OF CHOROIDAL MELANOMAS

The bulk of our knowledge regarding photocoagulation treatment of uveal melanomas comes from the statistical analyses of two series of cases treated by xenon photocoagulation. The first series, reported by Meyer-Schwickerath and Bornfeld [1], consists of 164 cases; the second series, reported by Jules François [2], consists of 122 cases. In these two series, the same photocoagulation technique was used. First, a circular atrophic photocoagulation scar was produced by a double row of confluent photocoagulation spots, after which an attempt was made to isolate the tumor from the choroidal circulation. In the second stage, progressive photoablation of the tumor was carried out in two to five sessions.

Reevaluation of the second series of cases by independent observers demonstrated that, after a follow-up period of at least 5 years, 43.75% of the cases were considered clinically cured, the tumor-related mortality was 12.5%, and 50% of the treated eyes were ultimately enucleated [3]. Late local recurrences, as long as 16 years after the treatment, did occur. Scleral invasion was present in 55% of the enucleated eyes, extrascleral extension was present in 35% of the cases, and invasion of the optic nerve was identified in 70% of the cases.

In the short term, in spite of some positive results, numerous complications that led to partial or total functional loss were described. The most common of these were tractional retinal detachment, preretinal fibrosis, vitreous hemorrhage, retinal vascular occlusion, cystic macular edema, and pigment dispersion into the vitreous body, as well as persistent inflammatory reaction and secondary cataract formation.

L'Espérance [4] and Shields *et al.* [5] have proposed a photocoagulation technique using the argon laser following the same therapeutic protocol introduced by Meyer-Schwickerath and Bornfeld [1] for xenon photocoagulation of melanomas. In a small series of cases, and after a follow-up ranging from 58 to 150 months, the local recurrence rate was much higher in cases treated with the argon laser (64%) than in cases treated with xenon photocoagulation (14%) [5]. Less pen-

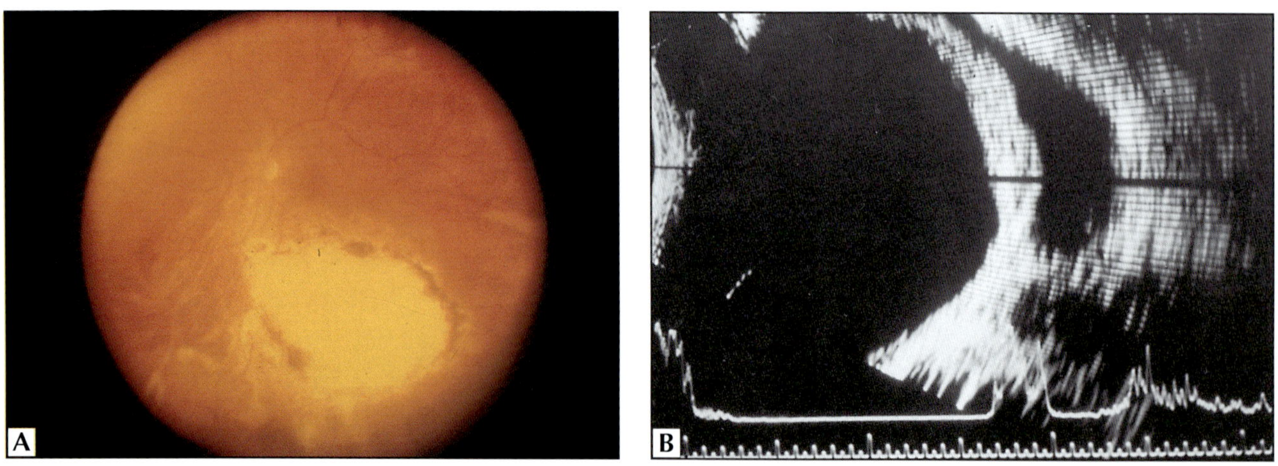

FIGURE 11-1. **A,** Wide-angle photograph of a chorioretinal scar 5 years after xenon photocoagulation of a uveal melanoma. **B,** Ultrasound of a large extraocular extension of tumor behind the atrophic chorioretinal scar.

etration of the blue-green argon light into the tumor mass behind the pigment epithelium, where most light is absorbed, may partially explain this difference. In addition, laser photocoagulation may cause microexplosions on the surface of the tumor, which could lead to hemorrhages as well as to a dispersion of viable tumor cells in the vitreous cavity. To reduce the risk of the latter, Foulds and Damato [6] proposed the use of argon or krypton lasers with low energy and long exposures. The follow-up period for small melanomas treated in this manner, as well as for recurrent melanomas similarly treated following local surgical excision, is relatively short.

Treatment of uveal melanomas by various forms of radiotherapy, such as brachytherapy or external beam irradiation with charged particles, at present offers greater security than photocoagulation does for the control of intraocular tumors (Fig. 11-1). For this reason, radiotherapy is almost always the treatment of choice, even in those situations in which a small tumor is located in the nasal part of the optic disc and photocoagulation presents less potential risk for functional loss (Fig. 11-2).

Currently, laser photocoagulation is used for the treatment of some side effects from ocular radiotherapy and for the treatment of marginal recurrences after radiotherapy. In cases of irradiation-induced retinal ischemia, sectorial or panretinal photocoagulation is quite effective in preventing or treating neovascular glaucoma and vitreous hemorrhage from epipapillary or preretinal new vessels (Fig. 11-3). Laser photocoagulation may be effective in eliminating small tumor recurrences following conservative treatment with either irradiation or local excision.

The combined use of argon laser or xenon photocoagulation with radiotherapy has been reported [7–10]. In various series, this combined therapy resulted in a more rapid and complete regression of the tumor, a more rapid reabsorption of the secondary exudative detachment of the retina, and a decreased rate of vitreous hemorrhages. The combination of these two therapeutic modalities did not, however, have any beneficial effect on visual function during follow-up.

More recently, Lee *et al.* [11] reported more rapid tumor regression after photocoagulation with a diode laser (630 to 680 nm) used in conjunction with applica-

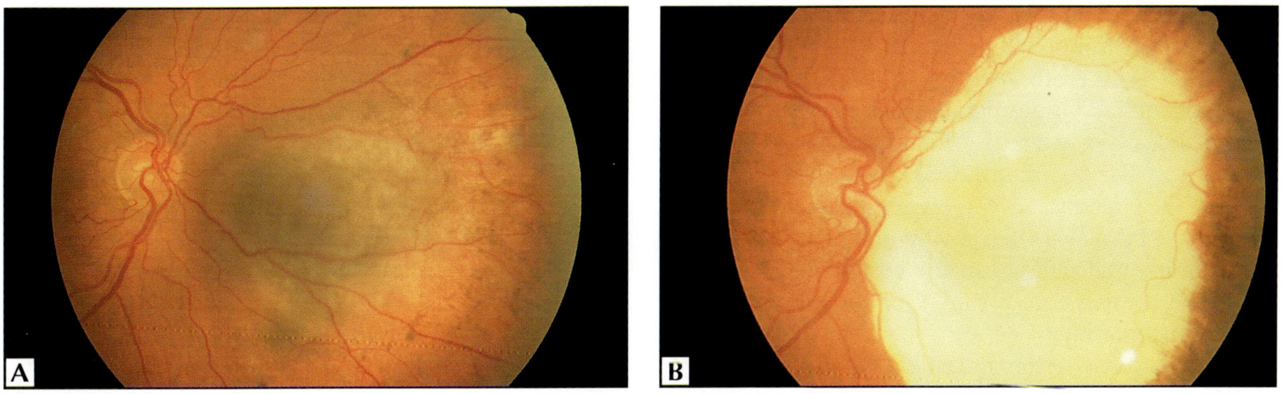

FIGURE 11-2. A, Small uveal melanoma localized in the nasal part of the disc and treated by a combination of krypton laser and xenon photocoagulation. **B**, At 2 years after treatment, an atrophic chorioretinal scar appears, containing a focus of pigmentation in its center. Visual acuity was 20/20.

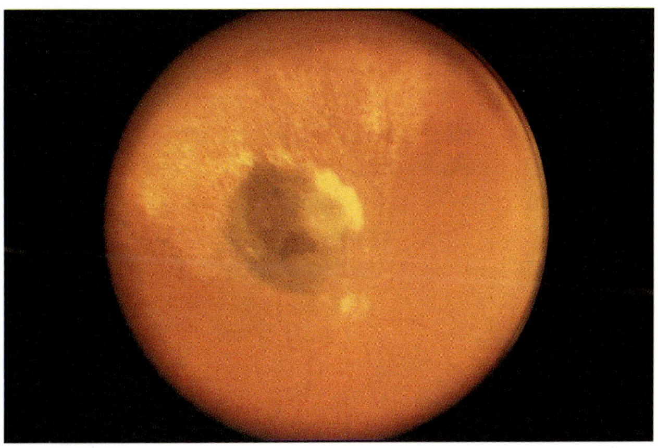

FIGURE 11-3. Sectorial photocoagulation of ischemic zones caused by arteriovenous occlusion following proton-beam irradiation of a uveal melanoma localized in the upper temporal quadrant. The retina overlying the tumor and the entire upper temporal quadrant are treated with confluent laser burns.

tion of radioactive iodine plaques. This rapid tumor regression may be related to deeper penetration of the light by the longer wavelengths. The diode laser can also be used in transscleral treatment of the base of the tumor. The efficacy of this laser when used after injection of indocyanine green dye, which increases the absorption of its light, was demonstrated in an animal experiment in which extensive necrosis was produced [12,13].

Diode lasers were also used at a low energy setting to increase intratumor temperature, such as in transpupillary hyperthermia, which is a new therapeutic approach currently under investigation for the treatment of uveal melanomas. Although initial results were encouraging [14,15], recent follow-up of patients treated early in the investigation showed 100% recurrence; thus, the investigators advised against using this method without combining it with radiation [16].

Photodynamic therapy (PDT) involves the use of photosensitizers that accumulate in and are retained by proliferating tissues. When these molecules are activated by light at the appropriate wavelength, active forms of oxygen and free radicals are generated, resulting in photochemical damage to cells in which the photosensitizer is present. Direct destruction of tumor cells may ensue [17], but damage to the tumor vasculature is also an important mechanism in tumor cell death [18,19]. Both injury to endothelial cells (with resulting platelet adhesion and degranulation) and irradiation of macrophages (with subsequent release of vasoactive mediators) play important roles in vascular occlusion [20,21]. Ischemia and tumor necrosis then follow. Several classes of photosensitizing agents have been evaluated in vitro and in animal models to determine their efficacy in the destruction of tumors. Most clinical experience has involved the porphyrin variants, hematoporphyrin derivative, and a combination of dihematoporphyrin esters and ethers, which is also known as Photofrin. These agents have been extensively studied in clinical trials for different cancers but their use has been limited by the small absorption peak and the prolonged period over which they induce skin photosensitivity. New photosensitizers, such as benzoporphyrin derivative, phthalocyanines, and chlorins, have absorption peaks at higher wavelengths and cause less skin photosensitivity, as compared with porphyrin variants [22].

Various investigators have studied the effect of PDT on experimental choroidal melanoma. Favorable results with PDT using phthalocyanines [23,24] and benzoporphyrin derivative [25] have been observed in the treatment of amelanotic Greene hamster melanoma in the rabbit eye. However, because most human choroidal melanomas are pigmented, the results of these studies have limited clinical application. Hu *et al.* [26] established a pigmented choroidal melanoma model that allows better assessment of PDT in treating pigmented melanomas [26]. Pigmented choroidal melanomas in the rabbit model had been treated with phthalocyanines and argon dye laser at 25 to 70 J/cm^2 and melanomas up to 4.8 mm showed regression [27]. PDT using benzoporphyrin derivative was performed in 18 rabbit eyes with pigmented melanoma; regression was seen in all tumors treated with 60 J/cm^2 [28]. Histologic examination showed acute vascular damage to the full thickness of the tumor, up to 4.6 mm [28], and necrosis with mononuclear and macrophage infiltration, which was prominent at 1-month follow-up [29].

Clinical studies using hematoporphyrin derivative with transpupillary or transcleral (or both) argon pumped dye laser light delivery at 630 nm have demonstrated a moderate response with small melanomas or melanomas that are slightly pigmented. In larger, heavily pigmented tumors, however, recurrence was common [30,31]. In addition, posttreatment complications included chemosis, iritis, cataract, vitritis, choroidal detachment, and exudative retinal detachment. Favilla *et al.* [32] treated 19 patients with choroidal melanomas of 7 to 10 mm in height. Six of these treated patients showed complete regression, but no regression was seen in eight tumors.

Clinical experience remains inconclusive in determining the role of PDT in the treatment of choroidal melanomas. Efforts to refine PDT are ongoing. Better patient selection and the development of second generation photosensitizers may achieve better results with lower toxicity. Advances using tumor-reactive monoclonal antibodies conjugated to a photosensitizer might increase delivery to the target tissue, promote more accurate tumor localization, enable lower dosing, and allow for use of a wider selection of photosensitizers that might possess more optimal photophysical properties but lack sufficient intrinsic tumor selectivity [33–35]. Combining PDT with other therapeutic modalities might also allow for synergistic effects. From experimental studies, it is thought that PDT and hyperthermia exhibit such effects [36,37]. Rapid vascular occlusion caused by PDT can hinder heat dissipation through circulation, which may then potentiate damage to cell membranes [38]. The combination of PDT with radiotherapy has also been considered. Several investigations have found synergistic effects between the two, particularly when radiotherapy precedes photodynamic therapy by 24 hours [38,39]. The combination of PDT and hyperbaric oxygen therapy has also been suggested, because PDT depends on the concentration of oxygen in the treated tissue and some tumors may contain relatively hypoxic regions that limit the damage caused by PDT [40]. Overall, present experimental studies, especially with the new photosensitizers, suggest that PDT holds promise for the treatment of uveal melanomas.

PHOTOCOAGULATION TREATMENT OF NEVI AND ATYPICAL MELANOCYTIC TUMORS OF THE CHOROID

In cases of choroidal nevi, laser photocoagulation may be used to treat the neovascular membranes that sometimes develop on the surface of these lesions (Fig. 11-4). The proliferation of a neovascular membrane on the surface of pigmented choroidal tumors is rare and in most cases is associated with a choroidal nevus close to the optic disc or the macula. The presence of such a neovascular membrane has no prognostic significance and does not indicate malignant transformation of the choroidal nevus. Visual prognosis in these eyes is excellent if the neovascular membrane is extrafoveal and can be eliminated completely by photocoagulation [41]. In even rare instances, spontaneous regression of the neovascular membrane may occur. This must be taken into account before performing photocoagulation treatment of a neovascular membrane located close to the fovea.

In most cases of atypical choroidal melanocytic tumors, an observation period is used to document the presence or absence of tumor growth before treatment is considered. Some of these lesions present with a small exudative retinal detachment that can involve the macula and affect central vision. In these cases, photocoagulation treatment may be applied on the surface of the tumor. Treatment should be light and restricted to the central area of the tumor. Close follow-up of patients is indicated as tumor growth may extend through photocoagulation-induced ruptures of Bruch's membrane, resulting in a mushroom-shaped lesion [42,43] (Fig. 11-5).

CONCLUSIONS

Laser photocoagulation alone is rarely used in ocular oncology. Rather, laser photocoagulation is most often used as a complementary treatment, mainly to manage the side effects of ocular irradiation and to prevent serious loss of vision. Although at present no concrete statistical data exist on the effects of new lasers in the treatment of intraocular pigmented tumors, preliminary clinical and experimental results are very promising.

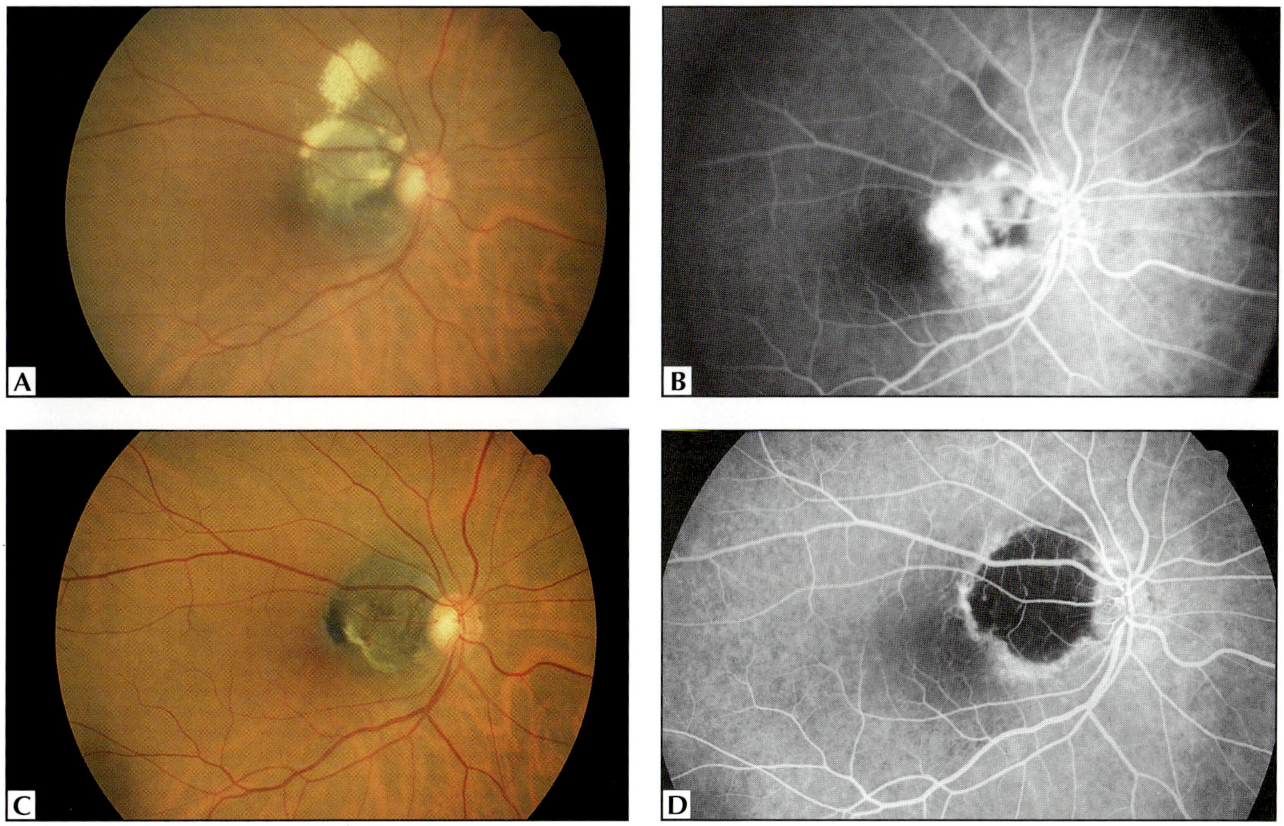

FIGURE 11-4. **A** and **B,** Clinical and angiographic photographs of an extrafoveal neovascular membrane on the surface of a localized choroidal nevus that is in contact with the optic disc. Note lipid deposits and serous detachment of the macula. Visual acuity was reduced to 20/200. **C** and **D,** Clinical and angiographic photographs 1 year after laser photocoagulation of the neovascular membrane. The retina is reattached and the lipid deposits have been reabsorbed. Visual acuity at this time had improved to 20/25.

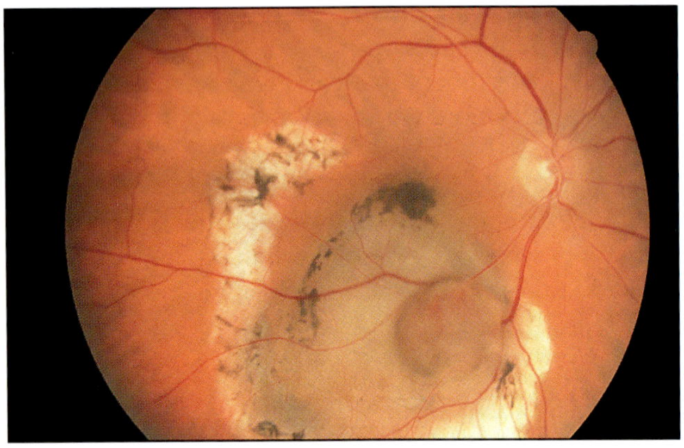

FIGURE 11-5. Mushroom-shaped choroidal melanoma after laser photocoagulation of the surface of small melanocytic lesion.

REFERENCES AND RECOMMENDED READING

Recently published papers of particular interest have been highlighted as:
- • Of interest
- •• Of outstanding interest

1. Meyer-Schwickerath G, Bornfeld N: Photocoagulation of choroidal melanomas: thirty years experience. In *Intraocular Tumors*. Edited by Lommatzsch PK, Blodi FC. Berlin: Akademie-Verlag; 1983:269–276.
2. François J: Treatment of malignant choroidal melanomas by xenon photocoagulation. In *Intraocular Tumors*. Edited by Lommatzsch PK, Blodi FC. Berlin: Akademie-Verlag; 1983:277–285.
3. De Lay JJ, Hanssens M, Ryckaert S: Photocoagulation of malignant melanomas of the choroid, a reappraisal. *Bull Soc Belge Ophthalmol* 1986, 213:9–18.
4. L'Espérance FA Jr: *Ocular Photocoagulation, A Stereoscopic Atlas*. St. Louis: CV Mosby; 1975:157–162.
5. Shields JA, Glazer LC, Mieler WF, *et al.*: Comparison of xenon arc and argon laser photocoagulation in the treatment of choroidal melanomas. *Am J Ophthalmol* 1990, 109:647–655.
6. Foulds WS, Damato BE: Low-energy long-exposure laser therapy in the management of choroidal melanoma. *Graefes Arch Clin Exp Ophthalmol* 1986, 224:26–31.
7. Zygoulska-Mach H, Maciejewski Z, Link E: Conservative treatment of choroidal melanomas combined use of cobalt plaques and photocoagulation. In *Intraocular Tumors*. Edited by Lommatzsch PK, Blodi FC. Berlin: Akademie-Verlag; 1983:417–423.
8. Zografos L, Gailloud CL: Traitement conservateur des mélanomes de la choroïde avec les applicateurs de cobalt 60 radioactifs. *Klin Monatsbl Augenheilkd* 1983, 182:499–501.
9. Moura RA, McPherson AR, Easley J: Malignant melanoma of the choroid: treatment with episcleral 198Au plaque and xenon-arc photocoagulation. *Ann Ophthalmol* 1985, 17:114–125.
10. Augsburger JJ, Kleineidam M, Mullen D: Combined iodine-125 plaque irradiation and indirect ophthalmoscope laser therapy of choroidal malignant melanomas: comparison with iodine-125 and cobalt-60 plaque radiotherapy alone. *Graefes Arch Clin Exp Ophthalmol* 1993, 231:500–507.
11. Lee KY, Sabates FN, Ziemianski MC, *et al.*: Combined iodine-125 plaque irradiation and laser photocoagulation in the treatment of choroidal malignant melanoma. In *Tumors of the Eye*. Edited by Bornfeld N, Gragoudas ES, Höpping W, *et al.* Amsterdam: Kugler; 1991:441–447.
12. Damato BE: An approach to the management of patients with uveal melanoma. *Eye* 1993, 7:388–397.
13. Chong LP, Özler SA, De Queiroz JM, Liggett PE: Indocyanine green-enhanced diode laser treatment of melanoma in a rabbit model. *Retina* 1993, 13:251–259.
14. Oosterhuis JA, Journée-de Korver HG, Kakebeeke-Kemme HM, Bleeker JC: Transpupillary thermotherapy in choroidal melanomas. *Arch Ophthalmol* 1995, 113:315–321.
15. Shields CL, Shields JA, De Potter P, Kheterpal S: Transpupillary thermotherapy in the management of choroidal melanoma. *Ophthalmology* 1996, 103:1642–1650.
16. Keunen JEE, Oosterhuis JA: Juxtapapillary melanomas and transpupillary thermotherapy. In *Proceedings of the Macula Society*, XXth Annual Meeting, Florence, Italy, June 18 to 21, 1997:140.
17. Henderson BW, Dougherty TJ: How does photodynamic therapy work? *Photochem Photobiol* 1992, 55:145–157.
18. vanGeel IP, Oppelaar H, Oussoren YG, Stewart FA: Changes in perfusion of mouse tumors after photodynamic therapy. *Int J Cancer* 1994, 56:224–228.
19. Nelson JS, Liaw LH, Orenstein A: Mechanism of tumor destruction following photodynamic therapy with hematoporphyrin derivate, chlorin, and phthalocyanine. *J Natl Cancer Inst* 1988, 80:1599–1605.

20. Catellani A, Pace GP, Concioli M: Photodynamic effect of hematoporphyrin on blood microcirculation. *J Pathol Bacteriol* 1963, 86:99–102.

21. Henderson BW, Donovan JM: Release of prostaglandin E2 from cells by photodynamic treatment. *Cancer Res* 1989, 49:6896–6900.

22. Levy JG, Waterfield E, Richter A: Photodynamic therapy of malignancies with benzoporphyrin derivative monoacid ring A. *Proc Soc Photo Optical Instr Eng* 1994, 2078:91–101.

23. Panagopoulos JA, Svitra PP, Puliafito CA, Gragoudas ES: Photodynamic therapy for experimental melanoma using chloroaluminum sulfonated phthalocyanine. *Arch Ophthalmol* 1989, 107:886–890.

24. Ozler SA, Nelson SJ, Liggett PE, *et al.*: Photodynamic therapy of experimental subchoroidal melanoma using chloroaluminum, sulfonated phthalocyanine. *Arch Ophthalmol* 1992, 110:555–561.

25. Schmidt-Erfurth U, Bauman W, Gragoudas E, *et al.*: Photodynamic therapy of experimental choroidal melanoma using lipoprotein-delivered benzoporphyrin. *Ophthalmology* 1994, 104:89–99.

26. Hu LK, Huh K, Gragoudas ES, Young LH: Establishment of pigmented choroidal melanomas in a rabbit model. *Retina* 1994, 14:264–269.

27. Gonzalez VH, Hu LK, Rheodossiadis PG, *et al.*: Photodynamic therapy of pigmented choroidal melanomas. *Invest Ophthalmol Vis Sci* 1995, 36:871–878.

28. Kim RY, Hu LK, Foster BS, *et al.*: Photodynamic therapy of pigmented choroidal melanomas of greater than 3-mm thickness. *Ophthalmology* 1996, 103:2029–2036.

29. Young LH, Howard MA, Hu LK, Gragoudas ES: Photodynamic therapy of pigmented choroidal melanomas using a liposomal preparation of benzoporphyrin derivative. *Arch Ophthalmol* 1996, 114:186–192.

30. Bruce RA Jr: Evaluation of hematoporphyrin photoradiation therapy to treat choroidal melanoma. *Lasers Surg Med* 1984, 4:59–64.

31. Murphree A, Cote M, Gomer CJ: The evolution of photodynamic therapy techniques in the treatment of intraocular tumors. *Photochem Photobiol* 1987, 46:919–923.

32. Favilla I, Barry WR, Gosbell A, *et al.*: Photodynamic therapy of posterior melanomas. *Br J Ophthalmol* 1991, 75:718–721.

33. Hu LK, Hasan T, Gragoudas ES, Young LH: Photoimmunotherapy of human melanomas cells. *Exp Eye Res* 1995, 61:385–391.

34. Jiang FN, Liu DJ, Neyndorff H, *et al.*: Photodynamic killing of human squamous cell carcinoma cells using a monoclonal antibody-photosensitizer conjugate. *J Natl Cancer Inst* 1991, 83:1218–1225.

35. Moan J, Berg K: Photochemotherapy of cancer: experimental research. *Photochem Photobiol* 1992, 55:931–948.

36. Mang TS, Dougherty TJ: Time and sequence dependent influence of in vivo photodynamic therapy survival by hyperthermia. *Photochem Photobiol* 1985, 42:533–540.

37. Waldow SM, Henderson BW, Dougherty TJ: Potentiation of photodynamic therapy by heat: effect of sequence and time interval between treatments in vivo. *Lasers Surg Med* 1985, 5:83–94.

38. Zhao FY, Zhang KH, Huang KH, *et al.*: Use of hematoporphyrin derivative as a sensitizer for radiotherapy of oral and maxillofacial tumors: a preliminary report. *Lasers Med Sci* 1986, 1:253–256.

39. Graschew G, Shopova M: Photodynamic therapy and gamma-irradiation: effect of tumor cell reoxygenation. *Lasers Med Sci* 1986, 1:193–195.

40. Jirsa M Jr, Pouckova P, Dolezal J, *et al.*: Hyperbaric oxygen and photodynamic therapy in tumor-bearing nude mice. *Eur J Cancer* 1991, 27:109.

41. Callanan DG, Lewis ML, Byrne SF, Gass JDM: Choroidal neovascularization associated with choroidal nevi. *Arch Ophthalmold* 1993, 111:789–794.

42. Folk JC, Weingeist TA, Coonan P, *et al.*: The treatment of serous macular detachment secondary to choroidal melanomas and nevi. *Ophthalmology* 1989, 96:547–551.

43. Erie JC, Robertson DM, Mieler WF: Presumed small choroidal melanomas with serous macular detachments with and without surface laser photocoagulation treatment. *Am J Ophthalmol* 1990, 109:259–264.

CHAPTER 12

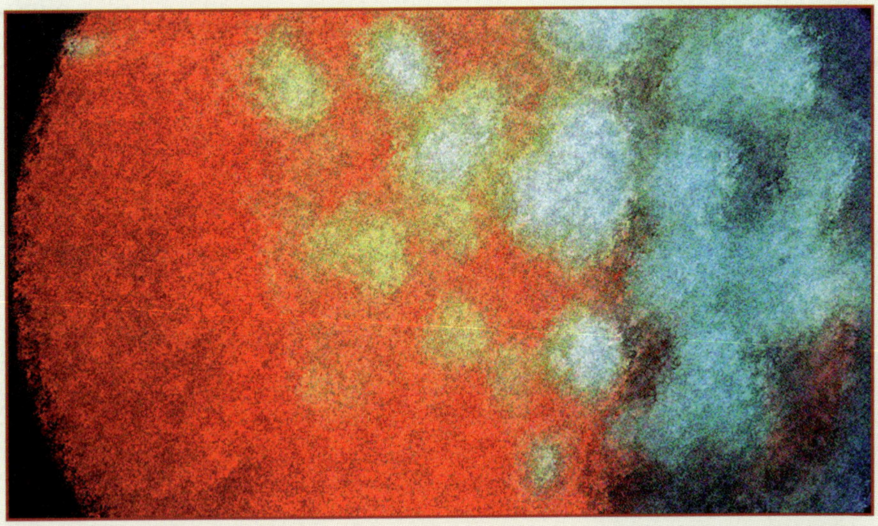

Lasers in Vitreous Surgery

SCOTT D. PENDERGAST
Z. NICHOLAS ZAKOV
MICHAEL A. NOVAK

Development of laser systems with the capability of intraocular delivery represents an important advance in vitreoretinal surgery. Prior to the advent of endophotocoagulation, chorioretinal adhesions could only be achieved intraoperatively by intraocular diathermy or cryotherapy. Although both these methods were effective in inducing chorioretinal adhesions during vitrectomy, direct contact with the retina was necessary and complications arising from inadvertent damage to the retina or choroid were not uncommon. In addition, the application of scatter or panretinal photocoagulation (PRP) was impractical. Xenon endophotocoagulation was developed by Charles [1] in the late 1970s, enabling surgeons to perform panretinal photocoagulation (PRP) intraoperatively. Endolaser photocoagulation using various wavelengths quickly emerged as an indispensable tool in vitreoretinal surgery, particularly for the treatment of proliferative diabetic retinopathy (PDR) associated with vitreous hemorrhage and neovascularization of the iris. Performing postoperative slit lamp PRP in an office setting was frequently difficult or impossible owing to patient discomfort and significant media opacity. Consequently, the retinal ischemic drive often persisted and patients continued to be at risk for the development of complications, such as recurrent vitreous hemorrhage or neovascularization of the iris and neovascular glaucoma. Before endolaser photocoagulation became widely available, the incidence of iris neovascularization following vitrectomy for PDR ranged from 5% to 23% in phakic eyes and 19% to 45% in aphakic eyes [2–5]. In addition, neovascular glaucoma developed postoperatively in 5% to 23% of eyes and occurred much more frequently in aphakic eyes [3–7]. Although prospective studies comparing the efficacy of intraoperative endolaser photocoagulation versus postoperative laser are lacking, it is generally accepted that endophotocoagulation has dramatically reduced the incidence of postoperative iris rubeosis and neovascular glaucoma. In addition to its important role in the management of PDR, endolaser photocoagulation is useful for retinopexy during retinal reattachment surgery for treating drainage retinotomy sites, retinal breaks, giant retinal tears, and panretinal photocoagulation. More recently, laser systems have been developed that are capable of cutting and segmenting vitreous bands or preretinal membranes. This chapter reviews the various laser systems and intraocular probes currently used as adjuncts in vitreoretinal surgery. In addition, the indications and complications of endophotocoagulation are highlighted at the end of the chapter.

LASER SYSTEMS FOR RETINAL PHOTOCOAGULATION

Laser wavelength

Various wavelengths have been used for endophotocoagulation during vitreoretinal surgery, including xenon, argon blue-green, krypton red, dye, diode, and continuous-wave neodymium:yttrium-aluminum-garnet (Nd:YAG) (Table 12-1). Xenon endophotocoagulation, first reported by Charles [1,8] in 1979, proved to play a valu-

TABLE 12-1 LASERS USED FOR FOCAL OR SCATTER PHOTOCOAGULATION

Laser	Wavelength, *nm*	Advantages	Disadvantages	Comments
Argon	488, 514	Excellent melanin absorption Coagulates bleeders directly Extensive clinical experience	488 nm—xanthophyll absorption Absorbed by hemorrhage	Most commonly used laser in vitreoretinal surgery
Diode	810, 670	Good melanin absorption Can penetrate hemorrhage Solid-state laser	Requires higher energy Increased risk of excessive burns or rupture of Bruch's membrane	Use is increasing
Dye	Tunable	Similar to argon	Absorbed by hemorrhage	No advantage over argon
Krypton	640	Similar to argon	Requires higher energy	No advantage over argon
Nd:YAG	1060	—	Cumbersome delivery Less efficacious than argon	Rarely used for photocoagulation
Xenon	400 to1600	—	Probe must be held close to retina	Superseded by more recent modalities

Nd:YAG—neodymium:yttrium-aluminum-garnet.

able role in vitreoretinal surgery. Xenon arc light is divergent and therefore necessitated positioning the probe within 0.1 to 0.5 mm of the retina. This requirement led to frequent iatrogenic retinal breaks and was time consuming, due to the probe's inability to fire rapidly. In addition, xenon arc light could not be used in air-filled eyes. These important limitations stimulated interest in developing endolaser systems that used wavelengths more amenable to vitreoretinal surgery.

In the early 1980s, several investigators reported results of argon-krypton, argon blue-green (488 nm), and argon green (514.5 nm) laser endophotocoagulation [9–12]. Argon laser intraocular photocoagulation afforded rapid, controlled application of burns at a safe distance from the retina (approximately 3 mm). In addition, laser could be applied in both fluid-filled and gas-filled eyes. Because of these significant advantages, xenon endolaser photocoagulation was quickly superseded by argon laser endophotocoagulation. Although continuous-wave Nd:YAG [13], krypton [9], and carbon dioxide [14,15] lasers have been proposed for endophotocoagulation, argon laser remains the type most frequently used in vitreoretinal surgery. Early studies reported favorable results of intraocular argon laser photocoagulation to treat retinal breaks and retinotomy sites and for the application of intraoperative PRP in eyes with PDR and proliferative vitreoretinopathy (PVR) [10–12]. Subsequent reports confirmed the efficacy of argon endolaser photocoagulation for application of PRP during diabetic vitrectomy [16,17], in the treatment of posterior retinal breaks associated with penetrating or perforating intraocular foreign bodies [18], and for the treatment of a choroidal bleeding site during submacular surgery [19]. More recently, tunable dye lasers with endophotocoagulation capability have become available. Although this laser system affords vitreoretinal surgeons more versatility in wavelength selection, tunable dye lasers offer little if any advantage over argon green lasers in most situations.

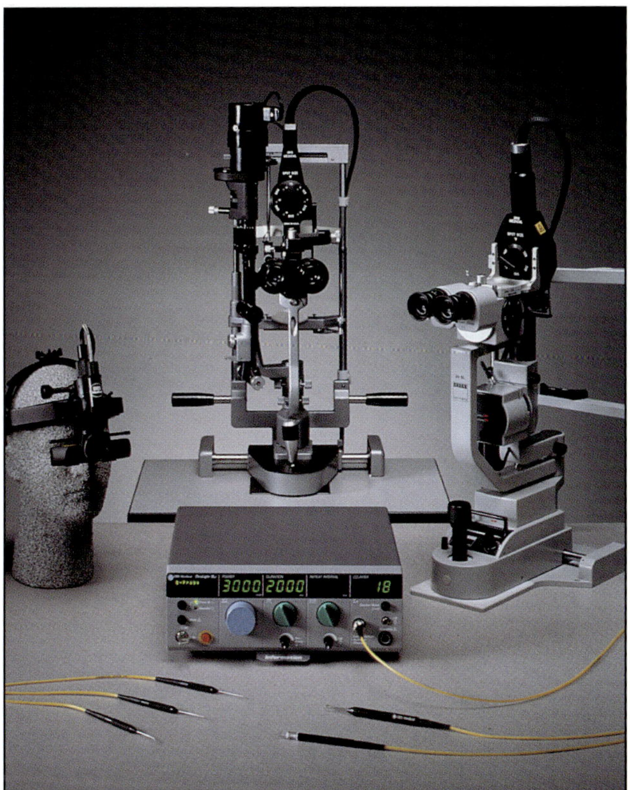

FIGURE 12-1. Diode laser (Iris Medical, Mountain View, CA) (810 nm) with laser indirect ophthalmoscope, slit lamp, endolaser, and transscleral delivery systems.

In 1987, Puliafito, *et al.* [20] developed an intraocular diode laser probe emitting a wavelength of 810 nm. This semiconductor device afforded important ergonomic advantages compared with argon-ion lasers, such as its compact size and portability, relatively low energy requirements, and durability (Fig. 12-1). Smiddy [21] demonstrated the efficacy of diode endolaser photocoagulation in 25 eyes undergoing vitrectomy for PDR and PVR. Histologic studies demonstrated a dose–response effect, with mild burns producing selective damage to the outer retina and retinal pigment epithelium (RPE), whereas more intense burns resulted in full-thickness retinal liquefaction [22]. Because near-infrared wavelengths produce deeper burns, tissue reaction is generally delayed and threshold lesions generally appear dull gray. Excessive burns can result in rupture of Bruch's membrane. Increasing burn duration rather than power during titration has been suggested to avoid this potential complication [22]. In a consecutive series of 226 eyes treated with diode endolaser photocoagulation during vitrectomy for PDR or PVR, Sasoh and Smiddy [23•] evaluated the clinical efficacy of diode endophotocoagulation. The intraoperative goals were achieved in 99% of cases and the surgical results were equivalent to those in 67 consecutive eyes treated with argon endophotocoagulation.

As semiconductor laser technology evolved, additional diode laser systems have recently been introduced. A 670-nm prototype diode laser with endolaser and transscleral delivery has recently been introduced for retinal and ciliary body photocoagulation [24]. The 670-nm wavelength combines the favorable absorption spectrum of krypton red wavelength with the ergonomic advantages inherent in semiconductor lasers. Results of this experimental study were encouraging but clinical studies are currently lacking. As discussed in Chapter 4, a diode-pumped solid state laser is now commercially available that produces a green wavelength (532 nm). This system uses a diode laser pump source to produce a near infrared wavelength of 808 nm. A laser crystal converts this wavelength to 1064 nm and a doubling crystal produces a final wavelength of 532 nm. In addition, Hoggatt *et al.* [25] recently developed a diode laser (810 nm) with a carbon dioxide–coated tip that can be used to perform retinectomy and retinotomy in a single step. Although this prototype diode-laser endoprobe successfully combined coagulation and vaporizing in rabbit eyes, extensive choroidal and scleral burns frequently resulted, particularly when longer durations were required. Further experimental and clinical studies will be required to establish the efficacy and safety of this endolaser.

Laser delivery systems

For argon, dye, and diode lasers, both endolaser probes and indirect ophthalmoscope delivery systems are currently available. Endolaser probes are the most commonly employed delivery system in vitreoretinal surgery and are used for treating retinal breaks, retinotomies, and PRP (Fig. 12-2). The laser indirect ophthalmoscope is useful for peripheral retinal ablation, particularly in treating the superior retina in phakic eyes and applying PRP following placement of an encircling scleral buckle. The diode laser is also capable of transscleral laser retinopexy owing to its ability to penetrate the sclera; diode transscleral laser probes are commercially available (Fig. 12-3). Previous studies have demonstrated the efficacy of transscleral laser retinopexy in experimental [24,26,27] and clinical studies [28–30]. In retinal detachment surgery, transscleral photocoagulation is an alternative to cryotherapy and potentially avoids or reduces dispersion of RPE cells and breakdown of the blood–retinal barrier associated with the latter modality [28]. Although transscleral retinopexy is not commonly used in vitreoretinal surgery, it could prove useful for peripheral retinopexy in eyes with significant media opacity undergoing scleral buckling or vitrectomy.

Endolaser probes

Over the past decade, endolaser probes have been developed that enhance the ability of the ophthalmic surgeon to perform photocoagulation in vitreoretinal surgery. In 1987, Peyman [31] introduced bent-tipped endolaser probes in which the final 3 to 4 mm of the tip is angled at 45° to 50°. This angulation permits photocoagulation in the vicinity of the superonasal and superotemporal sclerotomy sites as well as the superior retina—regions that are generally difficult to treat using conventional straight endolaser probes. Furthermore, angled endolaser probes facilitate complete PRP in phakic eyes and obviate the need to perform peripheral cryotherapy or photocoagulation using a laser indi-

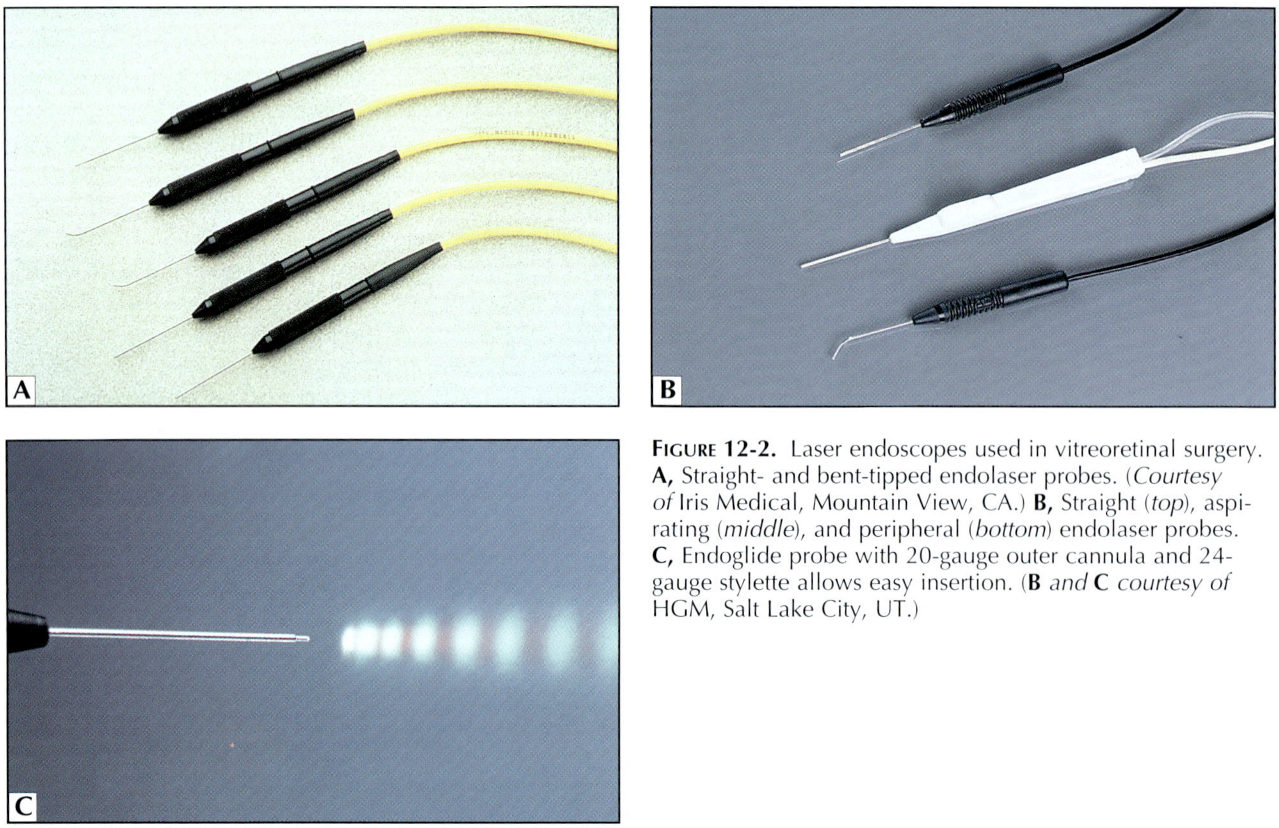

FIGURE 12-2. Laser endoscopes used in vitreoretinal surgery. **A,** Straight- and bent-tipped endolaser probes. (*Courtesy of* Iris Medical, Mountain View, CA.) **B,** Straight (*top*), aspirating (*middle*), and peripheral (*bottom*) endolaser probes. **C,** Endoglide probe with 20-gauge outer cannula and 24-gauge stylette allows easy insertion. (**B** *and* **C** *courtesy of* HGM, Salt Lake City, UT.)

rect ophthalmoscope [32]. The wide variety of angled endolaser probes currently available meet the needs of vitreoretinal surgeons (Fig. 12-2).

Multifunction endolaser probes have also proven useful in selected cases. A disposable endolaser probe with aspiration ability was developed by Peyman *et al.* [33]. This probe is particularly helpful in treating retinal breaks and retinotomies following air–fluid exchange because accumulated subretinal fluid can be aspirated immediately without exchanging instruments. Peyman and Lee [34] designed a multifunction endolaser probe consisting of endolaser, illumination, aspiration, and infusion capabilities. Combining these functions eliminates frequent instrument exchanges and permits efficient treatment of retinotomy sites following air–fluid exchange, allows PRP in eyes with preretinal hemorrhage, and frees the surgeon's other hand to perform other bimanual retinal manipulations. The primary disadvantage of this multifunction probe is its reduced fiber size owing to the presence of a parallel irrigation–aspiration tube that significantly limits the amount of available light. Awh *et al.* [35] have developed a simplified illuminating endolaser probe that provides excellent illumination and facilitates peripheral laser photocoagulation by allowing the operator to perform scleral depression with the other hand. Finally, Uram [36] introduced a laser endoscope that combines endolaser, illumination, and an endoscope in an 18- or 20-gauge endoscopic handpiece. This system affords an excellent view of anterior structures (*eg*, pars plana, ciliary body, posterior surface of iris), does not depend on media clarity, requires fewer instrument exchanges, and is potentially useful for anterior loop dissection and peripheral laser. However, this system is relatively expensive and the repertoire of retinal maneuvers is somewhat limited owing to the lack of stereopsis. Although the laser endoscope could prove to be useful in selected situations, the availability of other modalities, most notably wide-angle viewing systems, has curtailed its use.

LASER SYSTEMS FOR SEGMENTATION OF VITREOUS AND PRERETINAL MEMBRANES

Although mechanical vitrectomy with segmentation and delamination of preretinal tissue is highly successful in most cases, removal of highly adherent membranes remains challenging and can result in iatrogenic retinal tears and other complications. These considerations prompted investigators to develop photodisruptive laser systems capable of performing precise and near tractionless segmentation or delamination of preretinal membranes (Table 12-2). Early reports demonstrated that carbon dioxide lasers emitting at 10.6 µm were capable of cutting vitreous membranes [14,15,37]. However, a cumbersome delivery system and significant thermal damage to surrounding tissues have hindered its acceptance. More recent studies have shown that a variety of lasers with convenient delivery systems are effective in segmenting vitreous and preretinal membranes with minimal collateral damage. Although the Nd:YAG laser has recently been advocated for treatment of diabetic traction retinal detachment [38,39] and subhyaloid hemorrhage [40–43] as an office-based procedure, our discussion emphasizes lasers used as an adjunct to pars plana vitrectomy.

Excimer laser

Ultraviolet lasers are effective in cutting vitreous membranes as well as retinal tissue. An important theoretical advantage of excimer lasers is that absorption of ultraviolet wavelengths results in breaking of molecular bonds. Thus, ablation occurs through a photochemical pathway rather than by heating tissue. Accordingly,

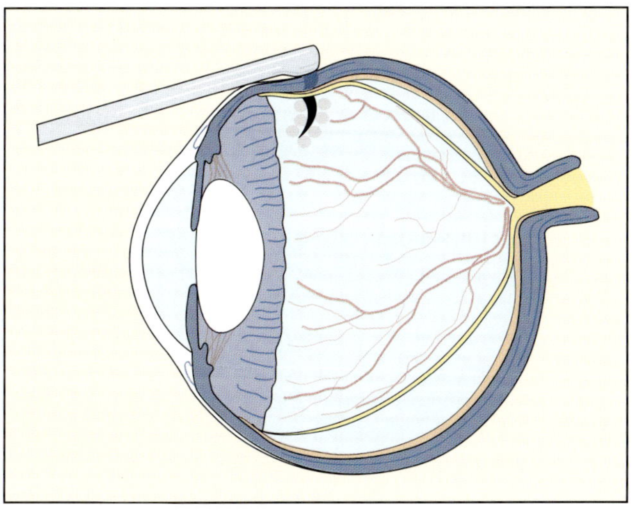

FIGURE 12-3. Transscleral retinopexy using the diode laser.

TABLE 12-2 LASERS USED FOR SURGICAL MANEUVERS IN VITREORETINAL SURGERY

Laser	Wavelength	Applications	Disadvantages
Carbon dioxide	10.6 µm	Transection of vitreous membranes External drainage of subretinal fluid	Significant collateral damage
Er:YAG	2.94 µm	Relaxing retinotomy, epiretinal membrane incision and ablation, vitreous membrane transection, subretinal membrane segmentation, capsulotomy (clinical studies) Production of choroidal shunt (CRVO)	Retinal hemorrhage in 16% of maneuvers Epiretinal membrane ablation difficult and inefficient
Excimer	193 nm	Highly precise ablation of retinal tissue in animal model	Expensive Cumbersome delivery Requires transmission through air (dry surface)
	308 nm	Transection of vitreous membranes	Ultraviolet radiation
Ho:YAG	2.2 µm	Transection of vitreous membranes in rabbits	Less precise than Er:YAG laser
Nd:YAG*	1060 nm	Evacuation of subhyaloid premacular hemorrhage Segmentation of fibrovascular proliferations in PDR with traction	 Relatively high energy required with significant collateral damage
Nd:YLF*	1053 nm	Segmentation of fibrovascular tissue and hyaloid near retina in PDR with traction	Endoprobes not yet available

*** Nd:YAG and Nd:YLF laser treatments are performed in the office using slit lamp delivery.**
CRVO—central retinal vein occlusion; Er:YAG—erbium:yttrium-aluminum-garnet; Ho:YAG—holmium:yttrium-aluminum-garnet; Nd:YAG—neodymiym:yttrium-aluminum-garnet; Nd:YLF—Neodymium:yttrium-lithium-fluoride; PDR—proliferative diabetic retinopathy.

this modality allows very precise, tractionless cutting of tissue with minimal damage to surrounding tissue. A 308-nm xenon chloride laser has been used to segment vitreous membranes [44], and a needle-guided 193-nm argon fluoride excimer laser accurately ablated retinal tissue with no evidence of damage to surrounding tissue [45]. However, these lasers are expensive and require cumbersome delivery systems. Moreover, ultraviolet wavelengths can only be transmitted through air, and the tissue surface must be kept dry during treatment. Because of the potential toxic, cataractogenic, and mutagenic effects of ultraviolet radiation, further studies will be necessary to establish the safety of excimer lasers.

Holmium:yttrium-aluminum-garnet laser

A pulsed (250-µs) holmium:YAG (Ho:YAG) laser emitting a wavelength of 2.12 µm has been used to transect experimental vitreous membranes in a rabbit model [46]. Using a commercial intraocular delivery system, the investigators transected or partially cut 35 membranes located 0.5 to 3.8 mm from the retina. Retinal injury, primarily consisting of nonhemorrhagic retinal burns, occurred in 58% of cases in which the bare optic fiber was employed. Use of a retinal-shielding pick significantly reduced the incidence of laser-induced retinal injury and allowed complete transection of vitreous membranes within 0.5 mm of the retina. The precision of the Ho:YAG laser is comparable to carbon dioxide laser incisions but is less precise than erbium:YAG (Er:YAG) lasers, producing a thermal zone of damage extending from 150 to 450 µm from the edge of the incision.

Erbium:yttrium-aluminum-garnet laser

The Er:YAG laser emits a wavelength of 2.94 µm that is strongly absorbed by water and allows precise ablation of tissue with minimal collateral injury. When an energy pulse is delivered to a target tissue, water within the tissues absorbs it so that the absorbed energy is converted to heat [47]. The delivery of high energy with extreme temporal and spatial focusing results in plasma heating and rapid expansion of a cavitation bubble with photovaporization of target tissue [48]. In 1989, Margolis *et al.* [49] developed an Er:YAG laser to transect experimental vitreous membranes. All vitreous membranes were effectively and precisely transected using a prototype Er:YAG laser with a thermal zone of damage of 18 to 60 µm in adjacent unablated tissue. However, the retina was injured in over 50% of cases, most commonly when the probe was held within 2000 µm of the retina. An early limitation of the Er:YAG laser involved difficulties with its delivery system. Both low hydroxyl-fused silica fibers and zirconium fluoride fibers encased in sapphire tips presented limitations that rendered their use impractical for vitreoretinal surgery.

Interest in the Er:YAG laser heightened following important innovations in the laser itself as well as the development of a more practical intraocular delivery system. Brazitkos *et al.* [47] used an Er:YAG laser equipped with a flexible fiber and endoprobes of varying sizes to perform retinotomies, epiretinal membrane incisions and ablations, and vitreous membrane transections as close as 0.5 mm from the retina. The laser was effective in both aqueous and air-filled eyes but was not effective in the presence of perfluoro-n-octane liquid due to progressive clouding during treatment. This modality proved efficient and precise, with retinal injury occurring in only 1 of 25 vitreous transections; subjacent thermal damage was 50 µm or less following ablation of epiretinal membranes. Although full-thickness incisions of epiretinal membrane could be performed with preservation of the underlying retina, retinal thermal damage or hemorrhage occurred in approximately 40% of the incisions.

The efficacy of Er:YAG laser for performing a variety of maneuvers in vitreoretinal surgery has recently been evaluated in two clinical studies [50••,51•]. D'Amico *et al* [51•] performed surgical manipulations using an Er:YAG laser with various 20-gauge endoprobes in 13 patients. Transections of elevated vitreous membranes and subretinal strands, incisions into vascularized diabetic preretinal membranes, retinotomies, and ablation of epiretinal membranes were successfully performed. Of the 48 maneuvers performed, complications occurred in two cases, involving an iatrogenic retinal break and damage to an intraocular lens during capsulotomy using a side-firing probe.

A prospective multicenter clinical trial was recently completed that evaluated the Er:YAG laser in 68 consecutive eyes of 66 patients undergoing vitreoretinal surgery for PDR, PVR, epiretinal membrane, and retinopathy of prematurity [50••]. Individual maneuvers judged to be most efficacious by surgeons included relaxing retinotomy, capsulotomy, and subretinal membrane transection. The Er:YAG laser was judged less efficacious for transecting elevated membranes and drainage retinotomies; moreover, it performed primary coagulation poorly. Intraoperative complications included retinal hemorrhage in 16% of maneuvers, retinal break or photocoagulation in 5% of epiretinal membrane incisions, and intraocular lens damage during two posterior capsulotomies. Although the results of these studies are promising, ablation of large regions of epiretinal membranes was time-consuming and difficult, and therefore most epimacular membranes were only partially removed. Based on investigations of scaling laws governing the thermal and mechanical effects of laser-tissue interactions, Berger and D'Amico [48] have postulated that using low pulse energies, high repetition rates, and small-diameter probe tips will maintain efficient ablation while minimizing mechanical injury.

A very recent application of the Er:YAG laser involves the production of a choroidal shunt for the treatment of central retinal vein occlusion. In a pilot study, Quiroz-Mercado [52] reported results in four patients undergoing vitrectomy followed by Er:YAG laser treatment of the main superonasal and inferonasal retinal veins. Burns were applied so as to produce retinal whitening, narrowing of the vein, and retinal perforation. Following treatment, intraretinal hemorrhage and macular edema decreased with improvement in visual acuity in each case. Further innovations and experience with the Er:YAG laser will further define the role of this modality in vitreoretinal surgery.

Neodymium:yttrium-lithium-fluoride picosecond laser

Neodymium:yttrium-lithium-fluoride (Nd:YLF) picosecond pulse laser is another recent innovation in photodisruptive laser technology [53]. As mentioned earlier, Nd:YAG laser has been used to treat diabetic traction retinal detachments [38,39] and premacular fibrosis [54] through slit lamp delivery. The Nd:YAG laser produces a short train of pulses with a duration of 10 nanoseconds and typically requires a pulse energy of 5 to 14 mJ to segment tissue. Owing to this comparatively high energy requirement, the Nd:YAG laser is ill-suited for transecting tissue in close proximity to the retina and has therefore failed to achieve widespread acceptance. The Nd:YLF laser emits a wavelength of 1053 nm and produces 1000 pulses per second for up to 10 seconds. The pulse duration of 60 picoseconds allows segmentation of tissue at lower energies, generally between 0.05 and 0.4 mJ. Cohen *et al.* [53] demonstrated that a prototype Nd:YLF laser could be used to segment fibrovascular tissue and contracted posterior hyaloid near the retinal surface in patients with traction retinal detachments related to proliferative diabetic retinopathy. Although this modality may obviate the need for vitrectomy with mechanical segmentation and delamination of preretinal membranes in a select group of patients, this laser could also prove to be a valuable adjunct to vitreoretinal surgery if an endoprobe delivery source becomes available.

INDICATIONS AND TECHNIQUES FOR LASERS IN VITREORETINAL SURGERY

Proliferative retinopathies

Proliferative retinopathies represent a broad spectrum of retinal vascular disorders characterized by neovascularization of the iris, disc, or retina in response to retinal ischemia. After neovascularization has developed, severe visual loss can ensue due to vitreous hemorrhage with or without traction retinal detachment. In most instances, laser photocoagulation can be performed in the office. Indications and treatment techniques are described in detail in Chapter 4. Intraoperative endophotocoagulation has proven indispensable for the treatment of proliferative retinopathies requiring vitrectomy because delivery of laser photocoagulation postoperatively can be difficult or impossible due to patient discomfort and media opacity (Table 12-3). Following vitrectomy and membrane dissection, laser treatment is applied in either a panretinal (*eg*, PDR) or scatter (branch retinal vein occlusion, proliferative sickle-cell retinopathy) pattern depending on the extent and distribution of retinal ischemia. A straight or bent-tipped endolaser probe is used in conjunction with argon, dye, or diode lasers. Burns of moderate intensity, and a spot size of approximately 500 µm are spaced one half to one full burn width apart. An exposure duration between 0.2 and 0.5 seconds is generally used. The size and intensity of burns can be modulated by adjusting the energy and pulse duration as well as by varying the distance of the endoprobe from the retina (*eg*, smaller and more intense burns result when the probe is moved closer to the retina). Peripheral laser photocoagulation can be accomplished using specialized endoprobes as discussed earlier, scleral depression, or laser indirect ophthalmoscopy. In addition, wide-angle viewing systems are useful in providing a panoramic view that facilitates peripheral endolaser photocoagulation in eyes filled with either fluid or air. Other applications for endolasers include direct treatment of bleeding vessels (argon green) (although endodiathermy is preferable) and production of chorioretinal adhesions around retinal breaks.

Retinal detachment surgery

Endolaser photocoagulation plays an important role in the management of complicated retinal detachments. Chorioretinal adhesions are produced to close retinal breaks and drainage retinotomies following air–fluid exchange or injection of perfluorocarbon liquids such as perfluoro-n-octane. Endophotocoagulation is particularly valuable in treating the posterior edge of giant retinal tears or relaxing retinotomies with several rows of closely spaced burns. Unusual forms of retinal detachments, such as those associated with colobomas [55], optic pits [56], peripheral angiomas associated with traction retinal detachment [57], and macular holes in myopic eyes have also been successfully man-

TABLE 12-3 INDICATIONS AND APPLICATIONS OF LASER PHOTOCOAGULATION IN VITREOUS SURGERY

Indication	Applications	Lasers	Delivery systems
Proliferative retinopathies	PRP Bleeders Flat neovascularization Retinopexy	Argon, diode, dye	ELP LIO Transscleral (diode)
Complicated retinal detachments	Retinal breaks Drainage retinotomies Relaxing retinotomies PRP on scleral buckle	Argon, diode, dye	ELP
Scleral buckling surgery	Retinopexy External drainage of subretinal fluid	Argon, diode, dye Carbon dioxide	LIO Transscleral (diode) external probe
Glaucoma	Cyclophotocoagulation	Argon, diode, dye	ELP Transscleral (diode) Laser endoscope

ELP—endolaser probe; LIO—laser indirect ophthalmoscope; PRP—panretinal photocoagulation.

aged by vitrectomy and endolaser photocoagulation [58]. Finally, the carbon dioxide laser has been used to perform external drainage of subretinal fluid in scleral buckling surgery and may reduce the incidence of choroidal and subretinal hemorrhage compared with conventional techniques [59].

Glaucoma

Occasionally, eyes with advanced glaucoma have been treated by vitrectomy and laser photocoagulation. Direct ablation of the ciliary body can be performed in aphakic or pseudophakic eyes using an endoprobe when scleral depression is performed. Alternatively, laser endoscopes have been used to allow direct visualization of anterior structures during treatment. These procedures are generally reserved for eyes with severe glaucoma in which conventional therapies have failed.

COMPLICATIONS

The major complications associated with laser photocoagulation have been highlighted in Chapter 4 and are largely independent of the delivery system used. However, certain complications specifically related to endophotocoagulation merit consideration here. Appropriate filters positioned in front of the objective lens are necessary to protect the eyes of the surgeon and assistant. Although modern microscopes are generally equipped with such filters, correct placement of the filter must be confirmed before commencing treatment. The most frequent complication associated with endophotocoagulation is excessive coagulation, which can result in retinochoroidal hemorrhage alone or in conjunction with the rupture of Bruch's membrane and subsequent subretinal choroidal or choriovitreal neovascularization. This complication usually occurs when the probe is inadvertently moved closer to the retina or in treatment areas containing preretinal or intraretinal hemorrhage. Direct treatment of retinal vasculature can result in focal attenuation or occlusion of the vessel. If the probe inadvertently strikes the retina, retinal breaks or choroidal hemorrhage can result. Finally, if the probe inadvertently touches the crystalline lens, cataract usually ensues.

CONCLUSIONS

The laser has emerged as an important tool in vitreoretinal surgery and is routinely used in various clinical settings. Endophotocoagulation can be applied in a safe and efficient manner and has dramatically reduced the incidence of postoperative rubeosis and neovascular glaucoma in eyes with PDR. In addition, intraoperative endolaser photocoagulation is widely used to treat complicated retinal detachments, given its efficacy in producing chorioretinal adhesions surrounding retinal breaks and relaxing retinotomies. Sundry endolaser probes are available that facilitate treatment and enable vitreoretinal surgeons to perform bimanual manipulations. Recent innovations in photodisruptive laser technology have expanded the role of lasers to include various surgical maneuvers, such as vitreous, preretinal, and subretinal membrane transections.

REFERENCES AND RECOMMENDED READING

Recently published papers of particular interest have been highlighted as:
- • Of interest
- •• Of outstanding interest

1. Charles S: Endophotocoagulation. *Retina* 1981, 1:117–120.
2. Blankenship G, Cortez R, Machemer R: The lens and pars plan vitrectomy for diabetic retinopathy complications. *Arch Ophthalmol* 1979, 97:1263–1267.
3. Machemer R, Blankenship G: Vitrectomy for proliferative diabetic retinopathy associated with vitreous hemorrhage. *Ophthalmology* 1981, 88:643–646.
4. Michels RG, Rice TA, Rice EF: Vitrectomy for diabetic vitreous hemorrhage. *Am J Ophthalmol* 1983, 95:12–21.
5. Blankenship GW, Machemer R: Long-term diabetic vitrectomy results. Report of 10 year follow-up. *Ophthalmology* 1985, 92:503–506.
6. The Diabetic Retinopathy Vitrectomy Study Research Group: Early vitrectomy for severe proliferative diabetic retinopathy in eyes with useful vision. Results of a randomized trial—Diabetic Retinopathy Vitrectomy Study Report 3. *Ophthalmology* 1988, 95:1307–1320.
7. The Diabetic Retinopathy Vitrectomy Study Research Group: Early vitrectomy for severe vitreous hemorrhage in diabetic retinopathy. Four-year results of a randomized trial: Diabetic Retinopathy Vitrectomy Study Report 5. *Arch Ophthalmol* 1990, 108:958–964.
8. Charles S: Endophotocoagulation. *Ophthalmology Times* 1979, 4:68–69.
9. Peyman GA, Grisolano JM, Palacio MN: Intraocular photocoagulation with the argon-krypton laser. *Arch Ophthalmol* 1980, 98:2062–2064.

10. Fleischman JA, Swartz M, Dixon JA: Argon laser endophotocoagulation. An intraoperative trans-pars plana technique. *Arch Ophthalmol* 1981, 99:1610–1612.

11. Peyman GA, Salzano TC, Green JL Jr: Argon endolaser. *Arch Ophthalmol* 1981, 99:2037–2038.

12. Landers MBI, Trese MT, Stefansson E, Bessler M: Argon laser intraocular photocoagulation. *Ophthalmology* 1982, 89:785–788.

13. Peyman GA, Conway MD, Ganti S, Viherkoski EP: A neodymium-YAG endolaser. *Ophthalmic Surg* 1983, 14:309–313.

14. Miller J, Smith MR, Boyer DS: Intraocular carbon dioxide laser photocautery. *Ophthalmology* 1980, 87:1112–1120.

15. Karlin D, Jakobiec F, Harrison W, *et al.*: Endophotocoagulation in vitrectomy with a carbon dioxide laser. *Am J Ophthalmol* 1986, 101:445–450.

16. Ramsay RC, Cantrill HL, Knobloch WH: Vitrectomy and endolaser for complications of proliferative diabetic retinopathy. *Can J Ophthalmol* 1986, 21:170–174.

17. Liggett PE, Lean JS, Barlow WE, Ryan SJ: Intraoperative argon endophotocoagulation for recurrent vitreous hemorrhage after vitrectomy for diabetic retinopathy. *Am J Ophthalmol* 1987, 103:146–149.

18. Vine AK: Endolaser photocoagulation in penetrating and perforating intraocular foreign bodies. *Eur J Ophthalmol* 1991, 1:119–122.

19. Thomas MA, Halperin LS: Subretinal endolaser treatment of a choroidal bleeding site. *Am J Ophthalmol* 1990, 109:742–744.

20. Puliafito CA, Deutsch TF, Boll J, To K: Semiconductor laser endophotocoagulation of the retina. *Arch Ophthalmol* 1987, 105:424–427.

21. Smiddy WE: Diode endolaser photocoagulation. *Arch Ophthalmol* 1992, 110:1172–1174.

22. Smiddy WE, Hernandez LAT: Histologic results of retinal diode laser photocoagulation in rabbit eyes. *Arch Ophthalmol* 1992, 110:693–698.

23.• Sasoh M, Smiddy WE: Diode laser endophotocoagulation. *Retina* 1995, 15:388–393.

Intraoperative surgical goals were achieved in 226 consecutive eyes undergoing vitrectomy with diode endolaser. Functional and anatomic results were similar to those in eyes treated with argon endophotocoagulation.

24. Immonen I, Viherkoski E, Peyman GA: Experimental retinal and ciliary body photocoagulation using a new 670-nm diode laser. *Am J Ophthalmol* 1996, 122:870–874.

25. Hoggatt JS, Pulido JS, Nash RW, *et al.*: The in vivo effects of a prototype diode laser coagulator/vaporizing endoprobe used to perform retinectomy and retinotomy in rabbits. *Ophthalmic Surg Lasers* 1997, 28:231–235.

26. Jennings T, Fuller T, Vulkich J, *et al.*: Transscleral contact retinal photocoagulation with an 810 nm semiconductor diode laser. *Ophthalmic Surgery* 1990, 21:492–496.

27. Peyman GA, Naguib KS, Gaasterland D: Transscleral application of a semiconductor diode laser. *Lasers Surg Med* 1990, 10:569–575.

28. Haller JA, Lim JI, Goldberg MF: Pilot trial of transscleral diode laser retinopexy in retinal detachment surgery. *Arch Ophthalmol* 1993, 111:952–956.

29. McHugh D, Schwartz S, Dowler J, *et al.*: Diode laser contact transscleral retinal photocoagulation: A clinical study. *Br J Ophthalmol* 1995, 79:1083–1087.

30. Seiberth V, Knorz MC: Transscleral diode laser photocoagulation in proliferative sickle cell retinopathy. *Invest Ophthalmol Vis Sci* 1997, 38 (Suppl 4):5258.

31. Peyman GA: A bent-tipped endolaser probe. *Ophthalmic Surg* 1987, 18:185–186.

32. Gross JG, Freeman WR: The 30 degree curved endolaser probe. *Ann Ophthalmol* 1990, 22:382–384.

33. Peyman GA, D'Amico DJ, Alturki WA: An endolaser probe with aspiration capability. *Arch Ophthalmol* 1992, 110:718.

34. Peyman GA, Lee KJ: Multifunction endolaser probe [letter]. *Am J Ophthalmol* 1992, 114:103–104.

35. Awh CC, Schallen EH, de Juan E Jr: An illuminating laser probe for vitreoretinal surgery. *Arch Ophthalmol* 1994, 112:553–554.

36. Uram M: Laser endoscope in the management of proliferative vitreoretinopathy. *Ophthalmology* 1994, 101:1404–1408.

37. Meyers SM, Bonner RF, Rodriques MM, *et al.*: Phototransection of vitreal membranes with the carbon dioxide laser in rabbits. *Ophthalmology* 1983, 90:563–568.

38. Brown GC, Benson WE: Treatment of diabetic traction retinal detachment with the pulsed neodymium:YAG laser. *Am J Ophthalmol* 1985, 99:258–262.

39. Jagger JD, Hamilton AMP, Polkinghorne PJ: Q-switched neodymium YAG laser vitreolysis in the therapy of posterior segment disease. *Graefes Arch Clin Exp Ophthalmol* 1990, 228:222–225.

40. Gabel VP, Birngruber R, Gunther-Koszka H, Puliafito CA: Nd:YAG laser photodisruption of hemorrhagic detachment of the internal limiting. *Am J Ophthalmol* 1989, 107:33–37.

41. Kaynak S, Eryildirim A, Kaynak T, *et al.*: Nd:YAG laser posterior hyaloidotomy in subhyaloid hemorrhage. *Ophthalmic Surg* 1994, 25:474–476.

42. Ezra E, Dowler JG, Burgess F, *et al.*: Identifying maculopathy after neodymium: YAG membranotomy for dense diabetic premacular hemorrhage. *Ophthalmology* 1996, 103:1568–1574.

43. Isaacs TW, Barry C, McAllister IL: Early resolution of premacular haemorrhage following Nd:YAG laser photodisruption of posterior hyaloid. *Aust N Z J Ophthalmol* 1996, 24:365–367.

44. Pellin MJ, Williams GA, Young CE, *et al.*: Endoexcimer laser intraocular ablative photodecomposition. *Am J Ophthalmol* 1985, 99:483–484.

45. Lewis A, Palanker D, Hemo I, *et al.*: Microsurgery of the retina with a needle-guided 193-nm excimer laser. *Invest Ophthalmol Vis Sci* 1992, 33:2377–2381.

46. Borirakchanyavat S, Puliafito CA, Kliman GH, *et al.*: Holmium-YAG laser surgery on experimental vitreous membranes. *Arch Ophthalmol* 1991, 109:1605–1609.

47. Brazitikos PD, D'Amico DJ, Bernal MT, Walsh AW: Erbium:YAG laser surgery of the vitreous and retina. *Ophthalmology* 1995, 102:278–290.

48. Berger JW, D'Amico DJ: Modeling of erbium:YAG laser-mediated explosive photovaporization: Implications for vitreoretinal surgery. *Ophthalmic Surg Lasers* 1997, 28:133–139.

49. Margolis TI, Farnath DA, Destro M, Puliafito CA: Erbium-YAG laser surgery on experimental vitreous membranes. *Arch Ophthalmol* 1989, 107:424–428.

50.•• D'Amico DJ, Blumenkranz MS, Lavin MJ, *et al.*: Multicenter clinical experience using an erbium:YAG laser for vitreoretinal surgery. *Ophthalmology* 1996, 103:1575–1585.

This clinical multicenter trial established the efficacy of Er:YAG laser in performing a variety of maneuvers in vitreoretinal surgery. This modality was particularly useful in segmenting vitreous, epiretinal, and subretinal membranes as well as creating relaxing retinotomies.

51.• D'Amico DJ, Brazitikos PD, Marcellino GR, *et al.*: Initial clinical experience with an erbium:YAG laser for vitreoretinal surgery. *Am J Ophthalmol* 1996, 121:414–425.

This initial clinical study suggested that Er:YAG laser may be useful in performing transections of vitreous, preretinal, and subretinal membranes.

52. Quiroz-Mercado H: Erbium YAG produces effective shunt in CRVO patients. *Ocular Surgery News* 1998, January 1:34–35.

53. Cohen BZ, Wald KJ, Toyama K: Neodymium:YLF picosecond laser segmentation for retinal traction associated with proliferative diabetic retinopathy. *Am J Ophthalmol* 1997, 123:515–523.

54. Tassignon MJ, Brihaye M, Stempels N: Nd-YAG laser treatment in preretinal macular fibrosis. *Graefes Arch Clin Exp Ophthalmol* 1987, 225:315–320.

55. McDonald HR, Lewis H, Brown G, Sipperley JO: Vitreous surgery for retinal detachment associated with choroidal coloboma. *Arch Ophthalmol* 1991, 109:1399–1402.

56. Brown GC, Brown MM: Repair of retinal detachment associated with congenital excavated defects of the optic disc. *Ophthalmic Surgery* 1995, 26:11–15.

57. McDonald HR, Schatz H, Johnson RN, *et al.*: Vitrectomy in eyes with peripheral retinal angioma associated with traction macular detachment. *Ophthalmology* 1996, 103:329–335.

58. Alexandridis E, Kohl-Eisenhut H: Treatment of retinal detachment with macular hole. *Graefes Arch Clin Exp Ophthalmol* 1986, 224:11–12.

59. Engel JM, Blair NP, Harris D, Baker DS: Use of carbon dioxide laser in the drainage of subretinal fluid. *Arch Ophthalmol* 1989, 107:731–734.

CHAPTER 13

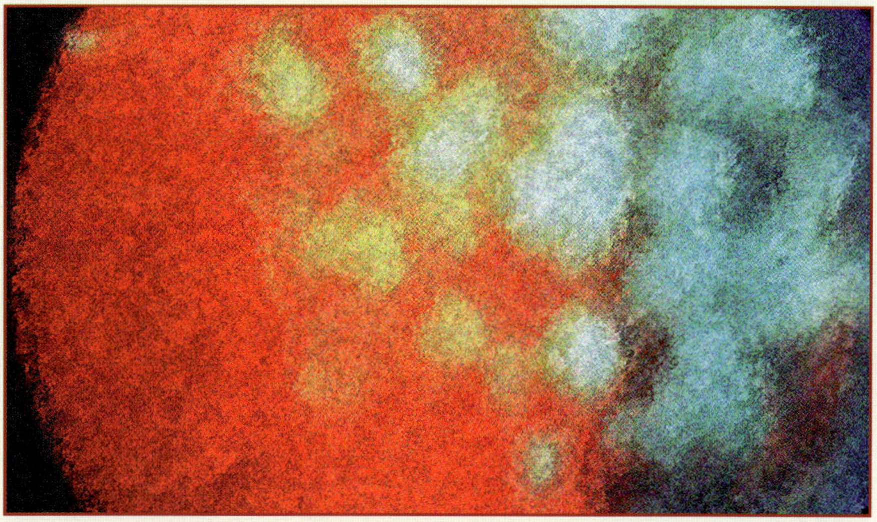

New Delivery Systems and New Uses of Lasers

JOEL M. KRAUSS
DAVID R. GUYER

New laser instruments and techniques are continually being developed, and few go untested for potential ophthalmic use. Diode lasers, aided by advances in endoprobes and indirect ophthalmoscopy and already being used to treat various vascular diseases, are becoming the treatment of choice for retinopathy of prematurity (ROP). Development of diode lasers at shorter wavelengths and pulse durations offers the potential for these devices to supplant many larger, more expensive ophthalmic lasers. Laser keratorefractive surgery is rapidly evolving, and ablation is also being studied for intraocular use. Although photodisruption, and increasingly ablation, have joined photocoagulation as established procedures, there is good reason to believe that the field of ophthalmic lasers is far from mature.

DIODE LASERS

Laser principles

Diode lasers emit radiation with exceptional electrical-to-optical efficiency (around 50%). They are much smaller, less expensive, and more portable than traditional ophthalmic lasers, and they require only a standard electrical outlet for clinical use. Such devices are constructed by joining n- and p-type semiconductors, which serve as electron donors and acceptors, respectively, creating a recombination region at their junction. The size of the band gap, across which photons jump and which thus establishes emission wavelength, is determined by the addition (doping) of other atoms. The band gap in gallium arsenide (GaAs) semiconductors is particularly well suited to producing radiation, with the application of an external electrical potential across the p–n junction creating an electron population inversion and the parallel GaAs crystal faces serving as semitransparent mirrors. Internally reflected light then stimulates further photon emission in the recombination region, ultimately resulting in coherent and monochromatic, albeit very divergent, output. Laser power is increased by constructing arrays of many diodes, with coupling between active zones making the total output spatially coherent.

Most diode lasers studied for ophthalmic use contain GaAs crystals doped with aluminum (GaAlAs), and emit between 780 and 850 nm (commercial versions are now generally 810 nm), although any given laser has only a single emission line and is not tunable. Radiation in this range is readily transmitted by the ocular media, but with less absorption than visible wavelengths by the retinal pigment epithelium (RPE) and choroid. Because this lower absorption requires higher laser power, clinically useful diode laser output is a relatively recent achievement.

Applications

Retina

In early clinical trials, McHugh *et al.* [1] and Balles *et al.* [2] demonstrated the potential efficacy of diode laser transpupillary photocoagulation, through a slit lamp biomicroscope, for treatment of such retinal vascular diseases as diabetic retinopathy, choroidal neovascular membranes, and branch and central retinal vein occlusion. The McHugh group achieved RPE photocoagulation even through a layer of blood about 150 µm thick. Neovascularization had regressed 6 weeks following treatment of diabetic retinopathy, with visual acuity changes similar to those associated with other lasers. Follow-up of all patients as much as 9 months later demonstrated the potential success of diode laser photocoagulation for these conditions.

The Balles group found that 4.5 times more energy, 2.5 times more power, and 1.8 times more irradiance and exposure duration were required to produce diode laser lesions that were clinically similar to those achieved with the argon laser, all consistent with the much lower absorption by the RPE of the longer wavelength. The deeper diode penetration, even greater than for krypton red light, necessitated retrobulbar anesthesia but resulted in only four cases of subretinal hemorrhage or rupture of Bruch's membrane in over 9000 treatment exposures. Penetration was excellent through macular edema and serous retinal thickening; transmission through cataracts and hemorrhages was much greater than for shorter-wavelength lasers, with less light scattering. Because the diode radiation is invisible, there were no complaints of bright flashes. Moreover, the permanent filter blocking the diode wavelength both permits continuous viewing throughout the procedure and eliminates the startling clicks often associated with movable shutters. However, the diode laser's greater beam divergence did require a greater intraocular focusing cone angle, which limited peripheral treatment.

Ulbig *et al.* [3] used a diode laser to close membranes in seven of nine eyes with parafoveal choroidal neovascularization secondary to age-related macular degeneration or angioid streaks, although four lesions required repeated treatment. A subsequent, larger study by Lanzetta *et al.* [4] yielded similar results. Another study Ulbig *et al.* [5] found at least partial resolution of macular edema in 27 of 33 eyes with diabetic retinopathy 6 months following transpupillary diode laser photocoagulation. They concluded that the diode laser has similar efficacy to the argon laser, as has recently been confirmed in a larger study directly comparing the two lasers [6]. In contrast to the Balles team, Ulbig's group found topical anesthesia sufficient for the diode treatments. It has also been suggested that the diode laser may be preferable to the argon laser for treating retinal vascular diseases associated with hypoxia, because under certain conditions the former causes a greater increase in the preretinal partial pressure of oxygen [7].

Given the experimental evidence that the diode laser can effectively produce chorioretinal adhesions, with less blood–retinal barrier destruction than with either cryotherapy or the argon laser [8], Haller *et al.* [9] performed transscleral diode laser retinopexy in conjunction with scleral buckling in a series of patients with rhegmatogenous retinal detachment. Mean power settings were 1162 mW for white patients and 342 mW for black patients, whereas exposure durations ranged from 1 to 9 seconds. Minor complications included a scleral thermal effect and presumed ruptures in Bruch's membrane in 30% of the patients, the ruptures accompanied by audible "pops." However, these problems were not encountered after the investigators used smaller, gray lesions as their endpoint. One logistic disadvantage was the longer procedure time compared with that of cryotherapy. Nine of 10 retinas were successfully attached at 6 months and the 10th redetached at 6 weeks secondary to proliferative vitreoretinopathy but responded to reattachment. In a similar study of transscleral diode laser photocoagulation, McHugh *et al.* [10] achieved chorioretinal adhesion in all 30 eyes treated for peripheral retinal breaks associated with retinal detachments and all six eyes with giant retinal tears. Although three eyes sustained punctate choroidal hemorrhages, it was thought that for giant retinal tears, in particular, this approach is less traumatic and less likely to cause proliferative vitreoretinopathy than is cryotherapy.

Glaucoma

Schuman *et al.* [11] reported the first human iridectomies produced with the diode laser, occasionally encountering the same mild anterior lens capsule opacity sometimes seen with the argon laser, especially with longer exposures and larger spot sizes. In a larger clinical series, Emoto *et al.* [12] employed a two-step method of circular burns to stretch the iris (200 mW, 0.2 seconds, 200 µm), followed by penetrating burns (1000 mW, 0.05 seconds, 75 µm), with a mean total of 152 burns. Iritis developed in all patients but responded to topical corticosteroids. Other complications included pupillary distortion (70%), transient anterior lens capsule opacification (60%), intraocular pressure (IOP) rise greater than 10 mm Hg (20%), and corneal endothelial lesions (5%). Focal cataract developed in 5% of eyes but resolved within 3 months. All openings remained patent at 9 months.

McHugh *et al.* [13] conducted a pilot clinical investigation of diode laser trabeculoplasty (LTP). Employing parameters of 0.8 to 1.2 W, 0.2 seconds, and 100 µm, and placing 50 burns for 180°, they noted that the desired exposure endpoint was a mild blanching of the pigmented portion of the trabecular meshwork. That these lesions were just above threshold was suggested by the absence of bubble formation, in contrast to that seen with the argon laser procedure. However, IOP was lowered just as much as with the more established laser (9.6 mm Hg at 6 months), with an even greater effect 2 to 4 weeks after the LTP, possibly as a result of the deeper penetration at 810 nm. Consistent with the lighter lesions and absence of bubbles, no IOP spike immediately followed treatment. As is sometimes seen with the argon laser, a mild IOP reduction was found in the fellow, untreated eye, suggesting that LTP may release chemical mediators. These researchers also showed that the trabecular meshwork damage is histologically similar whether LTP is performed with the diode or argon laser, further reflecting the procedure's independence of wavelength [14]. Indeed, in a direct clinical comparison, Brancato *et al.* [15] showed that patients undergoing diode LTP retained the same lowering of IOP through 12 months as those individuals treated with argon LTP. Moriarty *et al.* [16] noted only a small reversal in IOP decline, from 8.4 to 7.9 mm Hg, between 12 and 24 months after diode LTP, without the peripheral anterior synechiae seen in many argon LTP cases.

Initial clinical studies of contact diode laser cyclophotocoagulation by Gaasterland *et al.* [17] realized average IOP reductions from 36 mm Hg prelaser to 23 mm Hg at 3-month follow-up without any hypotony but with mild surface burns in 40% of patients. The lower scleral transmission at 810 versus 1064 nm can be largely overcome by employing scleral indentation with a probe [18].

In the latest and most comprehensive evaluation of contact diode laser transscleral cyclophotocoagulation to treat refractory glaucoma, Bloom *et al.* [19•] treated 210 eyes with 20 to 40 applications of 1.5 W for 1.5 seconds each over 180° to 360°, achieving a mean IOP reduction from 34.1 mm Hg to 20.1 mm Hg (two thirds below 22 mm Hg) at an average follow-up of 10 months. Approximately half the eyes required further treatments within several months of the first, up to a total of five treatments (mean 1.75). Visual acuity improved in 11% of eyes, remained unchanged in 60%, and decreased in 29%, whereas the number of required glaucoma medications decreased from an average of 2.3 to 1.7. Complications included one patient each with hypotony, phthisis, macular pucker, and combined hyphema/vitreous hemorrhage, and two with corneal graft decompensation. Whereas higher power settings may be more effective in lowering IOP and necessitate fewer re-treatments, they have also been found to cause more side effects [20]. The efficacy of diode laser cyclophotocoagulation is similar to that with the neodymium:yttrium-aluminum-garnet (Nd:YAG) laser [21] and somewhat less than that of drainage tube implants, albeit with fewer complications. Longer-term studies are needed to determine the duration of IOP lowering and the role of late re-treatments.

ENDOLASER

As clinical experience with the diode laser accumulates, concomitant progress has been made in refining both the laser itself and the means for delivering its output to the eye. This laser's compactness makes it particularly well suited to use with the endoprobe and indirect ophthalmoscope (Fig. 13-1). Numerous applications have been developed for endophotocoagulation since the technique was first introduced in the early 1980s. Smiddy [22] reported the first clinical use of diode endolaser photocoagulation, treating patients with proliferative diabetic retinopathy (PDR), proliferative vitreoretinopathy, complex retinal detachments, and retinal breaks. Exposure parameters were dictated by the specific pathology, always avoiding reaching the whitish lesions typically expected with the argon laser, which with the diode laser have been associated with iatrogenic choroidal folds [23]. As had been noted in other studies, treatment through small amounts of preretinal blood was facilitated by the diode's wavelength, but this had the corresponding disadvantage of preventing coagulation of bleeding stumps. Overall, it was believed that endophotocoagulation with the diode laser is as clinically efficacious as with the argon laser, but the former offers significant logistic and ergonomic advantages.

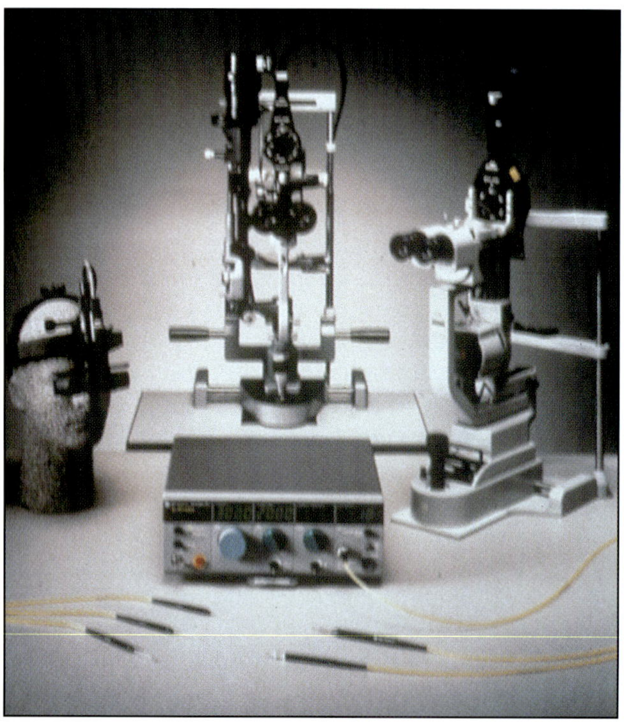

FIGURE 13-1. OcuLight SLx diode laser (Iris Medical Instruments, Mountain View, CA) has three modalities by which up to 2 W can be delivered to the eye: slit lamp biomicroscope, endoprobe, and indirect ophthalmoscope. The laser console measures 10 cm × 30 cm × 30 cm, weighs 5.5 kg, and runs on either 115 or 230 V without requiring external air or water cooling.

In the past few years, considerable advances have been made in probe technology, especially in conjunction with the diode laser, all aimed at maximizing functions that can be performed by a single probe. Peyman *et al.* [24] developed a couple of such 20-gauge devices, combining fiberoptic diode or argon lasers and aspiration and infusion capabilities, with one device also including fiberoptic illumination. These instruments can be used both to drain subretinal fluid and to photocoagulate the retinotomy site, thereby obviating repeated forays into the eye with separate instruments. Uram [25] also constructed 18- and 20-gauge probes incorporating diode laser and illumination fiberoptics, but rather than an aspiration–infusion capability, Uram's probe has a microendoscope with recording capability and a 75° (20-gauge) or 110° (18-gauge) field of view. These devices are able to deliver precisely titrated laser exposures to a specific number of ciliary processes under direct visualization, potentially enabling more effective treatment of certain forms of glaucoma—such as congenital glaucoma with displacement of the ciliary processes [26]—than is possible with a transscleral approach. Vitreoretinal endophotocoagulation is similarly facilitated, with the probe providing a clear view even when more anterior structures would obscure the view through an operating microscope, and permitting posttreatment inspection for retinal breaks without resorting to indirect ophthalmoscopy. Using a diode laser and coagulator/vaporizing endoprobe with a carbon-coated tip to perform retinectomies and retinotomies in rabbits, Hoggatt *et al.* [27] found that high power (500 to 750 mW) and short duration (100 ms) effectively created full-thickness retinal breaks and coagulation, whereas low power (100 to 200 mW) and long duration (500 ms) caused extensive choroidal and scleral burns.

LASER INDIRECT OPHTHALMOSCOPE

The laser indirect ophthalmoscope (LIO) is another instrument that has had increased use during the past decade [28•]. Unlike with slip lamp delivery, the spot size is impossible to standardize, because it depends on the power and position of the hand-held and headset lenses, the refractive power of the treated eye, and the presence of intraocular gas. Macular work is not recommended given the inherent limitations in aiming. However, the field of view is greater than with other laser modalities, and in conjunction with scleral depression, this technique reduces the laser power needed for photocoagulation, probably as a result of the stretched choroid's diminished ability to dissipate heat from the RPE. The LIO is useful in cases requiring far peripheral treatment, such as retinal tears or peripheral neovascularization, especially those with localized lens opacities or small pupils. It is essential for pneumatic retinopexy reattachment or laser treatment of ROP, and it has also been reported for treatment of retinoblastoma [29] and choroidal melanoma [30]. Complications include occasional choroidal hemorrhage from too-intense exposures, superficial burns of the iris and cornea [31], and melted Prolene haptics.

Retinopathy of prematurity is a potentially devastating condition affecting, to some extent, about two thirds of infants with birth weight below 1251 g. Cryotherapy has assumed an important role in treating ROP, almost halving the rate of unfavorable anatomic outcomes. Nevertheless, it is often ineffective, frequently requires intravenous sedation, and is associated with such complications as intraocular hemorrhage, retinal detachment, scleral trauma, apnea, bradycardia, and oxygen desaturation.

Although photocoagulation of ROP was first proposed almost 30 years ago, not until widespread use of the LIO did it become a viable alternative to cryotherapy. Landers *et al.* [32] reported the first use of this technique, and in another, more extensive investigation [33], they used an argon laser to create an average of 696 burns of 500 to 900 mW, 0.2 to 1.0 seconds, and 400 to 500 μm, resulting in favorable 6-month outcomes in 73% of infants with at least threshold, stage 3 "plus" disease. Iverson *et al.* [34] and McNamara *et al.* [35] conducted preliminary clinical trials directly comparing cryotherapy with argon LIO photocoagulation of threshold ROP. Both groups concluded that photocoagulation was at least as effective as cryotherapy, with less trauma to the eye.

Given its technical convenience, the diode laser has been the subject of most recent studies on photocoagulation of ROP [36–44]. Fleming *et al.* [36] used the diode LIO at 180 to 200 mW, 0.3 seconds, and approximately 676 μm to treat infants with prethreshold, posterior ROP. No complications arose, and all disease had subsided by 24 weeks. The researchers also indicated that the criteria for treating this condition should be less stringent than those for the less aggressive anterior form of ROP.

McNamara *et al.* [37] and Hunter *et al.* [38] performed randomized trials comparing diode LIO photocoagulation and cryotherapy for treatment of threshold ROP. In the McNamara study, exposure parameters were 120 to 600 mW and 0.3 seconds, with an average of 959 burns placed (Fig. 13-2). Transient vitreous hemorrhages were noted in 3.6% of the laser-treated eyes and 12.5% of the cryotherapy-treated eyes. Lid edema, conjunctival hyperemia, and chemosis lasting 1 to 3 days were found in all eyes treated with cryotherapy, whereas one laser-treated eye showed mild conjunctival hyperemia lasting only several hours. Pain was difficult to assess but appeared to be comparable with that seen in treatment with an argon laser and less than that with cryotherapy. In the laser-treated group, 25 of 28 eyes observed for 3 months and all seven of those receiving follow-up for 1 year showed regression; the corresponding numbers for the cryotherapy group were 20 of 24 eyes observed for 3 months and all seven of the 1-year group. Diode laser treatment was thus found at least as efficacious as cryotherapy and has the advantage over the argon laser of being portable, thus permitting treatment in neonatal units that might not have access to other lasers. Moreover, the diode laser's wavelength permits treatment through blood and minimizes damage or cataract formation in infants with persistent tunica vasculosa lentis [41]. Laser spots were placed one half burn width apart, sometimes necessitating re-treatment in "skip" areas. It has been suggested, however, that, as with cryotherapy, no such zones need be left untreated, given that photocoagulation appears at least as safe as cryotherapy [39].

Similar results were obtained by the Hunter group [38], despite employing a somewhat different photocoagulation strategy. Observing that, unlike in the treatment of subretinal neovascular disease in adults, the diode laser's deeper penetration and sparing of the inner retina with its capillary endothelial precursors

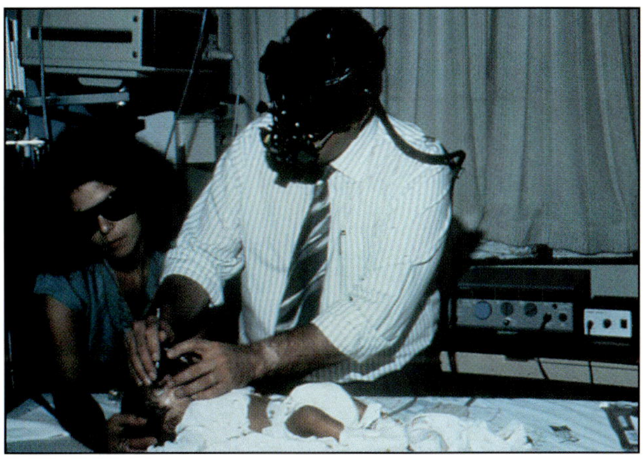

FIGURE 13-2. Diode laser indirect ophthalmoscope photocoagulation for retinopathy of prematurity. (*Courtesy of* Iris Medical Instruments, Mountain View, CA.)

may be a disadvantage in treating ROP, they used a clinical endpoint of creamy white lesions in attempting to extend the laser damage to the inner retina. In only one instance did this result in a subretinal hemorrhage consistent with a rupture of Bruch's membrane.

Studies over the past several years have consistently shown that photocoagulation, particularly with the diode laser is at least as good as and generally better than cryotherapy in treating various forms of ROP [40–44]. O'Keefe *et al.* [40] found that diode laser photocoagulation of the vascular retina posterior to the ridge caused regression in some infants with advanced stage 3 or stage 4A ROP who had previously received treatment to the avascular retina for threshold stage 3 disease. Laser treatment may have a greater advantage over cryotherapy in treating posterior zone I or II ROP than anterior–mid zone II ROP [42]. A long-term sequela of cryotherapy for ROP is the progressive development of myopia, perhaps because of damage to the developing sclera at an actively growing site. Most studies have shown much greater refractive stability up to 3 years following treatment with the diode (and argon) laser [43], although one smaller study found no significant difference [44].

ABLATION

The recent ophthalmic laser development with the most widespread potential applicability, and which has thus received the greatest public attention, is corneal ablation. Photorefractive keratectomy (PRK) with the excimer laser at 193 nm has become a highly successful clinical procedure some 15 years after the first experimental reports. Nevertheless, the technology and techniques are still evolving, and there have been many reports of potential alternatives to the excimer laser. Moreover, although the cornea remains the most common and suitable target for laser ablation, there has been considerable interest in extending the process to intraocular structures.

Cornea

Various excimer laser delivery systems and ablation strategies are continually being studied to optimize refractive outcome and minimize healing complications [45]. However, clinical considerations aside, the excimer laser's considerable size, cost, and energy requirement represent significant impediments to its widespread use. LaserSight's (Orlando, FL) Compak-200 Mini-Excimer laser operates from a 110-V outlet, is air cooled, and uses an excimer gas mixture containing only 0.19% fluorine. Because this device can generate sufficient fluences for ablation only over spot sizes 1.0 to 1.5 mm in diameter, it uses a computer-controlled "flying spot" system at 100 Hz to treat the cornea. Of the first 50 eyes treated in a US Food and Drug Administration (FDA) phase IIa study, over 80% had uncorrected visual acuity of at least 20/40 [46]. LaserSight recently introduced the LaserScan LSX (Fig. 13-3), which has a new ceramic laserhead and produces 10-nanosecond, 200-Hz output, and whose 0.8- to 1.0-mm flying spot yields fluences of 120 to 160 mJ/cm^2 when scanned over ablation zones up to 9 mm in diameter. The laser, which weighs less than 450 lb, also offers true active eye tracking.

For excimer laser PRK to realize its full potential, there must be disruption, if not obliteration, of what has traditionally been viewed as the inviolable Bowman's membrane. Although, in conjunction with steroids or antimetabolites, the cornea appears to heal with little or no residual scarring, the long-term implications of this procedure remain to be determined. Laser-assisted in situ keratomileusis (LASIK) avoids this problem, but the procedure is technically much more demanding than PRK. Moreover, there is concern about exposure to fluorine gas with any excimer laser procedure. Some researchers have thus proposed selective intrastromal ablation without damage to the anterior layers as an alternative to excimer laser anterior ablation. However, endeavors in this area with the Q-switched Nd:YAG laser at 500 to 2000 Hz and 100 nanoseconds [47]; the frequency-doubled Nd:YAG laser at 532 nm, 8 nanoseconds, 40 to 350 μJ [48]; and the Nd:yttrium-lithium-fluoride (Nd:YLF) laser at 1053 nm, 60 picoseconds, 20 to 350 μJ, and 10 to 1000 Hz [49] do not suggest that they are likely successors to the excimer.

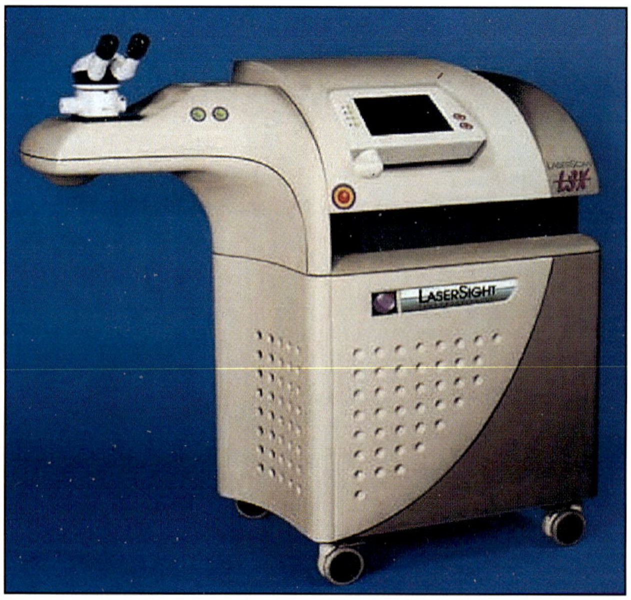

FIGURE 13-3. LaserScan LSX argon fluoride excimer laser (LaserSight, Orlando, FL).

Although extremely inefficient, the free electron laser is capable of generating a wide range of infrared wavelengths (approximately 2 to 9 μm) and allows independent variation of wavelength, energy, and pulse duration. Very preliminary studies achieved corneal ablation, but it remains to be determined whether this is preferable to any of the solid-state infrared lasers [50,51]. Early worries about possible mutagenesis with the argon fluoride excimer laser appear to have subsided, and, despite the achievement of infrared laser ablation, researchers have not been able to duplicate the precision achieved by the excimer [52,53]. As such, several groups are studying solid-state, ultraviolet alternatives. Researchers from the Bascom Palmer Eye Institute are collaborating with LaserSight on the use of the Nd:YAG fifth harmonic laser at 213 nm (achieved with a combination of cesium-dihydrogen-arsenate and barium borate crystals [54]) for possible ablation [55]. Tissue is removed by scanning a 0.5- to 1.0-mm beam across the cornea to achieve the desired profile [56]. Preliminary results revealed ablations similar to those of the excimer laser, with zones of damage less than 1 μm wide and without step-like transitions [57,58]. Photon Data (Winter Park, FL) is developing a system based on the frequency-quintupled Nd:YAG laser, although clinical trials have yet to begin and commercial availability is at least several years away [45]. The ultimate goal of this group is the development of a laser capable of generating several harmonics at various pulse durations, potentially also permitting photocoagulation and photodisruption [59].

Researchers at Tufts University and Schwartz Electro-Optics (Concord, MA) investigated ablation with the solid-state titanium-sapphire laser, using barium borate crystals to quadruple the frequency of its 10-nanosecond, 10-Hz output to 205 to 225 nm [60]. This laser, or perhaps a frequency-quintupled Nd:YLF laser [61], is at the heart of the LightBlade2 laser, which is manufactured by Novatec Laser Systems (Carlsbad, CA), and about which little technologic information is available (Fig. 13-4) [62, 63]. This solid-state laser with the most clinical refractive usage to date incorporates an eye-tracking system and produces fluences of 100 to 150 mJ/cm^2 with a 200 to 500 μm flying spot capable of ablating zones up to 12 mm in diameter. In FDA phase IIa studies, all 49 eyes treated for myopia of 1 to 6 diopters (D) had uncorrected visual acuity of at least 20/32, whereas 68.4% achieved 20/20 or better. Ablations were particularly smooth, probably as a result of both the precise scanning algorithm and the laser's operation in the fundamental mode, which eliminates the hot spots frequently experienced with multimode excimer lasers. Under an investigational device exemption, the LightBlade2 has been approved for FDA trials for myopia up to 12 D, with plans for studies of hyperopia, LASIK, and extremely high myopia.

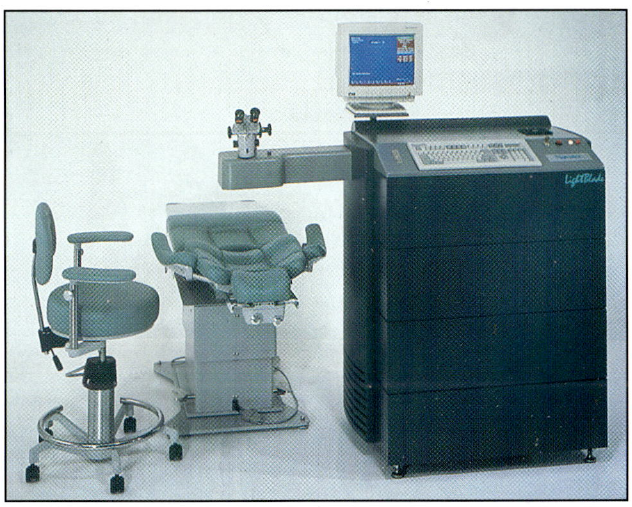

FIGURE 13-4. LightBlade laser workstation (Novatec Laser Systems, Carlsbad, CA).

Retina and vitreous

Although retinal photocoagulation was the first medical procedure to use lasers, practical applications of ablation in the posterior segment have been far more elusive. The carbon dioxide (CO_2) laser at 10.6 μm has had very limited experimental use, cannot be employed close to the retina, is large and inefficient, and requires an articulated arm. Selective RPE photocoagulation has been reported with the Q-switched Nd:YAG [64], micropulsed diode [65] and argon [66], and Nd:YLF [67] lasers. Stern *et al.* [68] have suggested that the use of pulses in the picosecond domain just above the ablation threshold may significantly reduce untoward thermal and mechanical effects, allowing safe cutting very near the retina. Indeed, Lin *et al.* [69] showed that 100-picosecond Nd:YAG laser pulses at 50 to 200 Hz achieved optical breakdown and efficient cutting in vitreous with only 70 μJ of energy, almost two orders of magnitude less than that used in nanosecond-level Nd:YAG lasers.

Borirakchanyavat *et al.* [70] attempted transection of experimental vitreous membranes using a 250-μs pulsed holmium:yttrium-aluminum-garnet (Ho:YAG) laser at 2.12 μm. When an optical fiber was used alone, only thin membranes could be sectioned at energy levels or repetition rates that permitted work near the retina. This problem was solved by encasing the fiber in a retinal-shielding pick, which allowed almost three quarters of the membranes, as close as 0.5 mm to the retina, to be completely transected. The laser directly caused one nonhemorrhagic retinal burn, whereas the pick caused two retinal injuries, including one with a small hemorrhage. Cutting precision was histologically comparable with that of the CO_2 laser, but an order of magnitude less than that of the erbium:yttrium-aluminum-garnet (Er:YAG) laser.

Margolis *et al.* [71] used a solid-state, fiberoptic-coupled, 250-μs pulsed Er:YAG laser at 2.94 μm—corresponding to an absorption peak of water—to cut experimental vitreous membranes in rabbits at distances of 500 to 3600 μm from the retina. All attempts at cutting the membranes were successful, although 53% resulted in some form of retinal lesion, as either hemorrhages or nonhemorrhagic burns. Nevertheless, the 200- to 300-μm size of the burns was not considered a contraindication to clinical application of the technique if the membranes occurred in extramacular sites. Lin *et al.* [72] showed that the Er:YAG output creates a bubble at the tip of the fiber through which it is transmitted, which can cause thermal and mechanical tissue damage. To minimize the size and movement of this bubble, and thus the resulting damage to the retina, they suggested reducing the pulse energy below 0.5 mJ and using a shielded tip. These steps may have their own adverse consequences, namely, requiring a higher repetition rate and decreasing some advantages of laser ablation over mechanical cutting for removal of membranes tightly adherent to the retinal surface, respectively.

Further studies have been conducted on Er:YAG vitreoretinal surgery [73,74,75•,76]. In 1996, D'Amico *et al.* [74] reported the first clinical trial, using an Er:YAG laser at 0.2 to 5.0 mJ, 300 μs, and 2 to 30 Hz, and a flexible fiberoptic and interchangeable 20-gauge endoprobes with tips ranging from 100 to 365 μm, to perform various procedures in both the posterior and anterior segments in 13 patients. Ablated areas were surrounded by a zone of thermal coagulation 15 to 40 μm thick, with rare and minor complications. In a larger, multicenter study employing the same Er:YAG laser apparatus and parameters, 66 patients underwent a total of 174 procedures [75•]. Among the results, 84% were deemed good or excellent, with a range of 100% for transection of subretinal membranes to 25% for coagulation of blood vessels. Minor bleeding from transected vessels occurred in 29% of retinotomies, intraocular lens damage in 18% of posterior capsulotomies, and retinal break or photocoagulation injury in 5% of epiretinal membrane incisions. High water absorption at 2.94 μm required holding the endoprobe tip very close to the tissue in fluid-filled eyes, whereas ablation was achieved across several millimeters in air-filled eyes. The precision of the laser approach exceeded that possible with conventional techniques, although critical work near the retina proceeded very slowly and visualization—such as of the macula in air-filled eyes—was difficult. A mathematical model suggests that Er:YAG ablation would be optimized and mechanical injury minimized by using small-diameter probe tips, low pulse energies, and repetition rates as high as 1000 Hz [76].

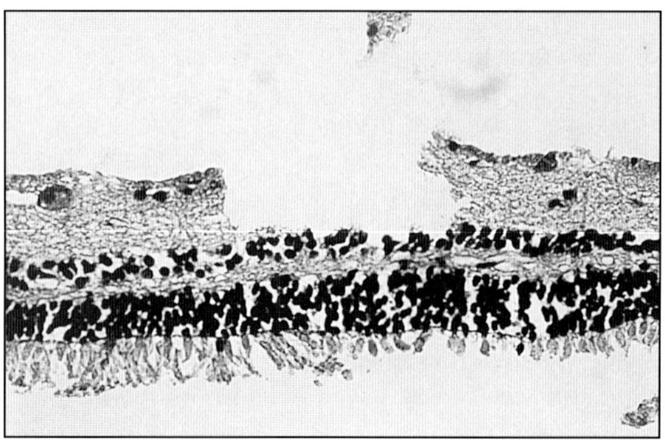

FIGURE 13-5. Ablation to the inner nuclear layer in a bovine retina, 40-μm deep, created with the argon fluoride excimer laser at 1.2 J/cm²/pulse. (*From* Lewis *et al.* [77]; with permission.)

A significant impediment to the intraocular use of 193-nm excimer laser radiation is the technical difficulty in transmitting it with the necessary accuracy. Lewis *et al.* [77] constructed a guide consisting of a fused silica lens of 1000-mm focal length and a rapidly tapered stainless steel tube whose outer diameter was that of an 18-gauge needle, with an inner diameter of 120 μm. They used this instrument to ablate bovine cadaver retinas and rabbit retinas in vivo following lensectomy and vitrectomy, employing pulses of 0.5 to 1.2 J/cm^2 and 120 μm, at 30 to 100 Hz. After a low pressure stream of air had been used to displace the thin layer of adherent fluid from the area to be treated, they were able to achieve retinal ablation with the precision typically associated with the cornea (Fig. 13-5). Possible applications include ablation of epiretinal membranes—as even a slight amount of underlying fluid would protect the retina—and the creation of precise retinotomies and retinectomies. Subsequent refinement of the delivery tip permitted ablation in a fluid environment, with tissue removal of 25 to 120 μm per pulse at energies of 0.075 to 0.17 mJ/pulse [78], and these researchers recently reported the first clinical application of this technique [79]. Using an energy of 0.12 ± 0.02 mJ/pulse, they performed tractionless cutting of preretinal and subretinal membranes in three patients with PDR or proliferative vitreoretinopathy without damaging adjacent tissue. Unlike radiation from the Er:YAG or CO_2 lasers, radiation from the excimer laser at 193 nm is not absorbed by water, nor does it penetrate tissue as deeply as the Nd:YAG output. Thus, ablation occurred only when the tip was in direct contact with the tissue and was precise and limited. The main drawbacks of this method were technical, and further improvements are expected. The articulated arm is heavy and has poor flexibility. Access was gained through relatively large 1.5-mm sclerotomies. Cutting of subretinal bands was performed through holes made in the retina, which were slightly larger than the tip diameter of 0.28 mm.

DIAGNOSTIC LASERS

Scanning laser ophthalmoscope

The scanning laser ophthalmoscope (SLO) uses a low-power laser beam to scan horizontally and vertically across the retina, creating a raster pattern that is used to map the retina or take highly localized measurements. The SLO also has excellent depth resolution and can produce three-dimensional, tomographic images that are particularly valuable in analyzing the optic disc in glaucoma [80] as well as edema, scars, and macular holes [81]. The SLO provides highly accurate and reproducible data, with whose variation from more traditional measurement techniques the clinician must nevertheless be familiar [82,83].

The contrast of the SLO image can be further enhanced by employing confocal optics [84]. Figure 13-6 shows a confocal SLO specifically designed to analyze the retinal nerve fiber layer (RNFL). It uses a polarization detector to produce a thickness map of the RNFL to document and follow glaucomatous and other changes [85–87]. Normal RNFLs have a symmetric, hourglass-shaped distribution that is gradually eroded as glaucoma progresses. The thickness of the form birefringent RNFL determines the degree to which the low-power diode laser beam is polarized [88]. The SLO obtains readings in less than 1 second, does not require pupil dilation, may be used in patients with cataracts, and avoids the flashes associated with conventional fundus photography. Because the RNFL does not ordinarily exceed 150 μm in thickness, but the optical depth resolution of the human eye is around 200 μm, the potential advantage of this method—with its resolution of 15 to 20 μm—over standard photographic techniques is apparent [89].

Figure 13-7 shows how a tomographic SLO is employed to perform topographic analysis of the retina. This device, which relies on specular reflection of laser light from the retina's internal limiting membrane, can be used to determine optic nerve head volume [90] and map the macula [91,92] and tumors. Unlike the confocal SLO, which measures thickness, the tomographic SLO assesses contour.

Visual evoked potentials can be measured more precisely with the SLO [93]. Visual function testing is performed by varying the SLO laser beam intensity to create patterns in the raster. The examiner sees the same pattern, localized to a specific portion of the retina, that

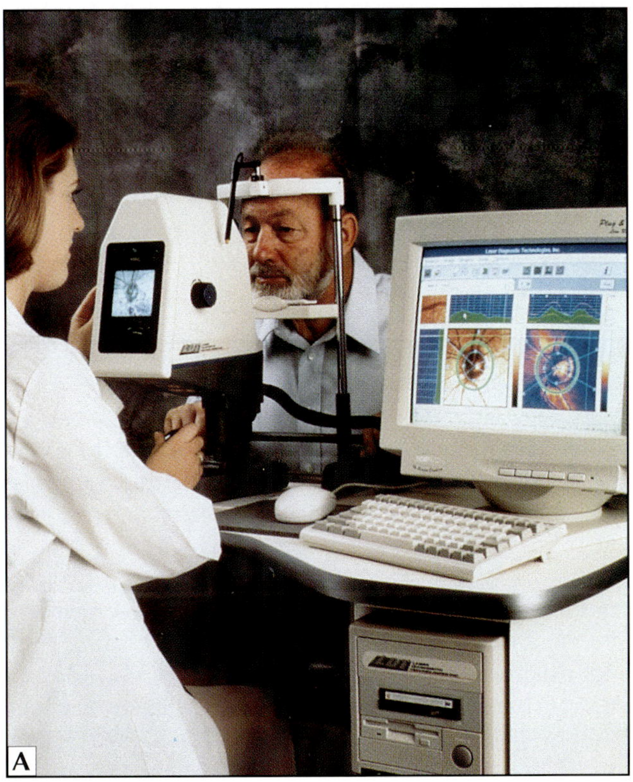
A

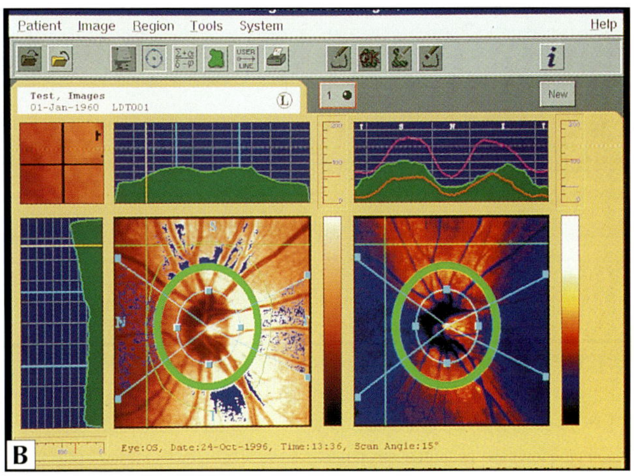

B

FIGURE 13-6. **A,** Instrument head of the GDx Nerve Fiber Layer Analyzer (Laser Diagnostic Technologies, San Diego, CA). An integrated monitor allows the physician to view the retina and maintain simultaneous eye contact with the patient. **B,** Fundus image and thickness map. Bright colors on the latter correspond to thick areas of the nerve fiber layer, whereas dark colors represent areas of thinning. The double-hump pattern above the thickness map shows the normal range and the specific thickness for the patient. In this case, the nerve fiber layer is within the normal range, but is very close to the lower limits in the inferonasal area.

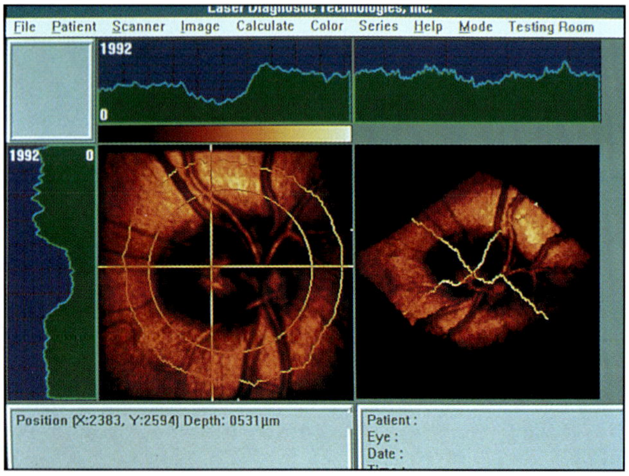

FIGURE 13-7. Display screen of the Topographic Scanning System (TopSS) (Laser Diagnostic Technologies, San Diego, CA). At *left* is an intensity image of an optic nerve head. *Above left,* horizontal and vertical cross sections, respectively, are shown through the optic nerve head. At *right* is a three-dimensional view of the same optic nerve head. The viewing angle can be adjusted by the physician. *Above right,* A peripapillary retinal contour of nerve fiber layer height along the circle superimposed around the optic nerve head is displayed.

the patient perceives, thus allowing the locus of fixation to be correlated with retinal pathology [94].

Angiography is another process that has been aided by the SLO. Less fluorescein is excited by an argon blue laser than is required with conventional angiography, yielding more and higher resolution images [95]. A method for stereoscopic video angiography has been described [96]. The SLO has been particularly important for indocyanine green (ICG) angiography, in which the low-fluorescence dye is excited by a diode laser to delineate subretinal neovascular membranes more precisely, as well as other retinal and choroidal pathology [97–100]. An alternate technique—combining slit lamp and helium-neon (He-Ne) 543-nm laser illumination—has been described to enhance visualization of fine vitreoretinal structures [101].

Laser flare and cell meter

Anterior segment inflammation, which may result from numerous types of intraocular pathology, causes breakdown of the blood–aqueous barrier and increased aqueous protein and cells. Fluorophotometry was the first method to quantify this process objectively but it is relatively time-consuming and requires intravenous injection of dye. In 1988, Sawa *et al.* [102] developed a slit lamp–based instrument, the Laser Flare Cell Meter (LFCM) (Kowa Acculas, San Jose, CA), that employed a low-power He-Ne or diode laser to detect the amount of protein and the number of cells in the anterior chamber (Fig. 13-8). Flare, produced by the Tyndall phenomenon, is linearly related to protein over a wide range of protein concentrations. Flare measurements with the LFCM are much more precise than with routine slit lamp biomicroscopy, are corrected for background scatter, are reproducible to within 8% [103], and take less than 1 second. These readings may be converted directly to protein concentration if the protein's type is known, but not in cases of heterogeneous scatterers such as low-molecular weight albumin and high-molecular weight globulins. Studies have revealed that flare has a diurnal variation [104] and tends to increase with age [105]. The LFCM has been used clinically to examine inflammation associated with uveitis of various etiologies [106], retinal detachment [107], cataract removal and intraocular lens insertion [108], posterior capsulotomy [109], and LTP [110]. Cytomegalovirus retinitis is a frequent finding in AIDS patients, and the LFCM's ability to detect slight increases in aqueous flare before any retinal changes are visible allows earlier institution of treatment [111].

To count cells, the laser beam is repeatedly scanned over a 0.465 mm^3 volume, with peaks further analyzed so that only leukocytes are registered. Cell count is less reproducible than flare measurement, especially with relatively few particles, whereas a spurious cell count in the clinical absence of cells may be caused by agglutination of proteins in high concentrations [112]. There is also less correlation with direct slip lamp measurements, which are made over larger volumes and longer periods, so that the clinical value of this application is less certain than that of flare.

Laser interferometer

The interference pattern produced with the laser interferometer is largely independent of the eye's various optical components. It offers the potential to assess visual acuity by projecting the pattern onto the retina and determining the greatest periodicity (corresponding to the closest fringe spacing) at which the subject is able to resolve discrete fringes [113]. Recently, laser interferometric techniques have been described for precise depth measurements of the cornea, retina, and other ocular structures. Both Fabry Perot and Michelson systems have been developed and offer the promise of highly accurate measurements in one and two dimensions [114–134].

Use of the laser Doppler principle allows considerably faster readings than can be achieved by interpretation of static interferometric images. Selection of intraocular lens refractive power is based largely on the eye's axial length, which the noncontact laser interferometric approach may determine more precisely and safely than the standard ultrasound method [134]. Although patient fixation is required with the laser, further technical enhancements should reduce scan time to under 1 second.

Optical coherence tomography

Researchers from Tufts University and the Massachusetts Institute of Technology have developed a new interferometric method of ocular tissue imaging. Known as optical coherence tomography (OCT) [116–132], it is a two-dimensional extension of laser interferometric ranging techniques that produces high-resolution, cross-sectional images of the eye [117,119]. OCT is similar to ultrasound B-mode imaging, except that the use of light rather than sound allows much higher image resolution with a noninvasive and noncontact measurement. Distance information is derived from the time-of-flight delay of light reflected from different structures within the eye using low-coherence interferometry. With this approach, interference fringes appear at a detector only when the path length of light reflected from the eye matches a reference path length to within the coherence length of the light source. A short coherence-length superluminescent diode light source enables a longitudinal resolution of around 10 μm. The transverse resolution is determined by the probe beam's spot size on the retina and can be made as small as a few μm. Optical heterodyne detection and the application of noise reduction techniques originally developed for optical communication achieve a high sensitivity to weakly reflected light.

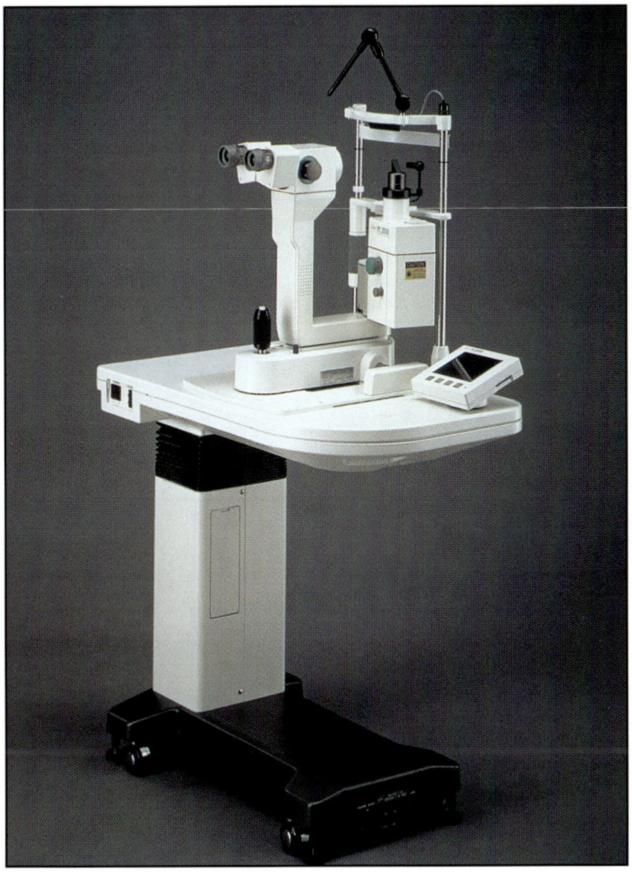

FIGURE 13-8. Kowa FC-2000 laser flare cell meter (Kowa Acculas, San Jose, CA).

The high resolution and sensitivity of OCT make it uniquely suited among current ophthalmic imaging modalities for tomography of the human retina. The available numeric aperture and ocular aberration limit the resolution at the retina of scanning confocal imaging devices, whereas acoustic attenuation makes the posterior segment unreachable by high frequency ultrasound. Figure 13-9 shows a false-color OCT tomograph obtained through the macula and optic disc of a human volunteer. Bright and dim colors correspond to regions of high and low relative optical reflectivity, respectively. The cross-sectional anatomy of the fovea and disc is evident, as is the layered structure of the retina. The posterior retina is bounded by a red layer corresponding to the choriocapillaris and RPE. Significantly reduced reflectivity from the photoreceptors is observed just anterior to this layer. The retinal nerve fibers are visible as a brightly back-scattering layer that increases in thickness toward the optic disc. OCT shows significant promise for the quantitative evaluation and monitoring of a variety of diseases of the macula and optic nerve head. Initial clinical studies [123–126, 128–131] have shown that OCT is useful in staging macular holes, evaluating vitreous detachments and traction of the vitreous on the retina, quantifying retinal thickness in macular edema and neovascularization, monitoring detachments of the neurosensory

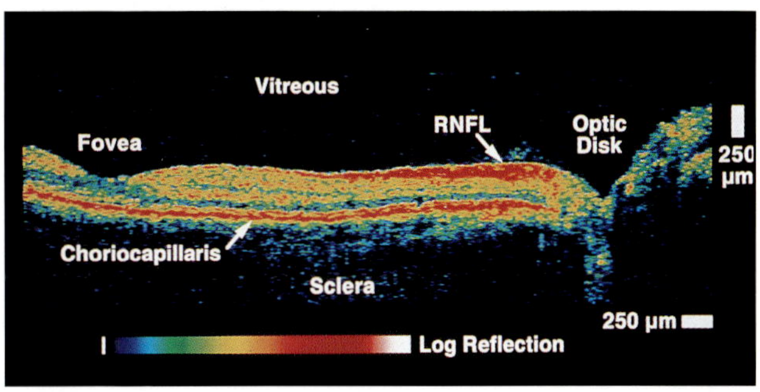

FIGURE 13-9. False-color optical coherence tomography image obtained through the macula and optic disc of a human eye. (*From* Krauss and Puliafito [135]; with permission.)

retina and RPE, measuring RNFL degeneration in glaucoma, and assessing the rapidly evolving retinal changes induced by laser photocoagulation.

OCT can also image the anterior eye [127]. The micrometer-scale resolution permits accurate biometry of large-scale ocular structures as well as the evaluation of changes in cellular morphology associated with pathologies of the cornea, iris, and lens. Figure 13-10 shows an OCT image of the anterior eye. Reflected signals are evident within both nominally transparent structures, such as the cornea and lens, and throughout opaque ones, such as the iris and sclera. Anterior chamber depth and angle, corneal thickness and curvature, and refractive power may be directly extracted from the image.

Laser Doppler velocimeter

The laser Doppler velocimeter (LDV) was developed over 25 years ago but is probably the least common type of ophthalmic diagnostic laser; it has been used almost exclusively for research purposes [136]. It typically combines a low-power He-Ne or diode laser with an SLO, a fundus camera, or a slip lamp biomicroscope, permitting simultaneous viewing and projection of an approximately 100-μm–diameter laser spot onto the desired vessel (Fig. 13-11). Light of frequency ν is scattered by erythrocytes; and autodyne optical mixing spectroscopy is employed to measure the resulting frequency shift of $\Delta\nu$ relative to the light scattered from the wall of the vessel containing the cells. Because there is a range of cell velocities, the LDV produces a spectrum indicating how many cells are moving at each velocity. This method measures only relative velocity, but absolute velocity can be determined by adding a second detector. Readings can be taken in patients with poor fixation or those who require particularly long study by using rapid calculation algorithms or techniques to compensate for eye movement [137]. The LDV has shown normal retinal blood flow to be about 80 μL per minute, which increases with antiglaucoma medication [138], hyperglycemia [139] and transition from dark-adaptation to light [140], and decreases after treatment with insulin [141], in cases of optic atrophy [142], and in PDR [143]. Regional abnormalities in blood flow detected by LDV in glaucomatous eyes [144–146] may help elucidate the pathogenesis of that disorder.

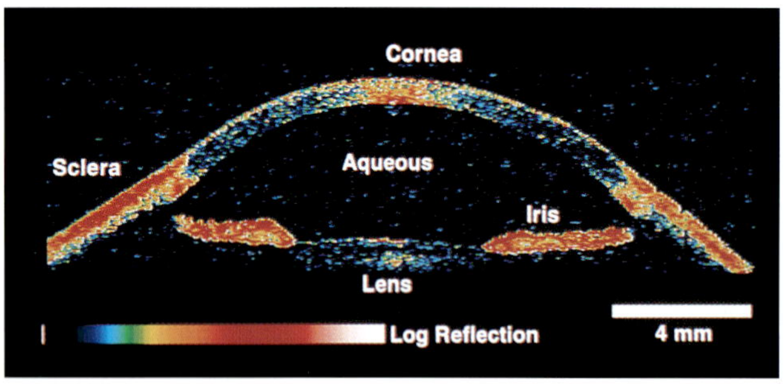

FIGURE 13-10. Optical coherence tomography image of the anterior human eye. (*From* Krauss and Puliafito [135]; with permission.)

LIPOSOMES

Zeimer *et al.* [147] and Khoobehi *et al.* [148–151] have conducted a series of studies on the intravenous injection of liposomes containing drugs or dye. Low-level irradiation with argon blue-green or dye yellow light is used to achieve heat-induced localized release in retinal vessels of those substances from the miniature

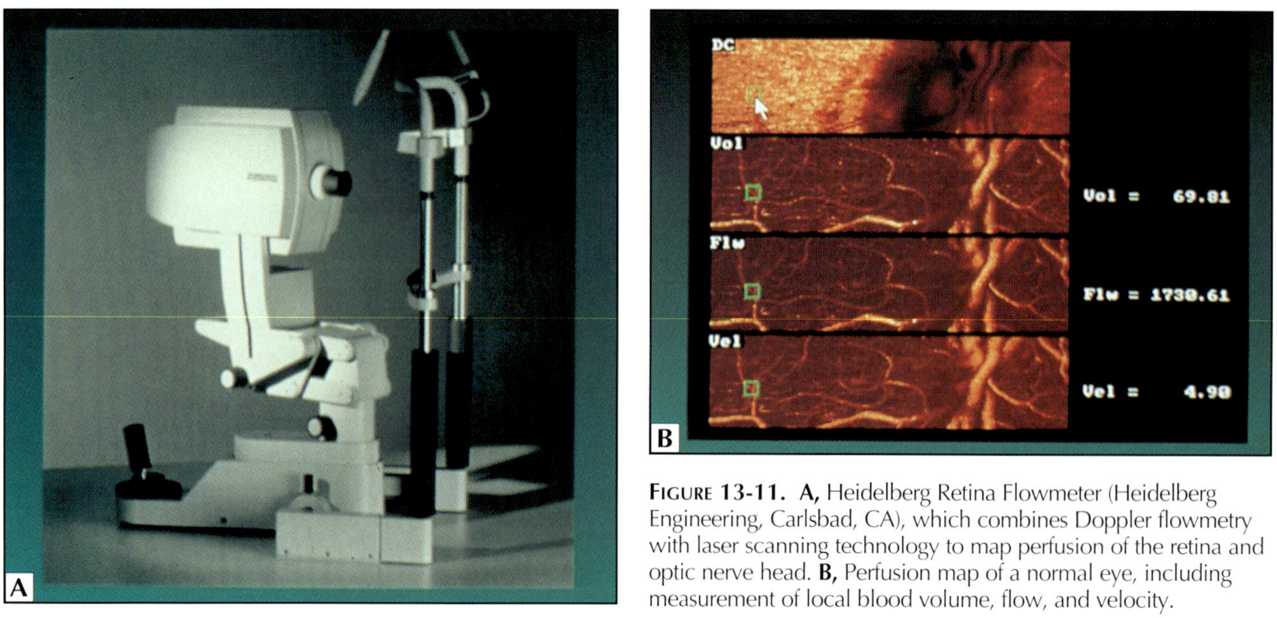

FIGURE 13-11. A, Heidelberg Retina Flowmeter (Heidelberg Engineering, Carlsbad, CA), which combines Doppler flowmetry with laser scanning technology to map perfusion of the retina and optic nerve head. **B,** Perfusion map of a normal eye, including measurement of local blood volume, flow, and velocity.

phospholipid containers with a transition temperature of 41°C. Potential applications include measurement of blood flow and selective angiography. Work on selective angiography [148] has shown that with a spot size of 1.5 to 2.0 mm centered on the optic disc and energy densities of 0.5 to 3.4 J/cm^2, it is possible to obtain multiple angiograms up to 3 hours after dye injection. Possible advantages of this technique include reduction of choroidal fluorescence, which permits optimal viewing of the retinal microcirculation, and clear separation of arterial and venous fluorescence. Selective angiography of a suspected leaking vessel could be documented by specifically targeting it with the laser.

Because targeted dye delivery requires the use of laser powers that might damage the retina, Khoobehi and Peyman [149] developed a fluorescent vesicle system in which a subquenched concentration of dye fluoresces inside the liposomes rather than being released and undergoing a dampening effect; they used this technique to measure retinal and choroidal blood velocity, without the signal attenuation by the RPE that complicates LDV measurements [149,151]. Noting that this approach had the disadvantage of not allowing leakage of fluorescent vesicles at sites of retinal or choroidal damage, Peyman *et al.* [150•] used an SLO with a combination of liposome-encapsulated and free dye and found that, with an optimal ratio of liposomal:free dye of 150:1 for fluorescein and 50:1 for ICG, they were able to realize the benefits of traditional angiography as well as to monitor directly the changes in retinal and choroidal circulation in response to various stimuli or treatments up to 2 hours after injection of the liposomes (Fig. 13-12). Blood flow could be monitored during and after laser treatment of tumors and angiomas. Before any clinical use, however, more extensive tissue damage studies are needed, as are data on the potential toxicity of the liposomes.

FUTURE DEVELOPMENTS

The diode laser is revolutionary more for economic and ergonomic reasons than because it provides fundamentally new laser–tissue interaction. Its low cost and easy portability will permit treatment in remote geographic areas, including many developing nations. Just as GaAlAs diode technology was gradually improved so that sufficient power is now available for many applications, the future holds the promise that, with new materials, useful diode output will be achieved at even lower, visible wavelengths, perhaps supplanting the much bulkier and less efficient argon, krypton, and dye lasers. Indeed, transscleral retinal and ciliary body photocoagulation was recently reported with a prototype diode laser at 670 nm, near the krypton red emission of 647 nm [152], and blue-light–emitting lasers based on gallium nitride diodes are in the early stages of development [153]. At present, diodes are beginning to replace flashlamps and other lasers as pumping sources for visible wavelengths. If sufficient energy can be generated by Q-switched diode lasers, they might be used in place of Nd:YAG laser photodisruption. Lesion variability—with the diode or other lasers—is unavoidable, but early work with a dynamic confocal reflectometer offers the possibility of reproducible retinal photocoagulation independent of pigmentation, media opacities, or optical aberrations [154].

Another possible improvement to the excimer itself is the addition of real-time tissue-depth monitoring, *ie*, topography; possible approaches include femtosecond (10^{-15} seconds) laser optical ranging [155] and optical coherence domain reflectometry [116]. This approach will likely be most valuable with the flying spot method, permitting the widest range of customized ablations of even the most irregular corneal surfaces.

Although laser removal of primary cataracts remains a popular misconception, reality may be

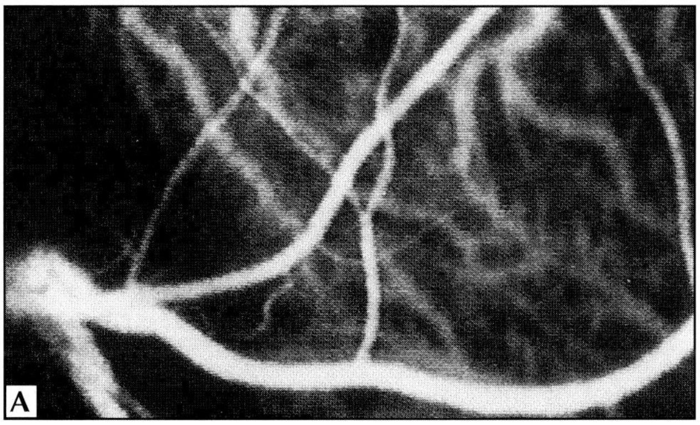

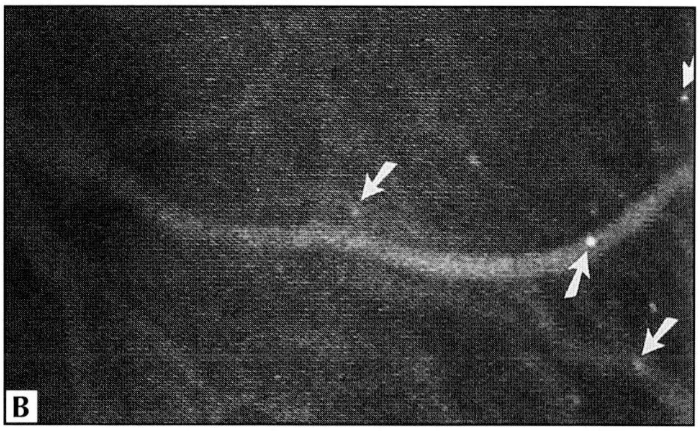

FIGURE 13-12. A, Arteriovenous-phase fluorescent vesicle angiogram using encapsulated and free indocyanine green (ICG) in a rhesus monkey, demonstrating the predominance of the free dye. **B,** Late-phase angiogram, same eye as *panel A*, demonstrating the fluorescent vesicles (*arrows*) flowing through the free ICG that highlights the vessels. (*From* Peyman *et al.* [150•]; with permission.)

catching up with myth. As discussed in Chapter 1, *photophacofragmentation* is the process of employing pulsed laser energy to soften a cataractous lens to facilitate aspiration at the time of surgery; studies employing the Nd:YAG [156] and Er:YAG [157,158] lasers have been reported. One possibility is the aspiration of lens remnants through a small incision, through which some polymer capable of reconstituting the lens—perhaps restoring accommodation [159]—could be injected.

REFERENCES AND RECOMMENDED READING

Recently published papers of particular interest have been highlighted as:
- • Of special interest
- •• Of outstanding interest

1. McHugh JDA, Marshall J, Ffytche TJ, *et al.*: Initial clinical experience using a diode laser in the treatment of retinal vascular disease. *Eye* 1989, 3:516–527.
2. Balles MW, Puliafito CA, D'Amico DJ, *et al.*: Semiconductor diode laser photocoagulation in retinal vascular disease. *Ophthalmology* 1990, 97:1553–1561.
3. Ulbig MW, McHugh DA, Hamilton AMP: Photocoagulation of choroidal neovascular membranes with a diode laser. *Br J Ophthalmol* 1993, 77:218–221.
4. Lanzetta P, Virgili G, Menchini U: Diode laser photocoagulation of choroidal neovascular membranes. *Int Ophthalmol* 1996, 19:347–354.
5. Ulbig MW, McHugh DA, Hamilton AMP: Diode laser photocoagulation for diabetic macular oedema. *Br J Ophthalmol* 1995, 79:318–321.
6. Akduman L, Olk RJ: Diode laser (810 nm) versus argon green (514 nm) modified grid photocoagulation for diffuse diabetic macular edema. *Ophthalmology* 1997, 104:1433–1441.
7. Funatsu H, Wilson CA, Berkowitz BA, *et al.*: A comparative study of the effects of argon and diode laser photocoagulation on retinal oxygenation. *Graefes Arch Clin Exp Ophthalmol* 1997, 235:168–175.
8. Sato Y, Berkowitz BA, Wilson CA, *et al.*: Blood-retinal barrier breakdown caused by diode vs argon laser endophotocoagulation. *Arch Ophthalmol* 1992, 110:277–281.
9. Haller JA, Lim JI, Goldberg MF: Pilot trial of transscleral diode laser retinopexy in retinal detachment surgery. *Arch Ophthalmol* 1993, 111:952–956.
10. McHugh DA, Schwartz S, Dowler JG, *et al.*: Diode laser contact transscleral retinal photocoagulation. *Br J Ophthalmol* 1995, 79:1083–1087.
11. Schuman JS, Puliafito CA, Jacobson JJ: Semiconductor diode laser peripheral iridotomy. *Arch Ophthalmol* 1990, 108:1207–1208.
12. Emoto I, Okisaka S, Nakajima A: Diode laser iridotomy in rabbit and human eyes. *Am J Ophthalmol* 1992, 113:321–327.
13. McHugh D, Marshall J, Ffytche TJ, *et al.*: Diode laser trabeculoplasty (DLT) for primary open-angle glaucoma and ocular hypertension. *Br J Ophthalmol* 1990, 74:743–747.
14. McHugh D, Marshall J, Ffytche TJ, *et al.*: Ultrastructural changes of human trabecular meshwork after photocoagulation with a diode laser. *Invest Ophthalmol Vis Sci* 1992, 33:2664–2671.
15. Brancato R, Carassa R, Trabucchi G: Diode laser compared with argon laser for trabeculoplasty. *Am J Ophthalmol* 1991, 112:50–55.
16. Moriarty AP, McHugh JDA, Ffytche TJ, *et al.*: Long-term follow-up of diode laser trabeculoplasty for primary open-angle glaucoma and ocular hypertension. *Ophthalmology* 1989, 100:1614–1618.
17. Gaasterland DE, Abrams DA, Belcher CD, *et al.*: A multicenter study of contact diode laser transscleral cyclophotocoagulation in glaucoma patients. *Invest Ophthalmol Vis Sci* 1992, 33(Suppl):1019.
18. Vogel A, Dlugos C, Nuffer R, *et al.*: Optical properties of human sclera and their consequences for transscleral applications. *Lasers Surg Med* 1991, 11:331–340.
19.• Bloom PA, Tsai JC, Sharma K, *et al.*: "Cyclodiode." Transscleral diode laser cyclophotocoagulation in the treatment of advanced refractory glaucoma. *Ophthalmology* 1997, 104:1508–1520.

This group treated 210 eyes, achieving a mean reduction in IOP from 34.1 to 20.1 mm Hg at an average follow-up of 10 months. Approximately 50% of the eyes required further treatments within several months of the first, up to a total of five treatments (mean, 1.75). Visual acuity improved in 11% of eyes, remained unchanged in 60%, and decreased in 29%, whereas the number of required glaucoma medications decreased from an average of 2.3 to 1.7. Complications were few, but included one patient each with hypotony, phthisis, macular pucker, and combined hyphema/vitreous hemorrhage, and two with corneal graft decompensation.

20. Brancato R, Carassa RG, Bettin P, *et al.*: Contact transscleral cyclophotocoagulation with diode laser in refractory glaucoma. *Eur J Ophthalmol* 1995, 5:32–39.
21. Ulbig MW, McHugh DA, McNaught AI, *et al.*: Clinical comparison of semiconductor diode versus neodymium:YAG noncontact cyclophotocoagulation. *Br J Ophthalmol* 1995, 79:569–574.
22. Smiddy WE: Diode laser photocoagulation. *Arch Ophthalmol* 1992, 110:1172–1174.
23. Diskin J, Maguire AM, Margherio RR: Choroidal folds induced with diode endolaser. *Arch Ophthalmol* 1992, 110:754.

24. Peyman GA, D'Amico DJ, Alturki WA: An endolaser probe with aspiration capability. *Arch Ophthalmol* 1992, 110:718.

25. Uram M: Ophthalmic laser microendoscope endophotocoagulation. *Ophthalmology* 1992, 99:1829–1832.

26. Mora JS, Iwach AG, Gaffney MM, *et al.*: Endoscopic diode laser cyclophotocoagulation. *Ophthalmic Surg Lasers* 1997, 28:118–123.

27. Hoggatt JS, Pulido JS, Nash RW, *et al.*: The in vivo effects of a prototype diode laser coagulator/vaporizing endoprobe used to perform retinectomy and retinotomy in rabbits. *Ophthalmic Surg Lasers* 1997, 28:231–235.

28.• Friberg TR: Laser photocoagulation using binocular indirect ophthalmoscope laser delivery systems. *Ophthalmic Surg Lasers* 1995, 26:549–559.
This article reviews LIO theory.

29. Shields CL, Shields JA, Kiratli H, *et al.*: Treatment of retinoblastoma with indirect ophthalmoscope laser photocoagulation. *J Pediatr Ophthalmol Strabismus* 1995, 32:317–322.

30. Augsburger JJ, Mullen D, Kleineidam M: Planned combined I-125 plaque irradiation and indirect ophthalmoscope laser therapy for choroidal malignant melanoma. *Ophthalmic Surg* 1993, 24:76–81.

31. Irvine WD, Smiddy WE, Nicholson DH: Corneal and iris burns with the laser indirect ophthalmoscope. *Am J Ophthalmol* 1990, 110:311–313.

32. Landers MB, Semple HC, Ruben JB, *et al.*: Argon laser photocoagulation for advanced retinopathy of prematurity. *Am J Ophthalmol* 1990, 110:429–431.

33. Landers MB, Toth CA, Semple HC, *et al.*: Treatment of retinopathy of prematurity with argon laser photocoagulation. *Arch Ophthalmol* 1991, 110:44–47.

34. Iverson DA, Trese MT, Orgel IK, *et al.*: Laser photocoagulation for threshold retinopathy of prematurity. *Arch Ophthalmol* 1991, 109:1342–1343.

35. McNamara JA, Tasman W, Brown GC, *et al.*: Laser photocoagulation for stage 3+ retinopathy of prematurity. *Ophthalmology* 1991, 98:576–580.

36. Fleming TN, Runge PE, Charles ST: Diode laser photocoagulation for prethreshold, posterior retinopathy of prematurity. *Am J Ophthalmol* 1992, 114:589–592.

37. McNamara JA, Tasman W, Vander JF, *et al.*: Diode laser photocoagulation for retinopathy of prematurity: Preliminary results. *Arch Ophthalmol* 1992, 110:1714–1716.

38. Hunter DG, Repka MX: Diode laser photocoagulation for threshold retinopathy of prematurity: A randomized study. *Ophthalmology* 1993, 100:238–244.

39. Drack AV, Burke JP, Pulido JS, *et al.*: Transient punctate lenticular opacities as a complication of argon laser photoablation in an infant with retinopathy of prematurity. *Am J Ophthalmol* 1992, 114:583–584.

40. O'Keefe M, Burke J, Algawi K, *et al.*: Diode laser photocoagulation to the vascular retina for progressively advancing retinopathy of prematurity. *Br J Ophthalmol* 1995, 79:1012–1014.

41. Seiberth V, Linderkamp O, Vardarli I, *et al.*: Diode laser photocoagulation for threshold retinopathy of prematurity in eyes with tunica vasculosa lentis. *Am J Ophthalmol* 1995, 119:748–751.

42. Noonan CP, Clark DI: Trends in the management of stage 3 retinopathy of prematurity. *Br J Ophthalmol* 1996, 80:278–281.

43. Laws F, Laws D, Clark D: Cryotherapy and laser treatment for acute retinopathy of prematurity: refractive outcomes, a longitudinal study. *Br J Ophthalmol* 1997, 81:12–15.

44. White JE, Repka MX: Randomized comparison of diode laser photocoagulation versus cryotherapy for threshold retinopathy of prematurity: 3-year outcome. *J Pediatr Ophthalmol Strabismus* 1997, 34:83–87.

45. Knauf III HP, Fouraker BD, Rowsey JJ: Next-generation excimer and solid-state refractive lasers. *Ophthalmol Clin North Am* 1997, 10:543–553.

46. Asbell P, Beyer CF, Nevitt MP: LaserSight Compak-200 mini-excimer laser. In *The Excimer Laser. A Clinician's Guide to Excimer Laser Surgery.* Edited by Talamo JH, Krueger RR. Boston: Little, Brown and Company, 1997:341–353.

47. Taboada J, Poirier RH, Yee RW, *et al.*: Intrastromal photorefractive keratectomy with a new optically coupled laser probe. *Refract Corneal Surg* 1992, 8:399–402.

48. Rowsey JJ, Bowyer BL, Margo CE, *et al.*: Intrastromal ablation of corneal tissue using a frequency doubled Nd:YAG laser. *Invest Ophthalmol Vis Sci* 1993, 34(Suppl):1247.

49. Gimbel HV, Coupland SG, Ferensowicz M: Review of intrastromal photorefractive keratectomy with the neodymium:yttrium-lithium-fluoride laser. *Int Ophthalmol Clin* 1997, 37:95–102.

50. Fowler WC, Wehrly SR, Imami NR, *et al.*: Keratorefractive change induced by circumferential infrared wavelength ablations utilizing the free electron laser in porcine corneas. *Invest Ophthalmol Vis Sci* 1994, 35(Suppl):2027.

51. Bende T, Walker R, Jean B: Thermal collateral damage in porcine corneas after photoablation with free electron laser. *J Refract Surg* 1995, 11:129–136.

52. Jean B, Kriegerowski M, Matallana M, *et al.*: Correction of myopia with Er:YAG laser fundamental mode photorefractive keratectomy. *J Refract Surg* 1995, 11:392–396.

53. Mrochen M, Seiler T: Midinfrared photorefractive surgery: technical standards and clinical aspects. *Int Ophthalmol Clin* 1996, 36:73–77.

54. Ren Q, Gailitis RP, Thompson K, *et al.*: Corneal refractive surgery using an ultra-violet (213 nm) solid state laser. *Proc Ophthalm Technol, SPIE* 1991, 1423:129–139.

55. Gailitis RP, Ren Q, Thompson KP, *et al.*: Solid-state ultraviolet laser (213 nm) ablation of the cornea and synthetic collagen lenticules. *Lasers Surg Med* 1991, 11:556–562.

56. Manns F, Ren Q, Parel J-M, *et al.*: Investigation of an algorithm for photorefractive keratectomy (PRK) using a scanning beam delivery system. *Invest Ophthalmol Vis Sci* 1993, 34(Suppl):800.

57. Ren Q, Simon G, Parel J-M, *et al.*: Ultraviolet solid-state laser (213-nm) photorefractive keratectomy. In vitro study. *Ophthalmology* 1993, 100:1828–1834.

58. Ren Q, Simon G, Legeais J-M, *et al.*: Ultraviolet solid-state laser (213-nm) photorefractive keratectomy. In vivo study. *Ophthalmology* 1994, 101:883–889.

59. Lin JT: A multiwavelength solid state laser for ophthalmic applications. *Proc Ophthalm Technol II, SPIE* 1992, 1644:266–275.

60. Feld JR, Lin CP, Woods WJ, *et al.*: Cornea ablation studies at wavelengths between 205 and 225 nm using a tunable solid state laser. *Invest Ophthalmol Vis Sci* 1992, 33(Suppl):1105.

61. Goelz S, Goetz MH, Kessler R, *et al.*: Comparative investigation of corneal ablation by different UV-laser sources at 193 nm and 211 nm. *Invest Ophthalmol Vis Sci* 1997, 38(Suppl):S540.

62. Swinger CA, Lai ST, Kornmehl EW: Novatec LightBlade. In *The Excimer Laser. A Clinician's Guide to Excimer Laser Surgery.* Edited by Talamo JH, Krueger RR. Boston: Little, Brown, 1997:369–380.

63. Swinger CA, Williams E, Chayet A, *et al.*: Results of the Novatec solid-state laser with active eye tracker for correction of compound myopic astigmatism. *Invest Ophthalmol Vis Sci* 1997, 38(Suppl):S412.

64. Huie TY, Chang CJ, TSO MOM: Localized surgical debridement of RPE by Q-switched neodymium:YAG laser. *Invest Ophthalmol Vis Sci* 1993, 34(Suppl):959.

65. Chong LP, Kohen L: A retinal laser which damages only the RPE: ultrastructural study. *Invest Ophthalmol Vis Sci* 1993, 34(Suppl):960.

66. Roider J, Michaud N, Flotte T, *et al.*: Selective RPE photocoagulation by 1 μsec laser pulses. *Invest Ophthalmol Vis Sci* 1993, 34(Suppl):960.

67. Roider J, Brinkmann R, Laqua H, *et al.*: Therapeutical bandwidth of selective RPE-photocoagulation treatment by repetitive μs-laser pulses (527 nm)—first clinical results. *Invest Ophthalmol Vis Sci* 1997, 38(Suppl):S83.

68. Stern D, Schoenlein RW, Puliafito CA, *et al.*: Corneal ablation by nanosecond, picosecond, and femtosecond lasers at 532 and 625 nm. *Arch Ophthalmol* 1989, 107:587–592.

69. Lin CP, Weaver YK, Birngruber R, *et al.*: Intraocular microsurgery with a picosecond Nd:YAG laser. *Lasers Surg Med* 1994, 15:44–53.

70. Borirakchanyavat S, Puliafito CA, Kliman GH, *et al.*: Holmium-YAG laser surgery on experimental vitreous membranes. *Arch Ophthalmol* 1991, 109:1605–1609.

71. Margolis TI, Farnath DA, Destro M: Erbium-YAG laser surgery on experimental vitreous membranes. *Arch Ophthalmol* 1989, 107:424–428.

72. Lin CP, Stern D, Puliafito CA: High-speed photography of Er:YAG laser ablation in fluid. *Invest Ophthalmol Vis Sci* 1990, 31:2546–2550.

73. Brazitikos PD, D'Amico DJ, Bernal M-T, *et al.*: Erbium:YAG laser surgery of the vitreous and retina. *Ophthalmology* 1995, 102:278–290.

74. D'Amico DJ, Brazitikos PD, Marcellino GR, *et al.*: Initial clinical experience with an erbium:YAG laser for vitreoretinal surgery. *Am J Ophthalmol* 1996, 121:414–425.

75.• D'Amico DJ, Blumenkranz MS, Lavin MJ, *et al.*: Multicenter clinical experience using an erbium:YAG laser for vitreoretinal surgery. *Ophthalmology* 1996, 103:1575–1585.

In this study, 66 patients underwent a total of 174 procedures. Of the results, 84% were deemed good or excellent, with a range of 100% for transection of subretinal membranes to 25% for coagulation of blood vessels. Minor bleeding from transected retinal vessels occurred in 29% of retinotomies, intraocular lens damage in 18% of posterior capsulotomies, and retinal break or photocoagulation injury in 5% of epiretinal membrane incisions. High water absorption at 2.94 μm required holding the endoprobe tip close to the tissue in fluid-filled eyes, whereas ablation was achieved across several mm in air-filled eyes. Precision of the laser approach exceeded that possible with conventional techniques, although critical work near the retina proceeded slowly and visualization—such as of the macula in air-filled eyes—was difficult.

76. Berger JW, D'Amico DJ: Modeling of erbium:YAG laser-mediated explosive photovaporization: implications for vitreoretinal surgery. *Ophthalmic Surg Lasers* 1997, 28:133–139.

77. Lewis A, Palanker D, Hemo I, *et al.*: Microsurgery of the retina with a needle-guided 193-nm excimer laser. *Invest Ophthalmol Vis Sci* 1992, 33:2377–2381.

78. Palanker D, Hemo I, Turovets I, *et al.*: Vitreoretinal ablation in fluid media with 193 nm excimer laser beam. *Invest Ophthalmol Vis Sci* 1994, 35:3835–3840.

79. Hemo I, Palanker D, Turovets I, *et al.*: Vitreoretinal surgery assisted by the 193-nm excimer laser. *Invest Ophthalmol Vis Sci* 1997, 38:1825–1829.

80. Dreher AW, Weinreb RN: Accuracy of topographic measurements in a model eye with the laser tomographic scanner. *Invest Ophthalmol Vis Sci* 1991, 32:2992–2996.

81. Sjaarda RN, Frank DA, Glaser BM, *et al.*: Assessment of vision in idiopathic macular holes with macular microperimetry using the scanning laser ophthalmoscope. *Ophthalmology* 1993, 100:1513–1518.

82. Zangwill L, Shakiba S, Caprioli J, *et al.*: Agreement between clinicians and a confocal scanning laser ophthalmoscope in estimating cup/disk ratios. *Am J Ophthalmol* 1995, 119:415–421.

83. Dichtl A, Jonas JB, Mardin CY: Comparison between tomographic scanning evaluation and photographic measurement of the neuroretinal rim. *Am J Ophthalmol* 1996, 121:494–501.

84. Woon WH, Fitzke FW, Bird AC, *et al.*: Confocal imaging of the fundus using a scanning laser ophthalmoscope. *Br J Ophthalmol* 1992, 76:470–474.

85. Uchida H, Brigatti L, Caprioli J: Detection of structural damage from glaucoma with confocal laser image analysis. *Invest Ophthalmol Vis Sci* 1996, 37:2393–2401.

86. Anton A, Zangwill L, Emdadi A, *et al.*: Nerve fiber layer measurements with scanning laser polarimetry in ocular hypertension. *Arch Ophthalmol* 1997, 115:331–334.

87. Zangwill L, Berry CA, Garden VS, *et al.*: Reproducibility of retardation measurements with the Nerve Fiber Analyzer II. *J Glaucoma* 1997, 6:384–389.

88. Weinreb RN, Dreher AW, Coleman A, *et al.*: Histopathologic validation of Fourier-ellipsometry measurements of retinal nerve fiber layer thickness. *Arch Ophthalmol* 1990, 108:557–560.

89. Dreher AW, Bille JF, Weinreb RN: Active optical depth resolution improvement of the laser tomographic scanner. *Applied Optics* 1989, 28:804–808.

90. Cioffi GA, Robin AL, Eastman RD, *et al.*: Confocal laser scanning ophthalmoscope: reproducibility of optic nerve head topographic measurements with the confocal laser scanning ophthalmoscope. *Ophthalmology* 1993, 100:57–62.

91. Weinberger D, Stiebel H, Gaton DD, *et al.*: Three-dimensional measurements of idiopathic macular holes using a scanning laser tomograph. *Ophthalmology* 1995, 102:1445–1449.

92. Hudson C, Charles SJ, Flanagan JG, *et al.*: Objective morphological assessment of macular hole surgery by scanning laser tomography. *Br J Ophthalmol* 1997, 81:107–116.

93. Katsumi O, Timberlake GT, Hirose T, *et al.*: Recording pattern reversal visual evoked response with the scanning laser ophthalmoscope. *Acta Ophthalmol* 1989, 67:243–248.

94. Timberlake GT, Van de Velde FJ, Jalkh AE: Clinical use of scanning laser ophthalmoscope retinal function maps in macular disease. *Lasers Light Ophthalmol* 1989, 2:211–222.

95. Wolf S, Arend O, Sponsel WE, *et al.*: Retinal hemodynamics using scanning laser ophthalmoscopy and hemorheology in chronic open-angle glaucoma. *Ophthalmology* 1993, 100:1561–1566.

96. Frambach DA, Dacey MP, Sadun A: Stereoscopic photography with a scanning laser ophthalmoscope. *Am J Ophthalmol* 1993, 116:484–488.

97. Kuck H, Inhoffen W, Schneider U, *et al.*: Diagnosis of occult subretinal neovascularization in age-related macular degeneration by infrared scanning laser videoangiography. *Retina* 1993, 13:36–39.

98. Bartsch D-U, Weinreb RN, Zinser G, *et al.*: Confocal scanning infrared laser ophthalmoscopy for indocyanine green angiography. *Am J Ophthalmol* 1995, 120:642–651.

99. O'Brart DPS, de Souza Lima M, Bartsch D-U, *et al.*: Indocyanine green angiography of the peripapillary region in glaucomatous eyes by confocal scanning laser ophthalmoscopy. *Am J Ophthalmol* 1997, 123:657–666.

100. Mueller AJ, Bartsch D-U, Folberg R, *et al.*: Imaging the microvasculature of choroidal melanomas with confocal indocyanine green scanning laser ophthalmoscopy. *Arch Ophthalmol* 1998, 116:31–39.

101. Kiryu J, Ogura Y, Shahidi M, *et al.*: Enhanced visualization of vitreoretinal interface by laser biomicroscopy. *Ophthalmology* 1993, 100:1040–1043.

102. Sawa M, Tsurimaki Y, Tsuru T, *et al.*: New quantitative method to determine protein concentration and cell number in aqueous in vivo. *Jpn J Ophthalmol* 1988, 32:132–142.

103. Shah SM, Spalton DJ, Smith SE: Measurement of aqueous cells and flare in normal eyes. *Br J Ophthalmol* 1991, 75:348–352.

104. Oshika T, Araie M, Masuda K: Diurnal variation of aqueous flare in normal human eyes measured with laser flare-cell meter. *Jpn J Ophthalmol* 1988, 32:143–150.

105. Oshika T, Kato S, Sawa M, *et al.*: Aqueous flare intensity and age. *Jpn J Ophthalmol* 1989, 33:237–242.

106. Herbort CP, Guex-Crosier Y, de Ancos E, *et al.*: Use of laser flare photometry to assess and monitor inflammation in uveitis. *Ophthalmology* 1997, 104:64–72.

107. Oshika T: Aqueous protein concentration in rhegmatogenous retinal detachment. *Jpn J Ophthalmol* 1990, 34:63–71.

108. Oshika T, Yoshimura K, Miyata N: Postsurgical inflammation after phacoemulsification and extracapsular extraction with soft or conventional intraocular lens implantation. *J Cataract Refract Surg* 1992, 18:356–361.

109. Altamirano D, Mermoud A, Pittet N, *et al.*: Aqueous humor analysis after Nd:YAG laser capsulotomy with the laser flare-cell meter. *J Cataract Refract Surg* 1992, 18:554–558.

110. Mermoud A, Pittet N, Herbort CP: Inflammation patterns after laser trabeculoplasty measured with the laser flare meter. *Arch Ophthalmol* 1992, 110:368–370.

111. Nussenblatt RB, de Smet M, Podgor M, *et al.*: The use of flarephotometry in the detection of cytomegalic virus retinitis in AIDS patients. *AIDS* 1994, 8:135–136.

112. Yoshitomi T, Wong AS, Daher E, *et al.*: Aqueous flare measurement with laser flare-cell meter. *Jpn J Ophthalmol* 1990, 34:57–62.

113. Green DG: Testing the vision of cataract patients by means of laser-generated interference fringes. *Science* 1970, 168:1240–1242.

114. Hitzenberger CK: Optical measurement of the axial eye length by laser Doppler interferometry. *Invest Ophthalmol Vis Sci* 1991, 32:616–624.

115. Hitzenberger CK, Drexler W, Fercher AF: Measurement of corneal thickness by laser Doppler interferometry. *Invest Ophthalmol Vis Sci* 1992, 33:98–103.

116. Huang D, Wang J, Lin CP, *et al.*: Micron-resolution ranging of cornea anterior chamber by optical reflectometry. *Lasers Surg Med* 1991, 11:419–425.

117. Huang D, Swanson EA, Lin CP, *et al.*: Optical coherence tomography. *Science* 1991, 254:1178–1181.

118. Swanson EA, Huang D, Hee MR, *et al.*: High-speed optical coherence domain reflectometry. *Optics Lett* 1992, 17:151–153.

119. Swanson EA, Izatt JA, Hee MR, *et al.*: In vivo retinal imaging by optical coherence tomography. *Optics Lett* 1993, 18:1864–1866.

120. Izatt JA, Hee MR, Huang D, *et al.*: Micron-resolution biomedical imaging with optical coherence tomography. *Optics Photonics News* 1993, Oct:14–18.

121. Izatt JA, Hee MR, Huang D, *et al.*: Ophthalmic diagnostics using optical coherence tomography. *Ophthalm Technol III, SPIE* 1993, 1877:136–144.

122. Hee MR, Izatt JA, Swanson EA, *et al.*: Optical coherence tomography of the human retina. *Arch Ophthalmol* 1995, 113:325–332.

123. Puliafito CA, Hee MR, Lin CP, *et al.*: Imaging of macular diseases with optical coherence tomography. *Ophthalmology* 1995, 102:217–229.

124. Schuman JS, Hee MR, Puliafito CA, *et al.*: Quantification of nerve fiber layer thickness in normal and glaucomatous eyes using optical coherence tomography: a pilot study. *Arch Ophthalmol* 1995, 113:586–596.

125. Hee MR, Puliafito CA, Wong C, *et al.*: Optical coherence tomography of macular holes. *Ophthalmology* 1995, 102:748–756.

126. Hee MR, Puliafito CA, Wong C, *et al.*: Optical coherence tomography (OCT) of central serous chorioretinopathy. *Am J Ophthalmol* 1995, 120:65–74.

127. Izatt JA, Hee MR, Swanson EA, *et al.*: Micrometer-scale resolution imaging of the anterior eye in vivo with optical coherence tomography. *Arch Ophthalmol* 1994, 112:1584–1589.

128. Hee MR, Puliafito CA, Wong C, *et al.*: Quantitative assessment of macular edema with optical coherence tomography. *Arch Ophthalmol* 1995, 113:1019–1029.

129. Rutledge BK, Puliafito CA, Duker JS, *et al.*: Optical coherence tomography of macular lesions associated with optic nerve head pits. *Ophthalmology* 1996, 103:1047–1053.

130. Hee MR, Baumal CR, Puliafito CA, *et al.*: Optical coherence tomography of age-related macular degeneration and choroidal neovascularization. *Ophthalmology* 1996, 103:1260–1270.

131. Toth CA, Birngruber R, Boppart SA, *et al.*: Argon laser retinal lesions evaluated in vivo by optical coherence tomography. *Am J Ophthalmol* 1997, 123:188–198.

132. Toth CA, Narayan DG, Boppart SA, *et al.*: A comparison of retinal morphology viewed by optical coherence tomography and by light microscopy. *Arch Ophthalmol* 1997, 115:1425–1428.

133. Prydal JI, Campbell FW: Study of precorneal tear film thickness and structure by interferometry and confocal microscopy. *Invest Ophthalmol Vis Sci* 1992, 33:1996–2005.

134. Hitzenberger CK, Drexler W, Dolezal C, *et al.*: Measurement of the axial length of cataract eyes by laser Doppler interferometry. *Invest Ophthalmol Vis Sci* 1993, 34:1886–1893.

135. Krauss JM, Puliafito CA: Lasers in ophthalmology. *Lasers Surg Med* 1995, 17:102–159.

136. Riva CE, Ross B, Benedek GB: Laser Doppler measurements of blood flow in capillary tubes and retinal arteries. *Invest Ophthalmol* 1972, 11:936–944.

137. Milbocker MT, Feke GT: Intensified charge-coupled-device-based eyetracker and image stabilizer. *Applied Optics* 1992, 31:3719–3729.

138. Grunwald JE: Effect of topical timolol on the human retinal circulation. *Invest Ophthalmol Vis Sci* 1986, 27:1713–1719.

139. Sullivan PM, Davies GE, Caldwell G, *et al.*: Retinal blood flow during hyperglycemia. A laser Doppler velocimetry study. *Invest Ophthalmol Vis Sci* 1990, 31:2041–2045.

140. Riva CE, Petrig BL, Grunwald JE: Near infrared retinal laser Doppler velocimetry. *Lasers Ophthalmol* 1987, 1:211–215.

141. Grunwald JE, Riva CE, Martin DB, *et al.*: Effect of an insulin induced decrease in blood glucose on the human diabetic retinal circulation. *Ophthalmology* 1987, 94:1614–1620.

142. Sebag J, Delori FC, Feke GT, *et al.*: Effects of optic atrophy on retinal blood flow and oxygen saturation in humans. *Arch Ophthalmol* 1989, 107:222–226.

143. Grunwald JE, Brucker AJ, Grunwald SE, *et al.*: Retinal hemodynamics in proliferative diabetic retinopathy: a laser Doppler velocimetry study. *Invest Ophthalmol Vis Sci* 1993, 34:66–71.

144. Riva CE, Cranstoun SD, Grunwald JE, *et al.*: Choroidal blood flow in the foveal region of the human ocular fundus. *Invest Ophthalmol Vis Sci* 1994, 35:4273–4281.

145. Michelson G, Langhans MJ, Groh MJM: Perfusion of the juxtapapillary retina and neuroretinal rim in primary open-angle glaucoma. *J Glaucoma* 1996, 5:91–98.

146. Nicolela MT, Hnik P, Drance SM: Scanning laser Doppler flowmeter study of retinal and optic disk blood flow in glaucomatous patients. *Am J Ophthalmol* 1996, 122:775–783.

147. Zeimer RC, Khoobehi B, Niesman MR, *et al.*: A potential method for local drug and dye delivery in the ocular vasculature. *Invest Ophthalmol Vis Sci* 1988, 29:1179–1183.

148. Khoobehi B, Peyman GA, Vo K: Laser-triggered repetitive fluorescein angiography. *Ophthalmology* 1992, 99:72–79.

149. Khoobehi B, Peyman GA: Fluorescent vesicle system: a new technique for measuring blood flow in the retina. *Ophthalmology* 1994, 101:1716–1726.

150.• Peyman GA, Moshfeghi DM, Moshfeghi AA, *et al.*: Fluorescent vesicle angiography with sodium fluorescein and indocyanine green. *Ophthalmic Surg Lasers* 1996, 27:279–284.

This group used an SLO with a combination of liposome-encapsulated and free dye, and found that with an optimal ratio of liposomal:free dye of 150:1 for fluorescein and 50:1 for ICG they were able to realize the benefits of traditional angiography as well as to monitor directly the changes in retinal and choroidal circulation in response to various stimuli or treatments up to 2 hours after injection of the liposomes.

151. Peyman GA, Khoobehi B, Shaibani S, *et al.*: A fluorescent vesicle system for the measurement of blood velocity in the choroidal vessels. *Ophthalmic Surg Lasers* 1996, 27:459–466.

152. Immonen I, Viherkoski E, Peyman GA: Experimental retinal and ciliary body photocoagulation using a new 670-nm diode laser. *Am J Ophthalmol* 1996, 122:870–874.

153. Markoff J: A race to catch a Japanese star of blue lasers. *The New York Times* 1997, October 27:D1,D4.

154. Inderfurth JHC, Ferguson RD, Frish MB, *et al.*: Dynamic reflectometer for control of laser photocoagulation of the retina. *Lasers Surg Med* 1994, 15:54–61.

155. Stern D, Lin W-Z, Puliafito CA, *et al.*: Femtosecond optical ranging of corneal incision depth. *Invest Ophthalmol Vis Sci* 1989, 30:99–104.

156. Sperber LTD: Neodymium:YAG laser lens ablation in a rabbit model. *J Cataract Refract Surg* 1996, 22:485–489.

157. Wetzel W, Brinkmann R, Koop N, *et al.*: Photofragmentation of lens nuclei using the Er:YAG laser: preliminary report of an in vitro study. *Ger J Ophthalmol* 1996, 5:281–284.

158. Gailitis RP, Patterson SW, Samuels MA, *et al.*: Comparison of laser phacovaporization using the Er:YAG and the Er:YSGG laser. *Arch Ophthalmol* 1993, 111:697–700.

159. Haefliger E, Parel J-M, Fantes F, *et al.*: Accommodation of an endocapsular silicone lens (phaco-ersatz) in the nonhuman primate. *Ophthalmology* 1987, 94:471–477.

SELECT BIBLIOGRAPHY

Krauss JM: Contemporary ophthalmic lasers. In *New Frontiers in Medical Device Technology*. Edited by Rosen A, Rosen HD. New York: John Wiley & Sons, 1995:155–251.

Puliafito CA, Schuman JS, Fujimoto J: *Optical Coherence Tomography of Ocular Diseases*. Thorofare, NJ: Slack, 1996.

Talamo JH, Krueger RR, eds: *The Excimer Manual. A Clinician's Guide to Excimer Laser Surgery*. Boston: Little, Brown, 1997.

CHAPTER **14**

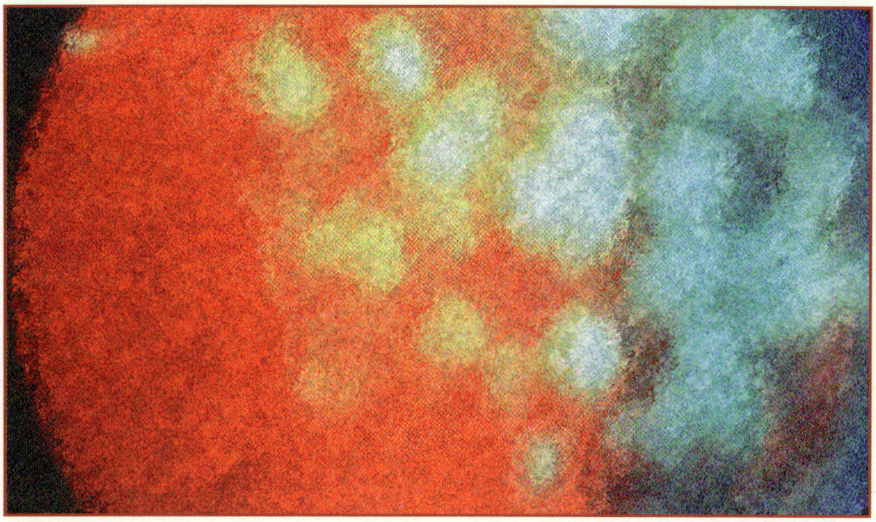

Argon Laser Trabeculoplasty

KATHLEEN A. LAMPING
GREGORY A. EIPPERT

HISTORY

It has been nearly 40 years since the concept of using photocoagulation in the anterior chamber angle for glaucoma control was introduced by Zweng and Flocks [1]. These initial studies reported reduced intraocular pressure (IOP) after selective coagulation of the filtering angles in cats, dogs, and monkeys.

A quiescent period of research of nearly a decade followed, until the early 1970s, when interest reemerged in laser treatment of the filtration angle. Krasnov [2,3], in the Soviet Union, studied a laser puncture technique to the anterior chamber angle termed *goniopuncture*. This initial technique consisted of full-thickness burns that allowed communication of aqueous humor from the anterior chamber to Schlemm's canal. Early results showed initially reduced IOP, followed soon after by diminished efficacy secondary to inflammation and fibrosis of the laser fistulas.

In 1979, Wise and Witter [4] initiated a pilot study for open-angle glaucoma. They used evenly spaced intervals of argon laser treatment to the trabecular meshwork; their treatment did not penetrate Schlemm's canal. With more predictable and encouraging results, this protocol became the basis for today's argon laser trabeculoplasty (ALT), the most commonly performed procedure to control IOP in primary and secondary open-angle glaucomas.

PATHOPHYSIOLOGY

Many theories have been proposed about and studies performed on the actual mechanism by which ALT reduces IOP. Fluorophotometric studies have shown no significant change in aqueous production after laser treatment [5–7]. The most convincing evidence has been produced using tonographic measurements and other techniques that arrive at the common denominator in gauging increased aqueous outflow facility [8–12]. The exact mechanism of this increased outflow facility is uncertain.

Wise and Witter [4] described a mechanism that suggests that thermal energy produced by the pigment absorption of laser light shrinks the collagen lamellae in the inner trabecular ring. This effect is thought to shorten the area of treated trabecular meshwork by separating the adjacent trabecular sheets, enlarging the spaces between treatment sites, and opening the aqueous channels. This "shrinking and shortening" of the trabecular beams may also reverse the pathologic collapse and laxity of the trabecular tissue that can occur with aging.

Van Buskirk *et al.* [13] extensively studied the mechanism of ALT. This report suggested that increased outflow facility is secondary to a biologic response by trabecular endothelial cells with increased synthesis of glycosaminoglycans. Van Buskirk [14] further suggested that ALT may eliminate certain unhealthy trabecular cells, stimulating new endothelial cells to migrate into the treatment zone; these more phagocytic cells thus reduce outflow resistance. Ferritin perfusion studies have been used to observe aqueous flow through treated areas of meshwork. Melamed and Epstein [15] showed in monkeys that a lack of flow through treated meshwork was accompanied by diversion of flow to adjacent, untreated areas, which alter structurally to accommodate this increased flow.

Trabecular cell division and repopulation of treated areas by adjacent cells have been areas of study in further understanding the pathophysiologic role of laser trabeculoplasty. Studies have evaluated thymidine incorporation into trabecular cells, comparing areas of treated and untreated trabecular meshwork. Untreated areas showed increased incorporation of thymidine, suggesting increased cell division in these areas adjacent to laser burns [16].

Our knowledge of the mechanism of ALT has matured greatly since the procedure was first described in 1961. Although the actual mechanism remains imprecisely understood, it likely involves a combination of structural, mechanical, and biochemical changes in the trabecular meshwork.

INDICATIONS

Argon laser trabeculoplasty is performed to attempt to lower IOP in primary and secondary open-angle glaucomas. Initial studies during the first decade of ALT therapy proved it to be effective as a supplement to maximally tolerable levels of medical therapy [17,18]. Potential postoperative complications of transient pressure elevation and the uncertainty of potential long-term damage to the trabecular meshwork were factors that precluded its earlier placement in glaucoma management. Today, with more data to prove the relative safety and efficacy of the procedure, timing of laser treatment earlier in the "medical regimen" has become more accepted; it is commonly being performed after a patient has tried or is using two or three antiglaucoma medications. ALT is virtually always indicated before filtration surgery for IOP control in open-angle glaucoma. The role of ALT as a primary treatment modality is currently being studied in the Glaucoma Laser Trial.

The definition of "maximal medical therapy" has evolved with the introduction of various new medications and the de-emphasis of others. Maximal medical therapy now often includes a topical β-blocker, prostaglandin analogue, α-2 agonist, carbonic anhydrase inhibitor, and cholinergic agent, although not necessarily in that order. With the recent introduction of a prostaglandin analogue (latanaprost) and new α-2 agonist (brimonidine), more options exist in choosing the initial treatment regimen. For this reason, the timing of ALT in the treatment spectrum remains subject to controversy. Most often, ALT is initiated after a trial of several medications but before systemic carbonic anhydrase inhibitors and before filtering surgery.

Although the above categories of medications have all proven efficacious in lowering IOP, they have potential side effects, both visual and systemic, that may contribute to decreased compliance. In patients with advanced cupping, uncontrolled IOP, and progressive visual field loss, ALT may reduce pressure sufficiently to stabilize glaucoma and prevent filtration surgery.

Because of its long track record, lack of drug-related side effects, and elimination of patient compliance issues, many short-term studies of ALT have proven the procedure safe and effective as initial therapy in glaucoma management [19,20]. Although ALT can be used in any form of open-angle glaucoma, the treatment is clearly more efficacious in certain diagnoses (Table 14-1). Spiegel *et al.* [21] reported that the types of glaucoma that seem to show the most significant IOP reduction are pigmentary glaucoma (31%), primary open-angle glaucoma (26%), and pseudoexfoliation glaucoma (19%) [21]. The response in pigmentary glaucoma seems to be proportional to the degree of trabecular meshwork pigmentation [22] and inversely proportional to age, with younger patients having a higher success rate [23]. Unfortunately, the initial success in pigmentary glaucoma reported in up to 53% by Lehto [24] can diminish rapidly to a 14% level at 3-month follow-up. A similar finding has been described for pseudoexfoliation. Threlkeld *et al.* [25] compared pseudoexfoliative and primary open-angle glaucomas, finding the failure rates at 1 year to be 18% and 40% respectively. At 3-year follow-up, failure rates were closer, at 47% for pseudoexfoliation and 58% for primary open-angle glaucoma. Although initial response to ALT was greater in the pseudoexfoliative group, the long-term outcome was similar in both groups.

Absolute contraindications to ALT include total angle closure or hazy media that preclude adequate visualization of the anterior chamber angle. Other potential contraindications include inflammatory glaucomas, which tend to show little effect from treatment; a history of increased IOP in one eye following ALT; and eyes requiring emergency IOP reduction that would be better accomplished by a filtering procedure (Table 14-2).

TECHNIQUE

Wise and Witter [4] originally described the application of between 100 and 120 evenly spaced, nonpenetrating burns to the posterior trabecular meshwork over 360° of the angle. Since then, many investigators have modified the technique; the variables include the degree of the angle treated, the power, and the placement of the burn (Table 14-3).

Regardless of the specific parameters used by the individual surgeon, a conscientious basic technique can maximize outcome and minimize complications.

One or both eyes are anesthetized topically. A preoperative discussion as to expectation can minimize patient anxiety. Either a three-mirror Goldmann lens or the Ritch trabeculoplasty lens, coated with methylcellulose solution, can be used (Fig. 14-1).

Identification of all angle structures preoperatively is crucial. An attempt is made to apply each burn equally over the angle circumference with continuous, precise focusing. The beam spot should be circular.

Placement of the burn

Since Wise and Witter [4] described the burn application to the posterior trabecular meshwork, many investigators have suggested placing the burns more anteriorly to prevent peripheral anterior synechiae formation [26]. Anterior placement of the burn may minimize early postoperative pressure spikes [27] (Fig. 14-2).

In many cases, the anterior portion of the trabecular meshwork is not easily discernible; therefore, treating

TABLE 14-1 FACTORS INCREASING SUCCESS RATES IN ARGON LASER TRABECULOPLASTY

Glaucoma diagnoses
Pigmentary glaucoma
Primary open-angle glaucoma
Pseudoexfoliative glaucoma
Pigmentation of trabecular meshwork
Absence of ocular inflammation
Patient age > 40 y

TABLE 14-2 CONTRAINDICATIONS TO ARGON LASER TRABECULOPLASTY

Total angle closure
Ocular inflammation
History of increased IOP following previous argon laser treatment
Eyes requiring emergent IOP reduction

IOP—intraocular pressure

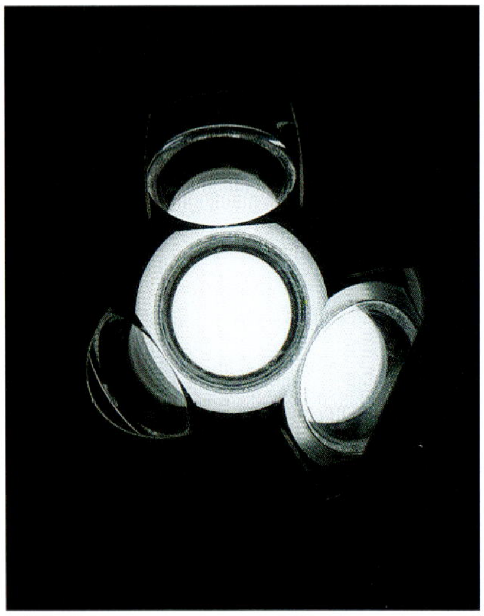

FIGURE 14-1. Three-mirror Goldmann lens.

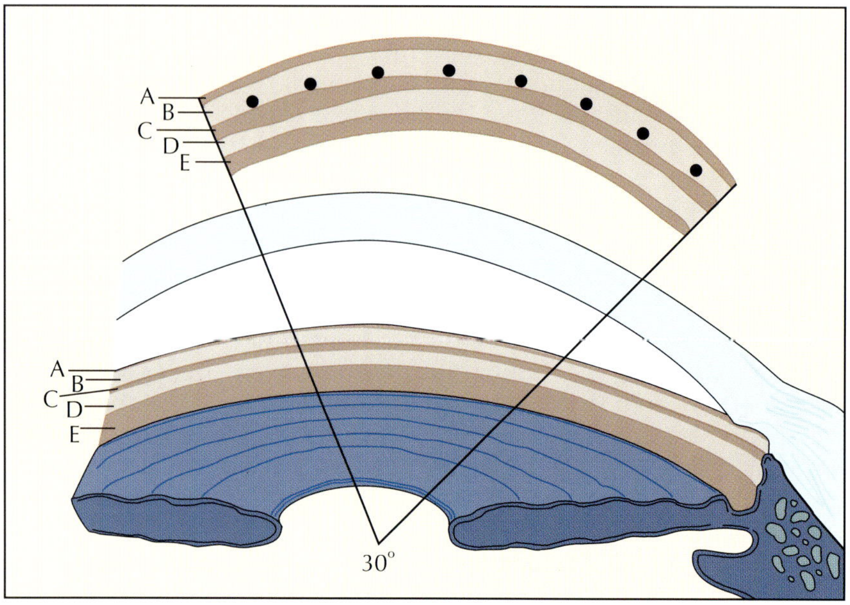

FIGURE 14-2. Gonioscopic view of argon laser trabeculoplasty treatment of the trabecular meshwork. **A**, Schwalbe's line; **B**, Nonpigmented trabecular meshwork; **C**, Pigmented trabecular meshwork; **D**, Scleral spur; **E**, Ciliary body.

the middle portion of the trabecular meshwork may ensure that the trabecular meshwork is being treated. In narrower angles, however, it may be advisable to treat the anterior trabecular meshwork to minimize peripheral anterior synechiae and postoperative inflammation.

Number of burns

Investigators have placed as few as 25 burns per 90° [28] to as many as 100 burns over 360° [29] with reported success. Long-term studies support the efficacy of 100 burns over 360° at one sitting. However, if 180° is treated at one sitting and additional pressure lowering is required, evidence shows that treating the remaining 180° of angle at another sitting is beneficial [30]. Fewer eyes treated with 180° developed an increase IOP spike postoperatively [17,31]. The postoperative use of apraclonidine, however, has greatly minimized the postoperative IOP spike seen after 360° of treatment [32–37]. The number of burns treated per sitting may be left to the judgment of the surgeon and may be individualized for each patient.

TABLE 14-3 ARGON LASER TRABECULOPLASTY LASER PARAMETERS AND PROTOCOL

Wavelength:	Argon blue-green
Spot size:	50 μm
Duration:	0.1 s
Power:	500 to 1200 mW
Treatment area:	180° or 360°
Number of laser burns:	40 to 50 per 180°

Laser power

General agreement exists that a spot size of 50 μm in diameter and a duration of 0.1 seconds should be used. Power settings vary, depending on the amount of pigment in the angle. The endpoint of treatment is between a blanch and a tiny bubble, and the power should be adjusted accordingly. The powers generally range from 500 to 1200 mW. Patients with greater pigmentation require less power, whereas those with less pigmentation require more power, to establish the desired effect. Many patients have variably pigmented angles and will thus require adjustments throughout the procedure.

Wavelength

Most investigators have used the argon blue-green light; however, no difference was noted with the argon green laser with respect to results and complications [38].

Laser trabeculoplasty using infrared energy emitted by diode semiconductor lasers has been encouraging. Patients treated with diode laser trabeculoplasty showed comparable success rates as compared with ALT [39–41]. Patients treated with diode laser trabeculoplasty to 180° of the trabecular meshwork, with 100 μm spot size, 0.2-second duration, and mean power of 1096 mW, showed a mean IOP reduction of 7.9 mm Hg at 24 months. No pressure spikes above 5.0 mm Hg were reported after treatment, and inflammation and discomfort were reported as minimal. No peripheral

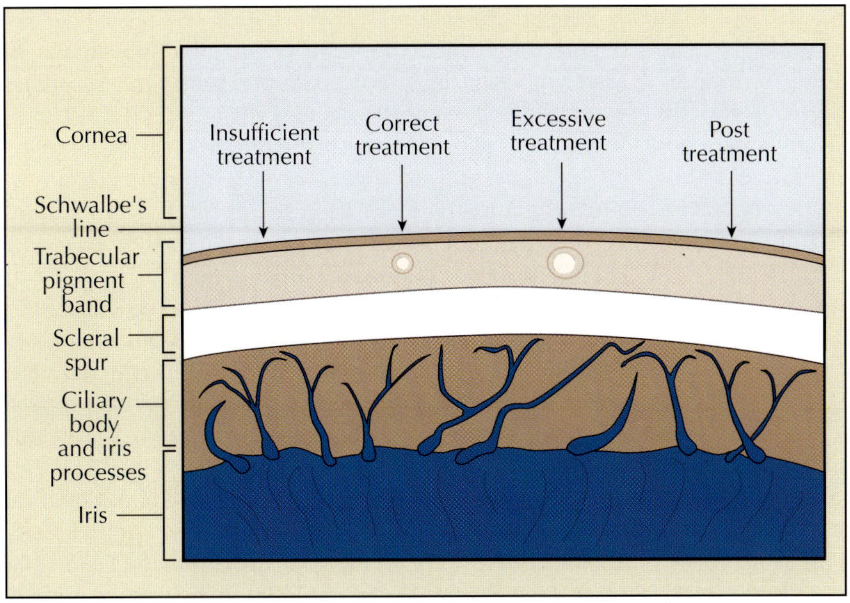

FIGURE 14-3. Treatment responses to variable laser power in argon laser trabeculoplasty (*Adapted from* Schwartz *et al.* [46]; with permission.)

anterior synechiae were identified [16]. Reduced inflammation after diode laser trabeculoplasty may result from less disruption of the blood-aqueous barrier [42]. The portable nature of these lasers makes them especially attractive.

The neodymium:yttrium-aluminum-garnet (Nd:YAG) laser is also being evaluated, especially in patients with lightly pigmented angles. Mermoud *et al.* [43] compared ALT with Nd:YAG laser treatment and found similar IOP lowering at 3 months; however, by 6 months, the Nd:YAG–treated group had higher IOP. Less inflammation was noted in patients treated with the Nd:YAG. Kwasniewska *et al.* [44] studied the long-term (mean follow-up 51 weeks) efficacy of continuous-wave Nd:YAG laser trabeculoplasty and reported a 71.5% success rate at 24 months with no serious inflammatory reactions.

Latina *et al.* [45] were able to attain selective targeting of trabecular cells in vitro using the pulsed and continuous wave Nd:YAG lasers. The ability to target trabecular cells selectively without coagulation while preserving the structural integrity of the meshwork is thought to be a useful approach for studying whether the biologic response to the noncoagulative damage to the trabecular meshwork and trabecular cells is similar to that seen in the coagulative damage to the trabecular meshwork that occurs with ALT [46] (Fig. 14-3). Future clinical studies in this area will be intriguing.

TABLE 14-4 COMPLICATIONS OF ARGON LASER TRABECULOPLASTY

Elevated intraocular pressure
Iritis
Peripheral anterior synechiae
Hypotony
Corneal abrasions and burns
Hyphema

COMPLICATIONS

Although complications may occur (Table 14-4), ALT remains perhaps one of the safest pressure-lowering procedures available.

Elevated postoperative pressure

With the advent of apraclonidine, this complication has been significantly minimized [32–37]. Both 0.5% and 1.0% apraclonidine are equally effective in preventing postoperative IOP spikes [32]. Perioperative apraclonidine with 360° ALT appeared to be as safe as 180° ALT without apraclonidine [36]. One drop of 1.0% apraclonidine instilled immediately after ALT prevented IOP rise 1 and 2 hours postoperatively as effectively as did instillation both 1 hour before and 1 hour after laser treatment [33]. In patients given perioperative apraclonidine, the percentages of patients with an IOP rise above 3 mm Hg at 1 hour, 1 day, and 1 month following ALT were 11.3%, 4.2%, and 5.2% respectively. IOP 1 day after ALT was rarely elevated and did not correlate with IOP elevation at 1 month [47].

We recommend instillation of one drop of 0.5% apraclonidine 30 minutes to 1 hour before ALT and immediately postoperatively. The IOP is checked 2 hours, 1 week, and 1 month postoperatively. Each case, however, is individual. If advanced cupping with field loss encroaching fixation is present, postoperative follow-up care is more frequent.

Perioperative apraclonidine administration is relatively ineffective in patients receiving long-term apraclonidine treatment [35]. Therefore, it is especially important in such patients to monitor postoperative IOP and to be prepared to treat postoperative spikes with agents other than apraclonidine. It may be advisable to treat 180° initially, especially if significant optic nerve damage exists.

Brimonidine has also been shown to reduce pressure spikes after ALT [48–51].

Iritis

Postoperative inflammation is generally mild and clears rapidly; it may persist for months, however, although this is more rare. Small, peaked peripheral anterior synechia are commonly seen after ALT and have no correlation to increased IOP [52] (Fig. 14-4). Diode laser treatment may be associated with less anterior chamber reaction [42]. Use of postoperative fluorometholone was ineffective in reducing inflammation and had no clinically significant impact on the outcome of ALT or on the incidence of postoperative pressure spikes [53].

One of the authors (KAL) noted a shallow anterior chamber postoperatively associated with moderate iritis and hypotony. Hypotony was presumed to be secondary to aqueous shutdown secondary to the inflammation. A suprachoroidal effusion has been reported after ALT [54].

Use of postoperative anti-inflammatory agents is no longer considered mandatory. In our practice, they are mainly given to minimize any postoperative patient discomfort.

Corneal complications

Corneal abrasions and burns are of little significance. There is one reported case of herpes simplex keratitis after ALT [55].

CONCLUSIONS

Argon laser trabeculoplasty is an effective means of lowering IOP in many patients who are receiving extended follow-up. However, up to one half of eyes within 5 years and two thirds of eyes within 10 years of ALT may require additional surgical intervention to control glaucoma [29]. As results of long-term studies become available, it is becoming more evident that ALT is a temporary solution [29,56].

In the United States, historically, ALT has been indicated after drug therapy has failed. In the Glaucoma Laser Trial [57], a multicenter clinical trial, 271 patients with newly diagnosed, previously untreated primary open-angle glaucomas were randomized into initial laser trabeculoplasty in one eye and timolol 0.5% in the other eye. The identical stepped regimen of additional medical therapy was administered in either eye as required. During the course of the Glaucoma Laser Trial and Glaucoma Laser Trial Follow-Up Study [58•], eyes treated initially with ALT had lower IOP and better visual field and optic disc status than did the fellow eyes that had been treated initially with topical medication. Considering the implications of decreased ocular blood flow secondary to topical β-blockers [59], the role of initial ALT compared with medical treatment is becoming more favorable.

The Advanced Glaucoma Intervention Study [60] was designed to examine the long-term clinical course of two sequences of surgical treatment in advanced glaucoma [60]. One sequence begins with ALT followed by trabeculectomy if ALT fails to control the disease. The other sequence begins with a trabeculectomy followed by ALT if the trabeculectomy fails. Results of this important study were not available at competition of this chapter. The Ocular Hypertensive Treatment Study, an ongoing multicenter clinical trial, is trying to determine whether topical medication is effective in preventing optic nerve damage and visual field loss in patients with ocular hypertension.

As the results of these studies unfold, the role of ALT will become more completely defined.

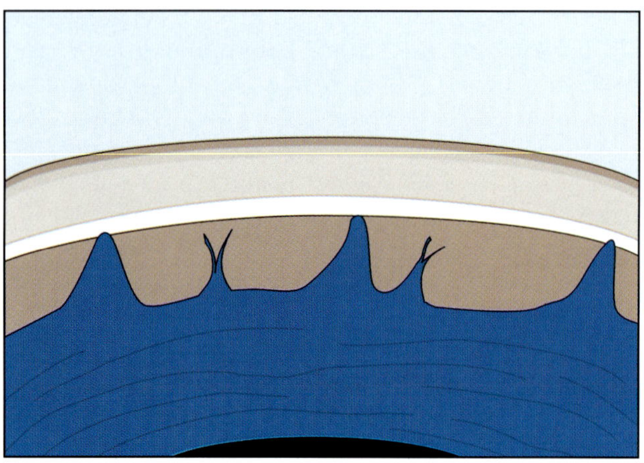

FIGURE 14-4. Gonioscopic view of angle with peripheral anterior synechiae. (*From* Richter [52]; with permission.)

REFERENCES AND RECOMMENDED READING

Recently published papers of particular interest have been highlighted as:
- • Of interest
- •• Of outstanding interest

1. Zweng HC, Flocks, M: Experimental photocoagulation of the anterior chamber angle. A preliminary report. *Am J Ophthalmol* 1961, 52:163
2. Krasnov MM: Q-switched laser goniopuncture. *Arch Ophthalmol* 1974, 92:37–41.
3. Krasnov MM: Laser puncture of the anterior chamber angle in glaucoma. *Vestn Oftal* 1972, 3:27–31.
4. Wise JB, Witter SL: Argon laser therapy for open-angle glaucoma. A pilot study. *Arch Ophthalmol* 1979, 97:319–322.
5. Brubaker RF, Liesegang TJ: Effect of trabecular photocoagulation on the aqueous humor dynamics of the human eye. *Am J Ophthalmol* 1983, 96:139–147.
6. Araie M, Yamamoto T, Shirato S, Kitazawa Y: Effects of laser trabeculoplasty on the human aqueous humor dynamics: a fluorophotometric study. *Ann Ophthalmol* 1984, 16:540–542.
7. Yablonski ME, Cook DJ, Gray J: A fluorophotometric study of the effect of argon laser trabeculoplasty on aqueous humor dynamics. *Am J Ophthalmol* 1985, 99:579–582.
8. Lichter PR: Argon laser trabeculoplasty. *Trans Am Ophthalmol Soc* 1982, 80:288–301.
9. Merte HJ, Denffer H, Hirsch B: Tonographic findings following argon laser trabeculoplasty. *Klin Monatsbl Augenheilkd* 1985, 186:220.
10. Aliseda PD, Fernandez VPC, Beneyto MP: Study of the aqueous humor flow measured by fluorophotometry after argon laser trabeculoplasty. *Int Ophthalmol* 1992, 16:315–319.
11. Wilensky JT, Jampol LM: Laser therapy for open angle glaucoma. *Ophthalmology* 1981, 88:213–217.
12. Yablonski ME, Cook DJ, Gray J: A fluorophotometric study of the effect of argon laser trabeculoplasty on aqueous humor dynamics. *Am J Ophthalmol* 1985, 99:579.
13. Van Buskirk EM, Pond V, Rosenquist RC, *et al.*: Argon laser trabeculoplasty: studies on mechanism of action. *Ophthalmology* 1984, 91:1005–1010.
14. Van Buskirk EM: Pathophysiology of laser trabeculoplasty. *Surv Ophthalmol* 1989, 33:264–272.
15. Melamed S, Epstein DL: Alterations of aqueous humour outflow following argon laser trabeculoplasty in monkeys. *Br J Ophthalmol* 1987, 71:776–781.
16. Acott TS, Samples JR, Bradley JMB, *et al.*: Trabecular repopulation by anterior trabecular meshwork cells after laser trabeculoplasty. *Am J Ophthalmol* 1989, 107:1.
17. Thomas JV, Simmons RJ, Belcher CD III: Argon laser trabeculoplasty in the presurgical glaucoma patient. *Ophthalmology* 1982, 89:187–197.
18. Sherwood MB, Lattimer J, Hitchings RA: Laser trabeculoplasty as supplementary treatment for primary open angle glaucoma. *Br J Ophthalmol* 1987, 71:188–191.
19. Rosenthal AR, Chaudhuri PR, Chiapella AP: Laser trabeculoplasty primary therapy in open-angle glaucoma. A preliminary report. *Arch Ophthalmol* 1984,102:699–701.
20. Tuulonen A, Koponen J, Alanko HI, Airaksinen PJ: Laser trabeculoplasty versus medication treatment as primary therapy for glaucoma. *Acta Ophthalmol* 1989, 67:275–280.
21. Spiegel D, Wegscheider E, Lund OE: Argon laser trabeculoplasty: long-term follow-up of at least 5 years. *Ger J Ophthalmol* 1992, 1:156–158.
22. Rouhianen H, Leino M, Terasvirta M: The effect of some treatment variables on long-term results of argon laser trabeculoplasty. *Ophthalmologica* 1995, 209:21–24.
23. Ritch R, Liebmann J, Robin A, *et al.*: Argon laser trabeculoplasty in pigmentary glaucoma. *Ophthalmology* 1993, 100:909–913.
24. Lehto I: Long-term follow up of argon laser trabeculoplasty in pigmentary glaucoma. *Ophthalmic Surg* 1992, 23:614–617.
25. Threlkeld AB, Hertzmark E, Sturm RT, *et al.*: Comparative study of the efficacy of argon laser trabeculoplasty for exfoliation and primary open-angle glaucoma. *J Glaucoma* 1996, 5:311–316.
26. Traverso CE, Greenridge KC, Spaeth GL: Formation of peripheral anterior synechiae following argon laser trabeculoplasty: a prospective study to determine relationship to position of laser burns. *Arch Ophthalmol* 1984, 102:861–863.
27. Lustgarten J, Podes SM, Ritch R, *et al.*: Laser trabeculoplasty: a prospective study of treatment parameters. *Arch Ophthalmol* 1984, 102:517–519.
28. Wilensky JT, Weinreb RN: Low-dose trabeculoplasty. *Am J Ophthalmol* 1983, 95:423–426.
29. Shingleton BJ, Richter CU, Dharma SK, *et al.*: Long-term efficacy of argon laser trabeculoplasty: a ten-year follow-up. *Ophthalmology* 1993, 100:1324–1329.
30. Horns DJ, Bellows AR, Hutchinson BT, Allen RC: Argon laser trabeculoplasty for open angle glaucoma: a retrospective study of 380 eyes. *Trans Ophthalmol Soc UK* 1983, 103:288–296.
31. Thomas JV, Simmons RJ, Belcher CD III: Complications of argon laser trabeculoplasty. *Glaucoma* 1982, 4:50.
32. Threlkeld AB, Assalian AA, Allingham RR, Shields MB. Apraclonidine 0.5% vs. 1% for controlling intraocular pressure elevation after argon laser trabeculoplasty. *Ophthalmic Surg Lasers* 1996, 27:657–660.

33. Ofner S, Sample JR, Van Buskirk EM: Apraclonidine and argon laser trabeculoplasty [letter]. *Am J Ophthalmol* 1992, 114:778–779.

34. Robin AL: Argon laser trabeculoplasty: medical therapy to prevent the intraocular pressure rise associated with argon laser trabeculoplasty. *Ophthalmic Surg* 1991, 22:31–37.

35. Chung HS, Shin DH, Birt CM, *et al.*:Chronic use of apraclonidine decreases its moderation of post-laser intraocular pressure spikes. *Ophthalmology* 1997, 104:1921–1925.

36. Allf BE, Shields MB: Early intraocular pressure response to laser trabeculoplasty 180° with apraclonidine vs. 360° with apraclonidine. *Ophthalmic Surg* 1991, 22:539–542.

37. Holmwood PC, Chase RD, Krupen T, *et al.*: Apraclonidine and argon laser trabeculoplasty. *Am J Ophthalmol* 1992, 114:19–22.

38. Smith J: Argon laser trabeculoplasty: comparison of biochromatic and monochromatic wavelengths. *Ophthalmology* 1984, 91:355–360.

39. Moriarty AP, McHugh JD, Ffytch TJ, *et al.*: Long-term follow-up of diode laser trabeculoplasty for primary open angle glaucoma and ocular hypertension. *Ophthalmology* 1993, 100:1614–1618.

40. Brooks AM, Gillies WE: Laser trabeculoplasty: argon or diode. *Aust N Z J Ophthalmol* 1993, 21:161–164.

41. Brancato R, Carassa R, Trabucchi G: Diode laser compared with argon laser for trabeculectomy. *Am J Ophthalmol* 1991, 112:50–55.

42. Moriarty AP, McHugh JD, Spalton DJ, *et al.*: Comparison of anterior chamber inflammatory response to diode and argon laser trabeculoplasty using a laser flare meter. *Ophthalmology* 1993, 100:1263–1267.

43. Mermoud A, Herbort CP, Schnyder CC, *et al.*: Comparison of argon laser and Nd:YAG laser trabeculoplasty. *Klin Monatsbl Augenheilkd* 1992, 200:404–406.

44. Kwasniewska AS, Fankhauser F, Larsen SE: The efficacy of CW Nd:YAG laser trabeculoplasty. *Ophthalmic Surg* 1993, 24:304–308.

45. Latina MA, Park C: Selective targeting of trabecular meshwork cells: in vitro studies of pulsed and CW laser interactions. *Exp Eye Res* 1995, 60:359–371.

46. Schwartz AL, Whitten ME, Bleiman B, *et al.*: Argon laser trabeculoplasty and uncontrolled phakic open angle glaucoma. *Ophthalmology* 1981, 88:203–212.

47. Mittra RA, Allingham RR, Shields MB: Follow-up of argon laser trabeculoplasty: is a day one postoperative IOP check necessary? *Ophthalmic Surg Lasers* 1995,26:410–413.

48. The Brimonidine-ALT Study Group: Effective brimonidine .5% on intraocular pressure spikes following 360° of argon laser trabeculoplasty. *Ophthalmic Surg Lasers* 1995, 26:404–409.

49. David R, Spaeth GL, Clevenger CE, *et al.*: Brimonidine in the prevention of intraocular pressure elevation following argon laser trabeculoplasty. *Arch Ophthalmol* 1993, 1111:1387–1390.

50. Greenfield DF, Liebmann JM, Ritch R, *et al.*: Brimonidine: a new alpha-II adrenoreceptor agonist for glaucoma treatment. *J Glaucoma* 1997, 4:250–258.

51. Barnebey HS, Robin AL, Zimmerman TI, *et al.*: Efficacy of brimonidine in decreasing elevations in intraocular pressure after argon laser trabeculoplasty. *Ophthalmology* 1993, 100:1083–1088.

52. Richter C: Laser therapy of open-angle glaucoma. In *Principles and Practice of Ophthalmology*. Edited by Albert D, Jakobiec F. Philadelphia: WB Saunders; 1994.

53. Shin DH, Frankel RE, David R, Cheetham JK: The effect of topical anti-inflammatory treatment on the outcome of laser trabeculoplasty. The Fluorometholone Laser Trabeculoplasty Study. *Am J Ophthalmol* 1996, 122:349–354.

54. Kennedy CJ, Roden DM, McAllister IL: Suprachoroidal effusion following argon laser trabeculoplasty. *Austr N Z J Ophthamol* 1996, 24:279–282.

55. Reed SY, Shin DH, Birt CM, Rhee RK: Herpes simplex keratitis following argon laser trabeculoplasty. *Ophthalmic Surg* 1994, 25:640.

56. Spaeth GL, Baez KA: Argon laser trabeculoplasty controls one-third of cases of progressive uncontrolled open angle glaucoma for five years. *Arch Ophthalmol* 1992, 110:491–494.

57. Beckman H, Meinert CL, Ritch R, *et al.*: The Glaucoma Laser Trial (GLT). 2. Results of argon laser trabeculoplasty vs topical medication. *Ophthalmology* 1990, 97:1403–1413.

58.• Beckman H, Meinert CL, Ritch R, *et al.*: The Glaucoma Laser Trial Research Group: The Glaucoma Laser Trial (GLT) and Glaucoma Laser Trial Follow-up Study. *Am J Ophthalmol* 1995, 120:718–731.

This follow-up study reports the results in 203 of 271 patients initially involved in the Glaucoma Laser Trial. Eyes treated initially with ALT had lower IOP and better visual field and optic disc status than did their fellow eyes treated initially with topical medication. Initial treatment with ALT was at least as efficacious as inital treatment with topical medication.

59. Kitaya N, Yoshida A, Ishiko S, *et al.*: Effective timolol and UF021 (a prostaglandin-related compound) on pulstaile ocular blood flow in normal volunteers. *Ophthalmic Res* 1997, 29:139–144.

60. The Advanced Glaucoma Intervention Study (AGIS): One study design in methods and baseline characteristics of study patients. *Controlled Clin Trials* 1994, 15:299–325.

CHAPTER **15**

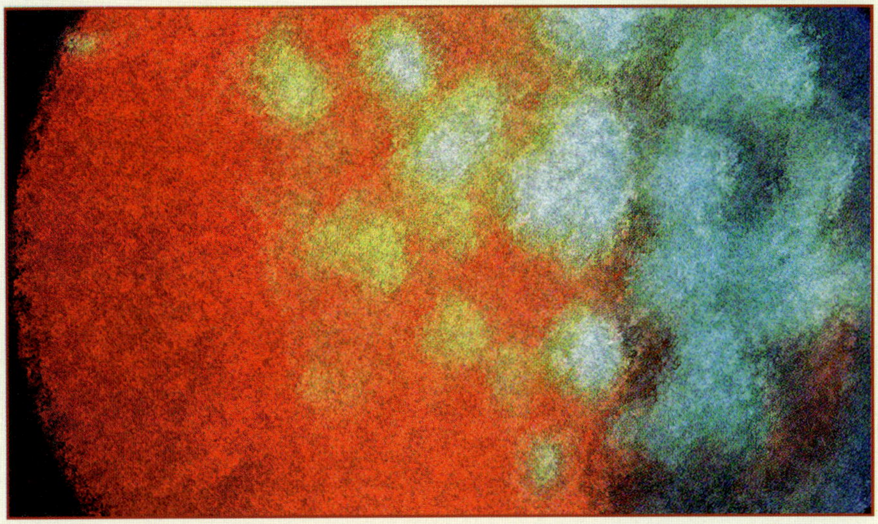

Laser Iridotomy and Peripheral Iridoplasty

Robert Ritch
Jeffrey Liebmann

This chapter discusses basic indications, techniques, and complications of laser iridotomy and argon laser peripheral iridoplasty (ALPI). Papers appearing in the literature since the last edition of this text are reviewed. Iridotomy is successful in eliminating the pupillary block component of angle-closure glaucoma and the reverse pupillary block component of pigment dispersion syndrome. ALPI is effective in treating angle-closure glaucoma caused by mechanisms other than pupillary block, such as plateau iris syndrome and phacomorphic glaucoma. The effectiveness of these procedures can be document ed by ultrasound biomicroscopy.

ANGLE-CLOSURE GLAUCOMA

Anatomic basis of angle-closure glaucoma

Angle-closure glaucoma is an anatomic disorder comprising a final common pathway of iris apposition to the trabecular meshwork resulting from various abnormal relationships of anterior segment structures. These in turn result from one or more abnormalities in the relative or absolute sizes or positions of anterior segment structures or posterior segment forces that alter anterior segment anatomy [1••]. Angle-closure results from blockage of the meshwork by the iris, but the forces causing this blockage may be viewed as originating at four successive anatomic levels (Fig. 15-1): the iris (pupillary block), ciliary body (plateau iris), lens (phacomorphic glaucoma), and posterior to the lens (malignant glaucoma) [1••]. The more posterior the level at which the angle-closure occurs, the more complex the diagnosis and treatment, because each level may have a component of the mechanism peculiar to each of the levels preceding it.

Gonioscopy

Accurate assessment and treatment of narrow or closed angles require indentation gonioscopy, which forces aqueous humor into the angle, thus widening it, when pressure is applied to the cornea. The presence and extent of synechial closure and the depth of the angle can be determined. Gonioscopy in a completely darkened room is of the utmost importance when assessing a narrow angle for occludability (Fig. 15-2). One should use the smallest square of light for a slit beam to avoid stimulating the pupillary light reflex. The quadrant of angle to be assessed is examined with a four-mirror lens without pressure on the cornea and with the patient

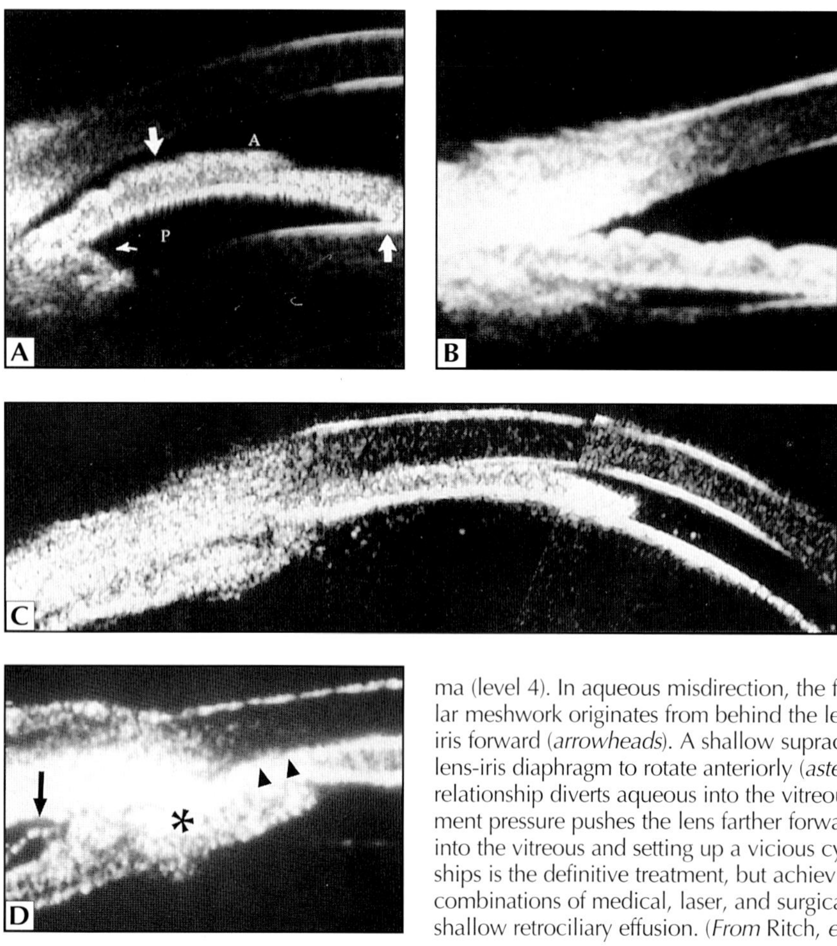

FIGURE 15-1. A, Pupillary block (level 1). The force producing iris apposition to the trabecular meshwork originates from the posterior chamber. Iridotomy provides definitive treatment. The *arrows* show narrowed iris approach and angle inlet. **B,** Plateau iris (level 2). The force producing iris apposition to the trabecular meshwork in this eye, which has already undergone laser iridotomy, originates from the anteriorly positioned ciliary processes holding the iris forward. Peripheral iridoplasty provides definitive treatment. **C,** Phako-morphic glaucoma (level 3). The force producing iris apposition to the trabecular meshwork originates from the intumescent lens, which pushes the ciliary processes and the iris forward. Peri-pheral iridoplasty can break an attack of acute angle-closure glaucoma. Iridotomy can be performed to eliminate any component of pupillary block to give the eye time to quiet and the media to clear so that lens extraction, the definitive procedure, can be safely performed. **D,** Malignant glaucoma (level 4). In aqueous misdirection, the force producing iris apposition to the trabecular meshwork originates from behind the lens, pushing the lens, ciliary processes, and iris forward (*arrowheads*). A shallow supraciliary detachment is present, causing the lens-iris diaphragm to rotate anteriorly (*asterisk*). As a result, the abnormal vitreociliary relationship diverts aqueous into the vitreous posteriorly. The increased posterior segment pressure pushes the lens farther forward, allowing more aqueous to be secreted into the vitreous and setting up a vicious cycle. Restoration of normal anatomic relationships is the definitive treatment, but achieving this can be difficult, entailing complex combinations of medical, laser, and surgical treatment. *Arrow* indicates presence of shallow retrociliary effusion. (*From* Ritch, *et al.* [2]; with permission.)

looking sufficiently far in the direction of the mirror so that the examiner can see as deeply into the angle as possible. The beam is then squared so that the pupil is not illuminated; the angle is observed while the pupil dilates in the dark. The narrowest quadrant is usually the superior angle (inferior mirror).

Pilocarpine paradox

Pupillary constriction induced by pilocarpine usually leads to opening of the angle. Pilocarpine, however, even in elderly patients, also increases axial lens thickness and causes anterior lens movement, further shallowing the anterior chamber [3]. The average eye with acute angle-closure has an anterior chamber depth of about 1.8 mm, which is 1.0 mm shallower than that of "normal" eyes [4]. Increased lens thickness accounts for 0.35 mm of this difference and a more forward lens position accounts for 0.65 mm. In certain cases, the effect of pilocarpine on these biometric parameters can be greater than that on the angle width. Patients with level 3 or level 4 block, in which the lens is directly involved in the angle-closure mechanism, are prone to worsening of the angle-closure when treated with pilocarpine. Paradoxic reactions to pilocarpine have been well documented.

Pupillary block

Pupillary block underlies most cases of angle-closure glaucoma. Aqueous humor flow from the posterior chamber to the anterior chamber is reduced by resistance to transpupillary flow by iridolenticular contact. This creates a relative pressure gradient between the two chambers and pushes the iris anteriorly, causing iris bowing and narrowing or closure of the angle. With sufficient aqueous flow through the pupil, the angle remains open.

Laser iridotomy eliminates the pressure differential between the anterior and posterior chambers and relieves iris convexity. The iris configuration becomes planar and the angle widens. It is the initial procedure of choice for all angle-closure glaucomas in which a component of pupillary block is present. Laser iridotomy deepens the peripheral anterior chamber and increases anterior chamber volume but does not alter central anterior chamber depth. The region of iridolenticular contact actually increases, because aqueous humor flows through the iridectomy rather than the pupillary space [5].

Plateau iris

In plateau iris, the ciliary processes are large or positioned anteriorly, supporting the iris root against the trabecular meshwork [6,7]. The anterior chamber is usually of medium depth and the iris surface slightly convex. On gonioscopy, the iris root angulates forward and then centrally. With indentation, the ciliary processes prevent posterior movement of the peripheral iris, resulting in a configuration in which the slit beam follows the curvature of the iris to its deepest point at the periphery of the lens where the ciliary processes begin, then rises again over the ciliary processes before dropping peripherally (the double hump sign) (Fig. 15-3) [7]. Greater force is needed to open the angle than in pupillary block because the ciliary processes must be displaced and the angle does not open as widely.

Phacomorphic glaucoma

Swelling of the lens may shallow the anterior chamber and precipitate acute angle-closure glaucoma. This is due to the pressing of the lens against the iris and ciliary body, which forces them anteriorly. Pilocarpine produces a paradoxic reaction, further shallowing the anterior chamber. Iridoplasty alone or with iridotomy in phacomorphic glaucoma allows the eye to quiet and corneal edema and anterior chamber inflammation to clear, improving visibility and reducing the possibility of complications at the time of cataract surgery [8]. Using iridotomy to eliminate any element of pupillary block, combined with iridoplasty to contract iris stroma physically at the site of apposition to the trabecular meshwork, we have been able to postpone surgery until the eye is quiet in virtually all patients with acute angle-closure resulting from phacomorphic glaucoma. This allows better assessment of intraocular pressure (IOP) control and the extent of peripheral anterior synechiae (PAS) so that a decision can be made regarding the possible need for a trabeculectomy at the time of cataract surgery.

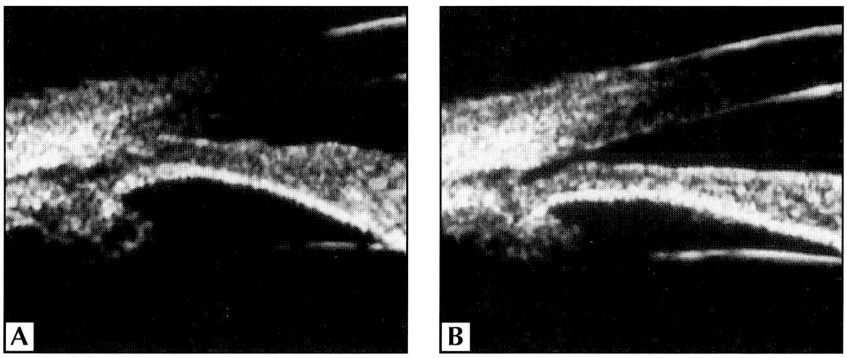

FIGURE 15-2. **A,** Ultrasound biomicrograph of the anterior chamber angle in bright illumination. The iris is slightly convex, consistent with relative pupillary block. Aqueous has access to the trabecular meshwork, which is between Schwalbe's line and scleral spur. **B,** In the dark the pupil dilates and the peripheral iris moves against the trabecular meshwork, closing the angle. (*From* Ritch *et al.* [2]; with permission.)

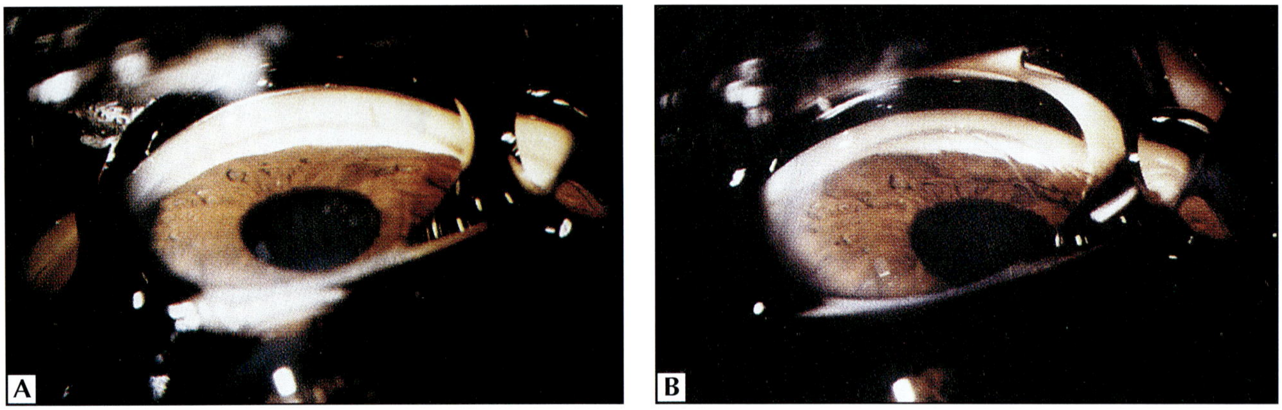

FIGURE 15-3. Gonioscopy in plateau iris syndrome. **A,** Angle postlaser iridectomy without indentation. **B,** With indentation. Note that the deepest point of depression of the iris surface occurs approximately two thirds of the distance between the center of the pupil and the periphery. (*From* Ritch [7]; with permission.)

Malignant glaucoma

Angle-closure caused by forces posterior to the lens that push the lens-iris diaphragm forward presents a great diagnostic and treatment challenge. Malignant (ciliary block) glaucoma is a multifactorial disease in which the following components may play varying roles: 1) previous acute or chronic angle-closure glaucoma, 2) anterior chamber shallowing, 3) forward lens movement, 4) pupillary block by the lens or vitreous, 5) zonular laxity, 6) anterior rotation or swelling of the ciliary body, 7) thickening of the anterior hyaloid, 8) expansion of the vitreous, and 9) posterior aqueous displacement into or behind the vitreous. Analogous to the situation in pupillary block, in which the angle is occluded by the iris because of a pressure differential between the posterior and anterior chambers, in ciliary block, a pressure differential is created between the vitreous and aqueous compartments by aqueous misdirection into the vitreous.

Approach to acute angle-closure glaucoma

The following list describes our approach to the treatment of acute angle-closure glaucoma:

1) Careful history of symptoms relating to intermittent angle-closure attacks, attacks in the fellow eye, prescription or nonprescription drugs that may precipitate attacks, and type of activity preceding the attack.
2) Examination of the affected eye and fellow eye with attention to central and peripheral anterior chamber depth as well as the shape of the peripheral iris.
3) Administration of oral isosorbide and one or more topical aqueous suppressants. Intravenous acetazolamide can be given according to the surgeon's preference.
4) Placement of the patient in a supine position to permit the lens to fall posteriorly with vitreous dehydration.
5) Reassessment of the status of the eye after 1 hour. IOP usually decreases, but the angle usually remains appositionally closed. One drop of pilocarpine 4% is administered and IOP and gonioscopy are reexamined 30 minutes later.

If IOP is reduced and the angle is open, a primary pupillary block (with or without plateau iris) is present (level 1 or level 2), and the patient may be treated medically with topical low-dose pilocarpine, aqueous suppressants, and steroids until the eye quiets and laser iridotomy can be performed.

If IOP is unchanged or elevated and the angle remains closed, lens-related angle-closure (level 3 or level 4) should be suspected, further pilocarpine withheld, and the attack broken using argon laser peripheral iridoplasty [8,9,10•].

Peripheral iridoplasty does not eliminate pupillary block and is not a substitute for laser iridotomy, which must be performed as soon as the eye is quiet. Even in eyes with extensive synechial closure, however, IOP is lowered sufficiently for a few days for the inflammation to resolve. Peripheral iridoplasty is much safer than attempting surgical iridectomy on an inflamed eye with elevated IOP. The risks of intraoperative surgery are avoided, and even if malignant glaucoma is present, the angle remains open long enough for inflammation to clear. The alternative of waiting and prolonging medical therapy for several days seriously increases the possibility of irreversible damage to the iris, lens, drainage pathways, and optic nerve head.

LASER IRIDOTOMY

Techniques of laser iridotomy

Argon laser

Various techniques were described in the 1970s and 1980s to penetrate different types of irides with the argon laser and to deal with certain unusual or complicated situations. Combinations of these techniques can virtually ensure 100% successful penetration in all types and colors of irides. A complete discussion of these techniques is beyond the scope of this chapter and has been thoroughly covered in an extensive review [9]. We ordinarily use the argon laser with a linear incision technique using a spot size of 50 µm, a duration of 0.01 to 0.02 seconds, and a power of 600 to 1200 mW. The linear incision technique allows the dilator muscle to assist in enlarging the opening. The short duration of each application results in a decreased incidence of iris charring, which is more common in dark irides. We prefer the argon laser because of efficient energy absorption, lower incidence of iris bleeding, and less pigment dispersion.

Neodymium:yttrium-aluminum-garnet laser

The neodymium:yttrium-aluminum-garnet (Nd:YAG) laser has become the most commonly used laser for performing iridotomy. The Nd:YAG laser creates a plasma of free ions and electrons at the site of optical breakdown. This photodisruption releases shock waves that mechanically cause tissue rupture, as opposed to the thermal effect of the argon laser. Iris color and density are much less important than with argon laser iridotomy.

Suggested settings for Nd:YAG iridotomy have varied from one to four pulses per burst and from 1 to 10 mJ per burst. Beginning with a single pulse of approximately 1.5 to 3 mJ allows the ophthalmologist to assess the initial response of the iris. An increase in energy to 4 to 6 mJ is often sufficient to create a patent iridotomy with one to three additional applications. We prefer a linear incision technique using lower power burns, on the order of 1 mJ [11]. One should never use more than a single pulse per burst. Precise focus on the anterior iris stroma produces maximal photodisruption and minimizes the possibility of lens injury. The incidence of lens injury is also decreased by choosing a peripheral location.

Sequential argon laser and neodymium:yttrium-aluminum-garnet laser iridotomy

The large variability of iris thickness and color must always be kept in mind when performing laser iridotomy. Thicker and darker irides are more difficult to penetrate and are associated with higher complication rates. Using argon laser techniques to thin the iris stroma and coagulate blood vessels followed by Nd:YAG completion of the iridotomy has been advocated as an approach with few complications, which takes advantage of the photothermal effects of the first and easier penetration achieved through photodisruption of the latter [12•]. The risk of operative hemorrhage is also reduced. Laser iridotomies may also be successfully created with combined dye and argon, diode, krypton, and picosecond lasers [13,14•].

Iris configuration and anterior chamber depth following laser iridotomy

Although the peripheral anterior chamber may deepen following iridotomy, central anterior chamber depth is generally unaffected. Any apparent deepening of the anterior chamber may result from postlaser use of cycloplegia and discontinuation of miotics and their respective effects on lens position. Jin and Anderson [15] showed a decrease in iris convexity following iridotomy using Scheimpflug photography.

Complications

Although laser iridotomy is generally safe, complications do occur. These are listed in Table 15-1. Visual blurring is common immediately after treatment; the causes include anterior segment inflammation, pigment dispersion, retinal pigment bleaching, and keratopathy from methylcellulose. More bothersome to the patient is prolonged glare or even diplopia as a result of the iridotomy's functioning as a second pupil. Iridotomies should always be placed superiorly and never nasally or temporally between the lid fissures.

Some patients complain of seeing a glaring horizontal line, especially when driving in bright sunlight. This phenomenon may result from possible spherical and chromatic aberration plus the diffractive interac-

TABLE 15-1	COMPLICATIONS OF LASER IRIDOTOMY
	Anterior uveitis (transient)
	Blurred vision (transient)
	Closure of the iridotomy
	Corneal epithelial and endothelial burns (argon laser)
	Corneal decompensation (argon laser)
	Cystoid macular edema
	Diplopia
	Glare
	Hyphema (Nd:YAG laser)
	Lens capsular rupture (Nd:YAG laser)
	Lens opacities (argon laser)
	Phacoanaphylactic endophthalmitis (Nd:YAG laser)
	Posterior synechiae
	Postlaser IOP elevation
	Pupillary peaking toward iridotomy (argon laser)
	Pupillary pseudomembrane
	Retinal damage
	Sterile hypopyon

IOP—intraocular pressure; Nd:YAG—neodymium:yttrium-aluminum-garnet.

tion of the eyelid or lashes with the iridotomy [16]. It is most common when the lid bisects the iridotomy and can be confirmed by raising or lowering the lid to expose the iridotomy completely or cover it, respectively. Weintraub and Berke [17] noted the occurrence of this phenomenon despite complete coverage of the iridotomy by the upper lid, with patients' symptoms disappearing when the lid was either raised or lowered sufficiently. They postulated a base-up prism effect of the tear meniscus formed by the edge of the upper lid, causing an upward bending of the light rays and resulting in the perceived extra image being displaced downward. Reassurance is the most important treatment, and most patients gradually stop noticing the phenomenon. If the problem persists, the iridotomy may sometimes be raised by placing contraction burns posterior to it, achieving complete coverage by the upper lid.

Corneal complications with the argon laser include epithelial and endothelial thermal burns, corneal edema, abrasions, and opacities. These rarely occur with the use of lower energy burns. Epithelial coagulation and whitening are transient, but may interfere with the delivery of laser energy and make the creation of a patent iridotomy difficult. Focal damage to the corneal endothelium or Descemet's membrane following laser iridotomy is usually transient. Progressive corneal edema requiring penetrating keratoplasty has been reported following iridotomy with both Nd:YAG and argon lasers. Risk factors appear to include preexisting guttata and excessive laser energy. We have seen one patient with preexisting Fuchs's endothelial dystrophy who developed bullous keratopathy following argon laser peripheral iridoplasty.

Although rare cases of lens capsule rupture with Nd:YAG iridotomy have been described, the earlier widespread fear of acute onset of cataract after Nd:YAG iridotomy caused by inadvertent rupture of the lens capsule has not been substantiated. Small ruptures of the anterior lens capsule after Nd:YAG iridotomy have been documented histopathologically in patients undergoing subsequent intracapsular cataract extraction [18]. Animal studies suggest that fibrous proliferation covers the small anterior capsular breaks [19].

Photocoagulation of the peripheral retina usually occurs when an opening is being enlarged after iris penetration has been achieved. The chance of this occurring is greatly reduced by the use of a contact lens. Inadvertent foveal photocoagulation, choroidal and retinal detachment, and nonrhegmatogenous retinal detachment in nanophthalmic eyes have also been reported. Microperforations of the retina may occur with the Nd:YAG laser if the beam is inadvertently focused to within 2 to 3 mm of the retina [20].

Acute postlaser rise of intraocular pressure

Transient postlaser pressure elevations lasting less than 24 hours are common, usually mild, and easily controlled. Rapid elevation of the pressure to high levels may, however, occur immediately after both argon and Nd:YAG iridotomies. Perioperative treatment with topical apraclonidine 1% decreases the duration and magnitude of the rise. Long-term use of apraclonidine decreases its effectiveness in controlling pressure spikes [21••]. This finding suggests that these patients should be more carefully monitored.

PERIPHERAL IRIDOPLASTY

Clinical applications

Argon laser peripheral iridoplasty is a simple and effective means of opening an appositionally closed angle in situations in which laser iridotomy either cannot be performed or does not physically eliminate appositional angle-closure because mechanisms other than pupillary block are present. The procedure consists of placing contraction burns (long duration, low power, and large spot size) in the extreme iris periphery to contract the iris stroma between the site of the burn and the angle, thus physically pulling open the angle (Fig. 15-4) [8,22,23]. ALPI is extremely useful in reversing an attack of angle-closure glaucoma when medical treatment fails [8,24].

Indications

Medically unbreakable attacks of angle-closure glaucoma

Argon laser peripheral iridoplasty is usually effective in breaking an attack of angle-closure glaucoma that is unresponsive to medical therapy or in which laser iridotomy is ineffective or cannot be performed because of corneal edema, anterior segment inflammation, or a shallow anterior chamber. As already mentioned, patients with acute angle-closure glaucoma who respond poorly to medical therapy usually have a component of lens-induced or phacomorphic angle-closure, which is worsened by the effect of miotics. In these cases, anterior chamber shallowing and increase in axial lens thickness overcome any tendency to open the angle by constricting the pupil. Frequent administration of pilocarpine causes further narrowing of the angle due to an increase in relative pupillary block or forward movement of the lens-iris diaphragm.

Circumferential treatment of the iris opens the angle in those areas in which no PAS are present. All published series have reported virtually 100% success. In a prospective study of 10 eyes with medically unbreakable attacks of 2 to 5 days' duration, mean prelaser IOP was 54.9 mm Hg and 2 to 4 hours postlaser IOP was 18.9 mm Hg [25]. Even when extensive PAS are present, the IOP is usually normalized within an hour or two, perhaps because of associated secretory hypotony. The effect lasts long enough for the cornea and anterior chamber to clear so that iridotomy can be performed. In cases in which an intumescent lens is responsible for the angle-closure attack, cataract extraction can be postponed until the intraocular inflammation has sufficiently resolved.

Weiss *et al.* [26] successfully treated 20 of 32 eyes with ALPI in which angle-closure glaucoma was not relieved by laser iridotomy. The median duration of angle-closure was 12 days in the 20 eyes treated successfully, compared with a median duration of 90 days in the 12 eyes that did not respond well. After a median follow-up period of 18 months, 19 of the 20 successfully treated eyes maintained an IOP $\leq$ 21 mm Hg. Although ALPI has been reported to break PAS [27], we have been unable to accomplish this.

Plateau iris syndrome

In plateau iris, a large or anteriorly positioned ciliary body maintains the iris root in proximity to the trabecular meshwork [6,7]. When indentation gonioscopy is performed in such an eye, the ciliary processes prevent posterior movement of the peripheral iris, producing the "double-hump" sign, in which the iris follows the curvature of the lens, reaches its deepest point at the lens equator, then rises again over the ciliary processes before dropping peripherally. Much more force is needed during gonioscopy to open the angle than in pupillary block, because the ciliary processes must be displaced and the angle does not open as widely.

Plateau iris syndrome refers to the development of angle-closure, either spontaneously or after pupillary dilation, in an eye with plateau iris despite the presence of a patent iridotomy. Some patients may develop acute angle-closure glaucoma [28]. The extent, or the "height" to which the plateau rises, determines whether the angle will close completely or only partially. In the complete plateau iris syndrome, the angle closes to the upper meshwork or Schwalbe's line, blocking aqueous outflow and leading to increased IOP. This situation is far less common than the incomplete syndrome, in which the angle closes only partially, leaving the upper portion of the filtering meshwork open, so that IOP will not rise. However, these eyes can develop PAS years after a successful iridotomy initially produces what appears as a widely opened angle. In addition, the angle can narrow further with age because of enlargement of the lens, so that an angle with plateau configuration that does not close after iridotomy may do so some years later. Periodic gonioscopy is required. Continued appositional angle closure in the presence of a patent iridotomy is an indication for ALPI.

Treatment must be targeted at the cause of angle closure, in this case the ciliary body and iris root. If pupillary block is either not a component mechanism of the angle closure or has been eliminated by iridotomy, it is necessary to find a way to eliminate the physical blockage of the angle. This is accomplished using ALPI, which compresses the iris root and creates a space where none existed before (Figs. 15-5 and 15-6).

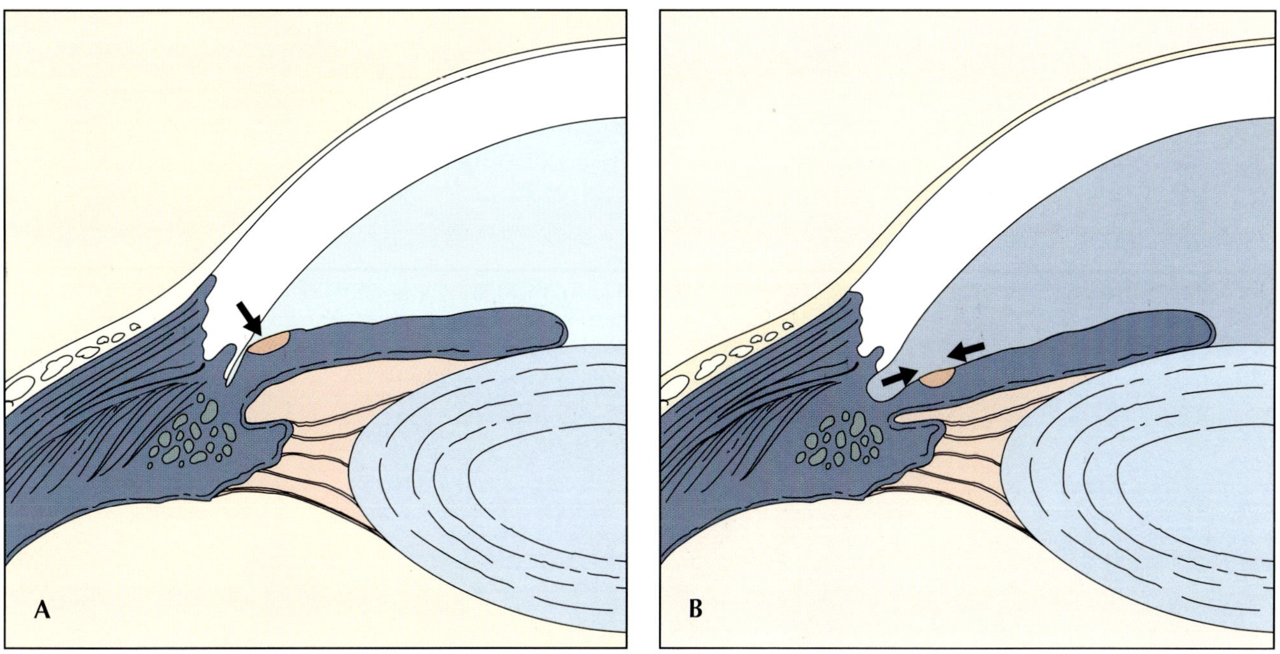

FIGURE 15-4. A, Iridoplasty contraction burns (*arrow*) placed on peripheral iris. **B,** Resulting contraction of peripheral iris stroma, opening the angle and relieving apposition of iris to trabecular meshwork. (*Adapted from* Ritch *et al.* [2]; with permission.)

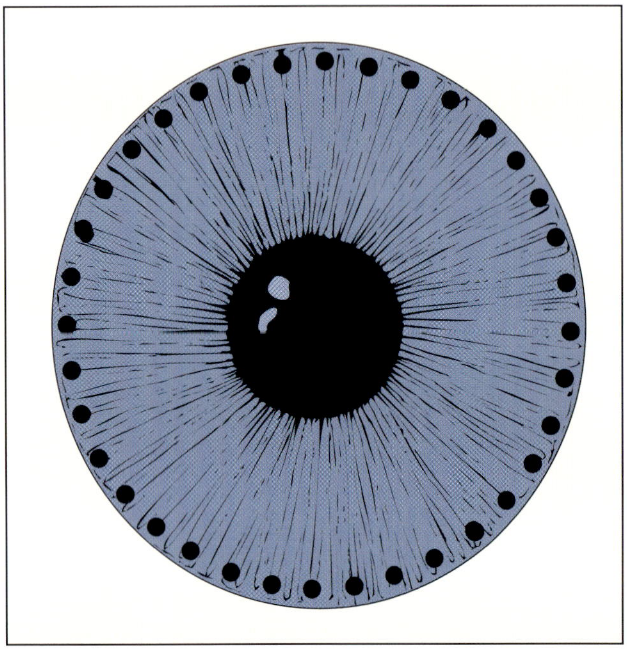

FIGURE 15-5. Technique of argon laser peripheral iridoplasty showing the placement of contraction burns circumferentially around the iris as far peripherally as possible. (*Adapted from* Ritch *et al.* [2]; with permission.)

Angle closure related to size or position of the lens

Angle closure caused by an enlarged lens or pressure posterior to the lens pushing it forward does not often respond to iridotomy, although a component of pupillary block may be present and should be eliminated by iridotomy. In situations in which the angle remains appositionally closed after laser iridotomy, the apposition can often be partially or entirely eliminated by ALPI [22,29–31]. After the angle has been opened and IOP reduced, cycloplegics may be given cautiously to ascertain the mechanism of the angle closure.

Nanophthalmos

Patients with nanophthalmos are anatomically predisposed to angle-closure glaucoma due to anterior chamber crowding. Angle-closure glaucoma usually appears between the ages of 20 and 50 years. Laser iridotomy is usually unsuccessful or only temporarily successful. Risks of surgical intervention include malignant glaucoma, expulsive suprachoroidal hemorrhage, and retinal detachment. Flattening of the peripheral iris by argon laser was first reported in 1979 by Kimbrough *et al.* [32]. Combined iridotomy and ALPI often bring the angle closure under control. Uveal effusions have been

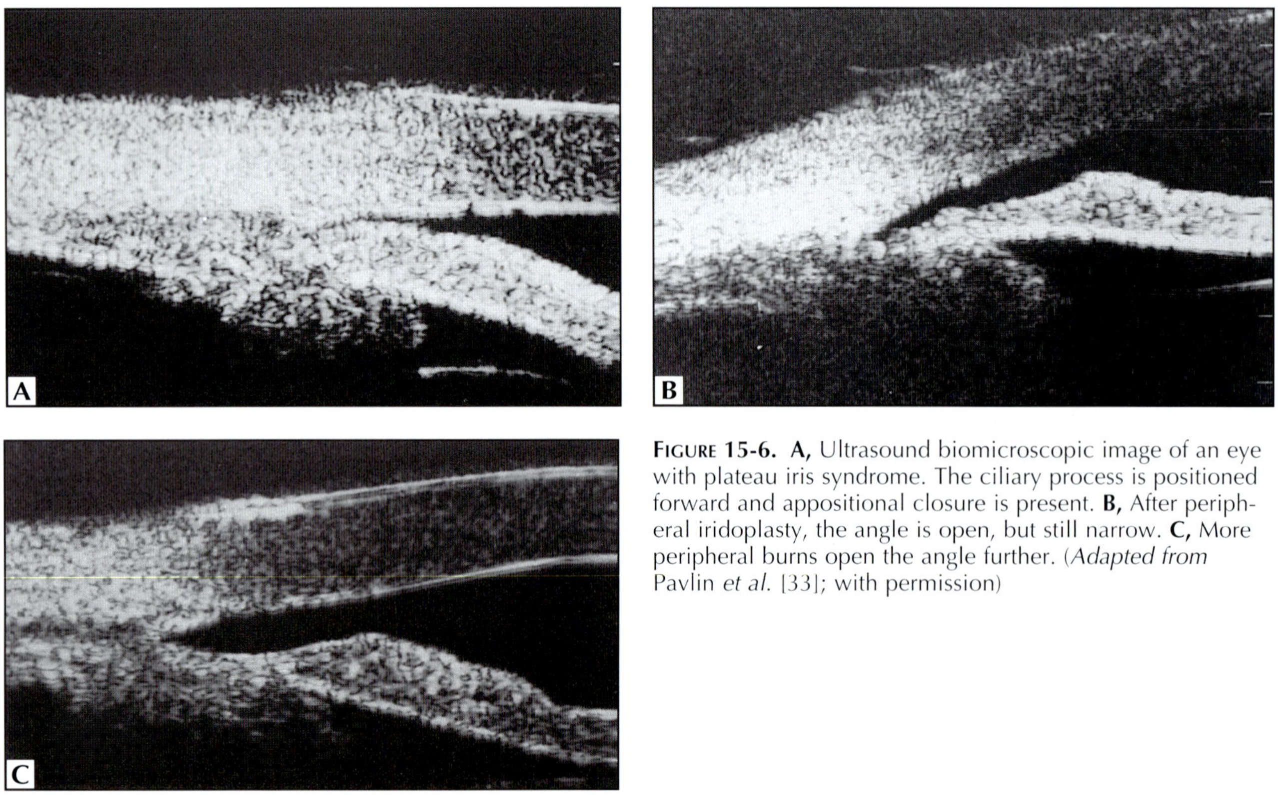

FIGURE 15-6. A, Ultrasound biomicroscopic image of an eye with plateau iris syndrome. The ciliary process is positioned forward and appositional closure is present. **B,** After peripheral iridoplasty, the angle is open, but still narrow. **C,** More peripheral burns open the angle further. (*Adapted from* Pavlin *et al.* [33]; with permission)

reported after both laser iridotomy [34] and argon laser trabeculoplasty [35].

Adjunct to laser trabeculoplasty

Argon laser peripheral iridoplasty can be used to widen a narrow angle to allow adequate visibility for spot placement for laser trabeculoplasty. Focal contraction burns may be used when iris irregularities or intraepithelial cysts obstruct the view of the trabecular meshwork. We have also found focal burns useful in cases where the iris stroma obstructs the internal ostium following trabeculectomy or ab interno sclerostomy. This must be performed relatively early in the postoperative course before the formation of permanent synechiae.

Contraindications to argon laser peripheral iridoplasty

Moderate degrees of corneal edema are not a contraindication to ALPI when it is performed to break a medically unresponsive attack of angle-closure glaucoma. Extensive corneal opacification may present difficulties, because higher powers necessary to cause contraction of the iris may injure the cornea as well. Glycerin may help clear the cornea temporarily.

If the anterior chamber is shallow, laser applications should be placed enough apart in time so that generated heat can dissipate. Corneal endothelial burns are generated by heating of the aqueous humor at the site of the laser burn and its reflux toward the corneal endothelium. If the iris is apposed to the cornea, any attempt at photocoagulation will result in damage to the corneal endothelium.

Because ALPI will not relieve synechial angle closure, it should not be used for this purpose, especially in eyes with uveitis, neovascular glaucoma, or iridocorneal-endothelial syndrome.

Techniques

Beginning approximately 45 minutes before treatment, 4% pilocarpine and 1% apraclonidine are applied topically to stretch the iris and to prevent a postlaser IOP spike, respectively. Topical anesthesia is administered, and an Abraham lens is used. We prefer a spot size of 500 µm, a duration of 0.5 seconds, and a low power setting of 200 to 400 mW, depending on iris color. These laser parameters allow condensation and compaction of the iris stroma but do not cause tissue vaporization or disruption. The spots are aimed through the periphery of the lens and 20 to 30 spots are placed at 360°, leaving two spot diameters between each spot and making certain radial iris vessels are avoided. Begin with 200 mW power in dark irides and 300 mW in light irides and adjust power as necessary to achieve contraction. It is important to treat as far peripherally as possible. It is also useful to allow a thin crescent of the aiming beam to overlap the sclera at the limbus and have the patient look in the direction of the aiming beam to obtain more peripheral spot placement.

We occasionally use a 200-µm spot size of 0.2-second duration and 100 to 250 mW. We find this to be more effective for causing contraction in light gray irides and for focal treatment when the iris root is plugging a trabeculectomy ostium or sclerostomy site. During these latter two situations, we prefer to treat the iris by focusing the laser through a goniolens, because this technique provides direct visualization of the problem and enables more accurate spot placement. When ALPI is performed using a goniolens, however, a more diffuse burn with less stromal contraction is obtained, because the laser strikes the iris surface more tangentially.

Another situation in which a goniolens is useful for iridoplasty is when a very sharp plateau configuration to the iris contour exists. Direct visualization of the area of apposition allows better spot placement. In patients with a very steep plateau, ALPI can be repeated to reach a more peripheral location following the first treatment; burns placed just inside the point of apposition pull the angle open and expose more peripheral iris stroma for a second application.

Immediately following ALPI, one drop of 1% apraclonidine and one drop of a topical corticosteroid are applied. Gonioscopy is performed and IOP is checked 1 hour postlaser. Topical steroids are prescribed for a few days.

If extensive PAS are present after ALPI, goniosynechialysis may be performed. In this procedure, PAS are surgically stripped from the angle wall to restore trabecular function. The procedure is successful only if the PAS have been present for less than 1 year [36], and it is effective both alone and in conjunction with other surgical procedures [37]. ALPI can be used postoperatively to flatten the peripheral iris further and prevent synechial reattachment [38].

Complications

A mild iritis is common (but usually transient) and responds well to topical steroids. Pupillary distortion rarely occurs and is more evident after focal treatment. Postlaser elevations in IOP may be related to inflammation or extensive synechial closure and usually respond well to medical therapy. Corneal endothelial burns can occur, especially in patients with a very shallow anterior chamber. These usually last a few days and are of no major consequence.

Pigment dispersion syndrome and pigmentary glaucoma

Pigment dispersion syndrome and pigmentary glaucoma are characterized by disruption of the iris pigment epithelium and deposition of the dispersed pigment granules throughout the anterior segment. The classic diagnostic triad consists of corneal pigmentation (Krukenberg spindle); slit-like, radial, midperipheral iris transillumination defects; and dense trabecular pigmentation. The iris insertion is typically posterior and the peripheral iris tends to have a concave configuration. Pigment dispersion syndrome is an inherited disorder of abnormal iridozonular contact that is exaggerated by physiologic pupillary movement and accommodation. This contact results in disruption of the iris pigment epilthelium cells and liberation of pigment [39]. Pigment liberation can be triggered by exercise and by pupillary dilation. Myopia predisposes to the phenotypic expression of pigment dispersion syndrome, which affects men and women equally, but men develop glaucoma 2 to 3 times more often than women and at an earlier age. Pigment dispersion begins in the teens or twenties and continues until about the mid-40s in most people, at which time a combination of relative pupillary block and presbyopia lead to gradual cessation of pigment liberation. After this, the visible signs of pigment loss can reverse and IOP control can improve. Older patients presenting for the first time with glaucomatous damage and normal IOP may be misdiagnosed as having normal tension glaucoma.

Anatomically, the iris appears unusually large for the eye and is inserted posteriorly, producing a characteristic concave midperipheral configuration. The concavity is accentuated by accommodation [33,40•]. When blinking is inhibited, the iris assumes a convex configuration that is immediately reversed on blinking, suggesting that the act of blinking acts as a mechanical pump to push aqueous humor from the posterior to the anterior chamber [41••]. Once in the anterior chamber, aqueous backflow is prevented by the abnormal iridolenticular contact, which produces a reverse pupillary block, further enhancing the iris concavity [42].

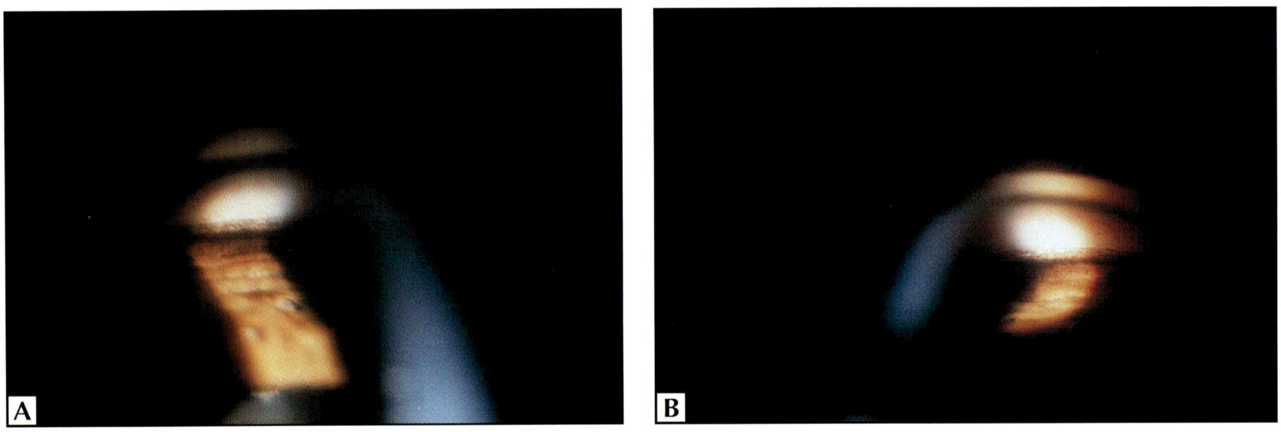

FIGURE 15-7. **A,** Gonioscopic photograph of an eye with pigment dispersion syndrome prior to argon laser iridotomy. Note the midperipheral iris concavity. **B,** Following laser iridotomy, resolution of an iris concavity is noted.

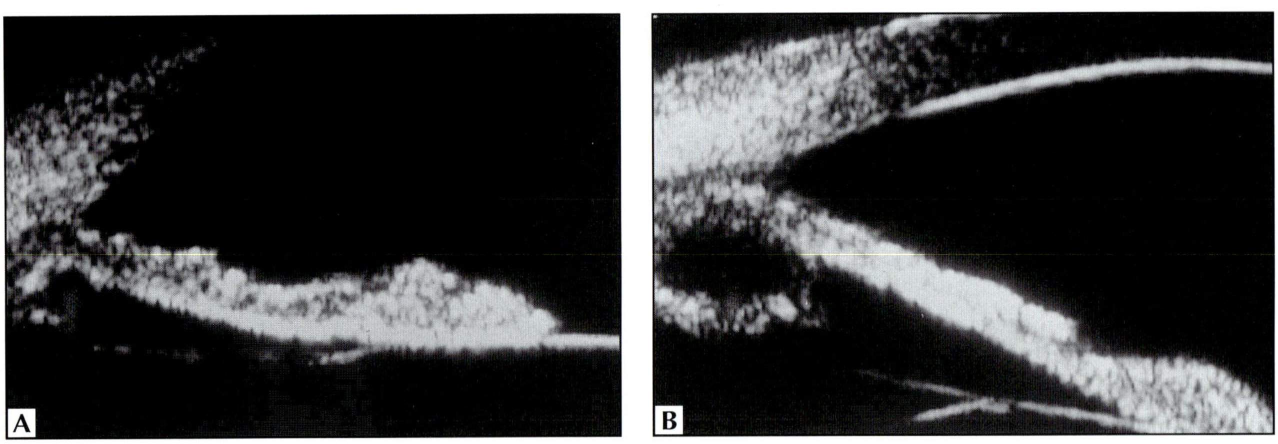

FIGURE 15-8. **A,** Ultrasound biomicrograph from a patient with pigment dispersion syndrome. Note the marked iris concavity and iridozonular contact. **B,** Following laser iridotomy, the iris has assumed a planar configuration and iridozonular contact has resolved.

Laser iridotomy eliminates the component of reverse pupillary block in pigment dispersion syndrome, just as it relieves forward pupillary block, by allowing equilibration of aqueous humor between the anterior and posterior chambers, eliminating the pressure differential across the iris (Figs. 15-7 and 15-8) [43,44,45••]. Pigment liberation from the iris is largely, but not entirely, eliminated [46].

Probably only a minority of patients with pigment dispersion syndrome or pigmentary glaucoma should undergo iridotomy. Patients who have uncontrolled glaucoma and are facing surgery are poor candidates for laser iridotomy, because years are required to achieve functional reconstitution of the trabecular meshwork. By preventing pigment liberation from the iris, the meshwork should have time to clear itself of pigment already deposited and reduce or eliminate further deposition. Therefore, patients should still be in the pigment liberation stage.

As a rule of thumb, we have restricted iridotomy thus far to patients under 45 years of age who have elevated IOP with either no damage or early glaucomatous damage. Although iridotomy has been reported to prevent a rise in IOP when eyes receiving iridotomy were compared with the fellow eye [47], we have not found anywhere near the percentage of fellow eyes having a rise in IOP in so short a time as reported. Clinical trials are needed to determine whether Ocuserts (Ciba Vision, Duluth, GA) or iridotomy can normalize IOP in eyes with glaucomatous damage, prevent glaucomatous damage in eyes with elevated IOP, and prevent elevated IOP in normotensive eyes. Because not all patients with pigment dispersion syndrome go on to develop elevated IOP, and because the iridotomy procedure itself results in significant pigment liberation, we do not advocate treating normotensive eyes at the present time.

REFERENCES AND RECOMMENDED READING

Recently published papers of particular interest have been highlighted as:
- • Of interest
- •• Of outstanding interest

1.•• Ritch R, Liebmann J, Tello C: A construct for understanding angle-closure glaucoma: the role of ultrasound biomicroscopy. *Ophthalmol Clin North Am* 1995, 8:281–293.

A new concept of classification of angle-closure glaucoma based on mechanisms elucidated by ultrasound biomicroscopy allows more precise diagnosis and treatment.

2. Ritch R, Shields MB, Krupin T: *The Glaucomas*. St. Louis: Mosby; 1989.

3. Abramson DH, Franzen LA, Coleman DJ: Pilocarpine in the presbyope: demonstration of an effect on the anterior chamber and lens thickness. *Arch Ophthalmol* 1973, 89:100–102.

4. Lowe RF: Primary angle-closure glaucoma: a review of ocular biometry. *Aust J Ophthalmol* 1977, 5:9–17.

5. Caronia RM, Liebmann JM, Stegman Z, *et al.*: Iris-lens contact increases following laser iridotomy for pupillary block angle-closure. *Am J Ophthalmol* 1996, 122:53–57.

6. Pavlin CJ, Ritch R, Foster FS: Ultrasound biomicroscopy in plateau iris syndrome. *Am J Ophthalmol* 1992, 113:390–395.

7. Ritch R: Plateau iris is caused by abnormally positioned ciliary processes. *J Glaucoma* 1992, 1:23–26.

8. Ritch R: Argon laser treatment for medically unresponsive attacks of angle-closure glaucoma. *Am J Ophthalmol* 1982, 94:197.

9. Ritch R, Solomon IS: Laser treatment of glaucoma. In *Ophthalmic Lasers*, vol. 2, edn 3. Edited by L'Esperance FAJ. St Louis: CV Mosby; 1989:650–748.

10.• Ritch R, Liebmann JM: Argon laser peripheral iridoplasty: a review. *Ophthalmic Surg Lasers* 1996, 27:289–300.

A recent review of indications, techniques, and results.

11. Wise JB: Low-energy linear-incision neodymium:YAG laser iridotomy versus linear-incision argon laser iridotomy: a prospective clinical investigation. *Ophthalmology* 1987, 94:1531.

12.• Lim L, Seah SKL, Lim ASM: Comparison of argon laser iridotomy and sequential argon laser and Nd:YAG laser iridotomy in dark irides. *Ophthalmic Surg Lasers* 1996, 27:285–288.

The total argon laser energy used can be reduced by 2.65 times using the sequential laser iridotomy technique.

13. Frangie JP, Park SB, Aquavella JV: Peripheral iridotomy using Nd:YLF laser. *Ophthalmic Surg* 1992, 23:220–221.

14.• Oram O, Gross RL, Severin TD, *et al.*: Picosecond neodymium:yttrium lithium fluoride (Nd:YLF) laser peripheral iridotomy. *Am J Ophthalmol* 1995, 119:408–414.

The picosecond Nd:yttrium-lithium-fluoride laser seems to be an effective instrument for reliably performing peripheral iridotomies of precise size and shape using low energy per pulse levels. This laser can easily make a larger iridotomy than is often possible with the Nd:YAG laser.

15. Jin JC, Anderson DR: The effect of iridotomy on iris contour. *Am J Ophthalmol* 1990, 110:260–263.

16. Murphy PH, Trope GE: Monocular blurring: a complication of YAG laser iridotomy. *Ophthalmology* 1991, 98:1539–1542.

17. Weintraub J, Berke SJ: Blurring after iridotomy [letter]. *Ophthalmology* 1992, 99:479–480.

18. Welch DB, Apple DJ, Mendelsohn AD, *et al.*: Lens injury following iridotomy with a Q-switched neodymium:YAG laser. *Arch Ophthalmol* 1986, 194:123.

19. Gaasterland DG, Rodrigues MM, Thomas G: Threshold for lens damage during Q-switched Nd:YAG laser iridectomy: a study of Rhesus monkey eyes. *Ophthalmology* 1985, 92:1616.

20. Jampol LM, Goldberg MF, Jednock N: Retinal damage from a Q-switched YAG laser. *Am J Ophthalmol* 1983, 96:326.

21.•• Chung HS, Sin DH, Birt CM, *et al.*: Chronic use of apraclonidine decreases its moderation of post-laser IOP spikes. *Ophthalmology* 1997, 104:1921–1925.

Patients treated chronically with apraclonidine have more frequent and greater magnitude of postlaser rises in IOP when given apraclonidine perioperatively.

22. Ritch R, Solomon IS: Glaucoma surgery. In *Ophthalmic Lasers* edn 3. Edited by L'Esperance FA. St. Louis: CV Mosby; 1989:650–748.

23. Ritch R: Argon laser peripheral iridoplasty: an overview. *J Glaucoma* 1992, 1:206–213.

24. Lim AS, Tan A, Chew P, *et al.*: Laser iridoplasty in the treatment of severe acute angle closure glaucoma. *Int Ophthalmol* 1993, 17:33–36.

25. Chew P, Chee C, Lim A: Laser treatment of severe acute angle-closure glaucoma in dark Asian irides: the role of iridoplasty. *Lasers Light Ophthalmol* 1991, 4:41–42.

26. Weiss HS, Shingleton BJ, Goode SM, *et al.*: Argon laser gonioplasty in the treatment of angle-closure glaucoma. *Am J Ophthalmol* 1992, 114:14–18.

27. Wand M: Argon laser gonioplasty for synechial angle closure. *Arch Ophthalmol* 1992, 110:353–367.

28. Wand M, Grant WM, Simmons RJ, *et al.*: Plateau iris syndrome. *Trans Am Acad Ophthalmol Otol* 1977, 83:122.

29. York K, Ritch R, Szmyd LJ: Argon laser peripheral iridoplasty: indications, techniques, and results. *Invest Ophthalmol Vis Sci* 1984, 25(Suppl):94.

30. Burton TC, Folk JC: Laser iris retraction for angle-closure glaucoma after retinal detachment surgery. *Ophthalmology* 1988, 95:742–748.

31. Koster HR, Liebmann JM, Ritch R, *et al.*: Acute angle-closure glaucoma in a patient with acquired immunodeficiency syndrome successfully treated with argon laser peripheral iridoplasty. *Ophthalmic Surg* 1990, 21:501–502.

32. Kimbrough RL, Trempe CS, Brockhurst RJ, *et al.*: Angle-closure glaucoma in nanophthalmos. *Am J Ophthalmol* 1979, 88:572.

33. Pavlin CJ, Harasiewicz K, Foster FS: Posterior iris bowing in pigmentary dispersion syndrome caused by accommodation. *Am J Ophthalmol* 1994, 118:114–116.

34. Karjalainen K, Laatikainen L, Raitta C: Bilateral nonrhegmatogenous retinal detachment following neodymium:YAG laser iridotomies. *Arch Ophthalmol* 1986, 104:1134.

35. Good WV, Stern WH: Recurrent nanophthalmic uveal effusion syndrome following laser trabeculoplasty. *Am J Ophthalmol* 1988, 106:234–235.

36. Campbell DG, Vela A: Modern goniosynechialysis for the treatment of synechial angle-closure glaucoma. *Ophthalmology* 1984, 91:1052–1060.

37. Shingleton BJ, Chang MA, Bellows AR, *et al.*: Surgical goniosynechialysis for angle-closure glaucoma. *Ophthalmology* 1990, 97:551–556.

38. Tanihara H, Nagata M: Argon-laser gonioplasty following goniosynechialysis. *Graefes Arch Clin Exp Ophthalmol* 1991, 229:505–507.

39. Campbell DG: Pigmentary dispersion and pigmentary glaucoma: a new theory. *Invest Ophthalmol Vis Sci* 1979, 20(Suppl):25.

40.• Pavlin CJ, Macken P, Trope G, *et al.*: Accommodation and iridotomy in the pigment dispersion syndrome. *Ophthalmic Surg Lasers* 1996, 27:113–120.

Accommodation increases iris concavity in some patients with pigment dispersion syndrome. The most likely explanation is an accommodation-induced relative increase in anterior chamber pressure secondary to anterior movement of the lens surface. Iridotomy prevents change in the iris profile with accommodation.

41.•• Liebmann JM, Tello C, Chew S-J, *et al.*: Prevention of blinking alters iris configuration in pigment dispersion syndrome and in normal eyes. *Ophthalmology* 1995, 102:446–455.

Increased iris concavity appears related to increased iridolenticular contact, creating an anatomic configuration that predisposes to reverse pupillary block. The accumulation of aqueous in the posterior chamber, when blinking is prevented, alters iris position in pigment dispersion syndrome and in healthy eyes and increases iridozonular and iridociliary-process distances while minimizing iridolenticular contact. Normal blinking appears to create transient vector forces that promote aqueous humor flow from the posterior to anterior chamber.

42. Karickhoff JR. Pigmentary dispersion syndrome and pigmentary glaucoma: a new mechanism concept, a new treatment, and a new technique. *Ophthalmic Surg* 1992, 23:269–277.

43. Potash SD, Tello C, Liebmann J, *et al.*: Ultrasound biomicroscopy in pigment dispersion syndrome. *Ophthalmology* 1994, 101:332–339.

44. Pavlin CJ, Macken P, Trope G, *et al.*: Ultrasound biomicroscopic features of pigmentary glaucoma. *Can J Ophthalmol* 1994, 29:187–192.

45.•• Lagréze WD, Funk J: Iridotomy in the treatment of pigmentary glaucoma: documentation with high resolution ultrasound. *Ger J Ophthalmol* 1995, 4:162–166.

Yttrium-argon-garnet-laser iridotomy is a prophylactic treatment in pigmentary glaucoma for a subgroup of patients in whom an iris concavity with iris-zonular rubbing can be demonstrated by high-resolution ultrasound or equivalent methods.

46. Haynes WL, Alward WLM, Tello C, *et al.*: Incomplete elimination of exercise-induced pigment dispersion by laser iridotomy in pigment dispersion syndrome. *Ophthalmic Surg Lasers* 1995, 26:484–486.

47. Gandolfi SA, Vecchi M: Effect of a YAG laser iridotomy on intraocular pressure in pigment dispersion syndrome. *Ophthalmology* 1996, 103:1693–1695.

CHAPTER 16

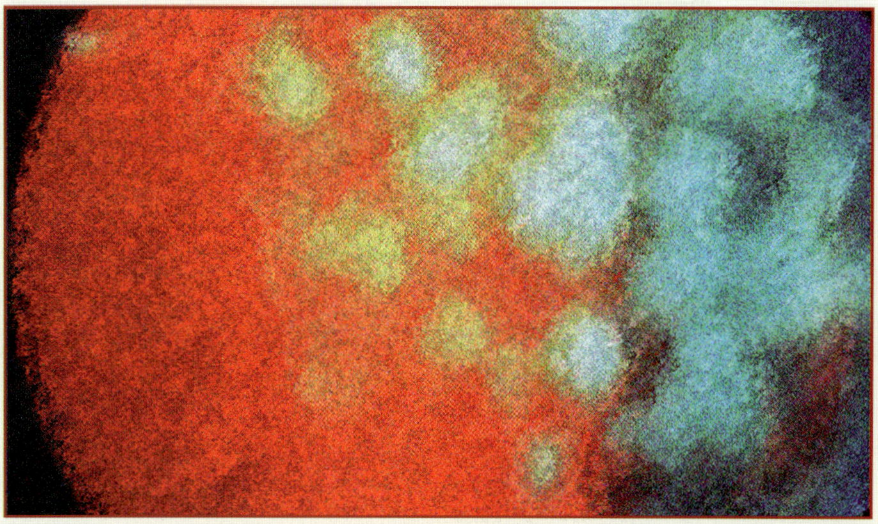

Laser Cyclophotocoagulation

DOUGLAS J. RIPKIN
PAUL N. SCHACKNOW

Cyclodestructive procedures for controlling intraocular pressure (IOP) are indicated when traditional medical, laser, and surgical procedures have proved inadequate to preserve the patient's vision or comfort in a case of advanced glaucoma. Early experience with cyclodestructive modalities (diathermy, β-irradiation, cyclocryotherapy, cycloelectrolysis, partial cyclectomy, and therapeutic ultrasound) revealed poor titration of effect ranging from inadequately controlled IOP to anterior segment necrosis, phthisis bulbi, sympathetic ophthalmia, and blind painful eyes [1–3].

Most patients selected for laser cyclodestructive therapy will have uncontrolled IOP on maximum tolerated medical therapy and will have failed prior filtration surgery with a poor prognosis for further glaucoma surgery, including the use of antimetabolites and shunt implants. Other patients will have a type of glaucoma that is very likely to fail filtering surgery (*eg*, neovascular, inflammatory, postpenetrating keratoplasty, postscleral buckling, and some aphakes and pseudophakes) or will be offered laser cyclodestruction for comfort or because they cannot tolerate filtering surgery for other, more general medical reasons.

Traditionally, cyclodestructive procedures were reserved for those patients with very poor visual potential, who had little chance of visual rehabilitation. Today, because modern laser cyclodestructive procedures have reduced the risk of complete aqueous shutdown, even eyes with useful vision may be considered for these treatments. The improved perioperative comfort and titratability of the laser procedures have allowed them to replace cyclocryotherapy for appropriate patients if the technology is available to the ophthalmic surgeon.

Cyclophotocoagulation instruments have used Xenon arc lamps and ruby, argon, neodymium (Nd) glass, Nd:yttrium-aluminum-garnet (YAG), and solid-state diode lasers. Current techniques employing Nd:YAG and solid-state lasers are more titratable and sometimes may be repeated. These techniques differ in their routes of delivery of the laser energy to the ciliary body and in their degree of invasiveness. Transpupillary cyclophotocoagulation requires direct visualization and treatment of the ciliary processes. Intraocular cyclophotocoagulation uses an endolaser probe to apply energy directly to the ciliary processes. Transscleral cyclophotocoagulation requires either focusing the laser through a slit lamp delivery system at the level of the ciliary body or application of a hand-held diode laser directly to the eye wall.

HISTOLOGIC AND PATHOLOGIC FINDINGS

Interest has increased greatly over the past several years regarding how laser cyclodestructive procedures lower IOP at anatomic and histopathologic levels. It has become clinically evident that aqueous production decreases after cyclodestruction. An increasing body of evidence is demonstrating that the histologic characteristics of laser cyclodestruction include tissue damage, principally to the ciliary epithelium. There is a single case report of pathologic assessment of an eye from a 72-year-old patient who died of pneumonia 3 days after transscleral diode cyclodestruction [4]. Treatment spots were placed 0.5 mm posterior to the surgical limbus externally. Gray-white circular lesions, correlating with the laser spots, were reported as present at the pars plicata, with no other damage noted during gross examination. Microscopic examination of the treated

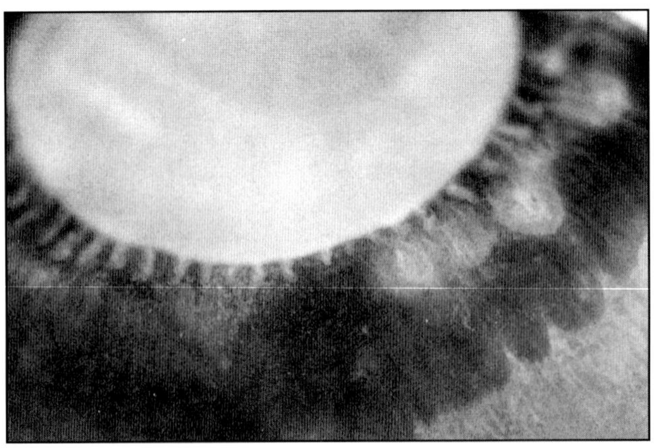

FIGURE 16-1. Gray white lesions seen at pars plicata and pars plana after cyclophotocoagulation (*From* Feldman *et al.* [4]; with permission.)

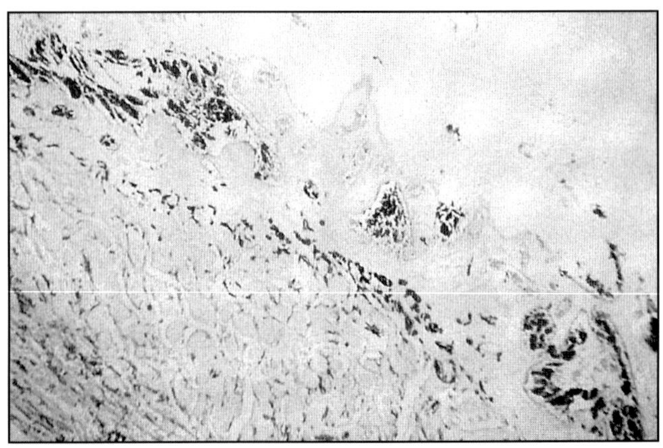

FIGURE 16-2. Photomicrograph showing nonpigmented and pigmented epithelium obliterated directly under laser probe. From an approximate 1-mm distance, the changes cannot be differentiated from autolysis preceding fixation (hematoxylin and eosin, × 100). (*From* Feldman *et al.* [4]; with permission.)

region showed sparse inflammatory infiltrate in the episclera. The sclera and the ciliary body revealed coagulative necrosis without inflammatory cells. Both pigmented and nonpigmented epithelia were obliterated in treated areas. It was also reported that normal cellular detail was lost in the treated area. Tissue adjacent to the treated areas, however, was normal with no perceived distant effects from laser treatment (Fig. 16-1 and 16-2).

Another study described histopathologic changes from three eyes that were enucleated at 2 weeks, 8 weeks, and 17 months after noncontact Nd:YAG cyclodestruction [5]. At 2 weeks, there was destruction of the nonpigmented and pigmented ciliary body epithelium, occlusion of the capillaries of the ciliary processes, and ciliary body stromal necrosis in the region of the ciliary processes. At 8 weeks and at 17 months, findings included hyperplasia of the pigmented and nonpigmented epithelium, fibrosis and near-total atrophy of the ciliary epithelium, fibrosis and near-total atrophy of the ciliary processes, and partial atrophy of the ciliary muscles. Treatment directed at the corneoscleral limbus destroys the pars plicata, which translates to histologic destruction of the ciliary processes, which, in turn, leads to decreased aqueous production.

These studies show that the ciliary epithelium is destroyed by the laser procedures themselves, regardless of the mode of delivery of the laser energy. It is also evident that the tissues adjacent to the treatment areas show very little damage. We would expect this to lead to reduced incidence of phthisis bulbi, compared with the cyclodestruction caused by cyclocryotherapy. Moreover, reduced laser-related pressure has been observed even when the laser lesions were applied posterior to the pars plicata. Other mechanisms of action may include ciliary vascular disruption, which may decrease aqueous production, and chronic inflammation, which may either reduce inflow or increase uveoscleral outflow (Figs. 16-3 and 16-4) [6–8].

CYCLODESTRUCTIVE PROCEDURES FOR CONTROLLING INTRAOCULAR PRESSURE

Transpupillary cyclophotocoagulation

Transpupillary cyclophotocoagulation employs the familiar argon laser to blanch the ciliary processes visible using gonioscopy. Direct visualization of the ciliary processes and ciliary ridges is often limited in patients with glaucoma, especially those who have been receiving long-term therapy with miotic agents. Patients with sector iridectomies or retracted irides from neovascularization may have excellent exposure of at least some ciliary processes. Scleral indentation, occasionally employing special contact lenses, may rotate the ciliary processes into more visible locales, but the inability to find adequate access for the argon beam is a major limitation of this technique.

The procedure itself is straightforward. Standard retrobulbar or peribulbar anesthesia is administered to the eye to be treated. After placing the gonioprism on the eye, all visible parts of the ciliary process are treated, using blanching and pigment dispersion as the visible endpoint. The laser settings, using the green light, are typically 800 to 1000 mW, 0.1 to 0.2 seconds, with

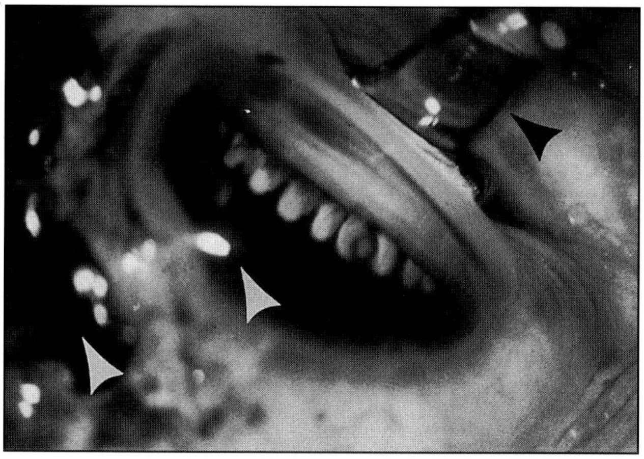

FIGURE 16-3. Intraocular cyclophotocoagulation with transpupillary visualization. Ciliary processes are brought into view with scleral depressor (*black arrow*) and treated with laser endophotocoagulator (*white arrows*) through a pars plana incision. (*From* Shields *et al.* [7]; with permission.)

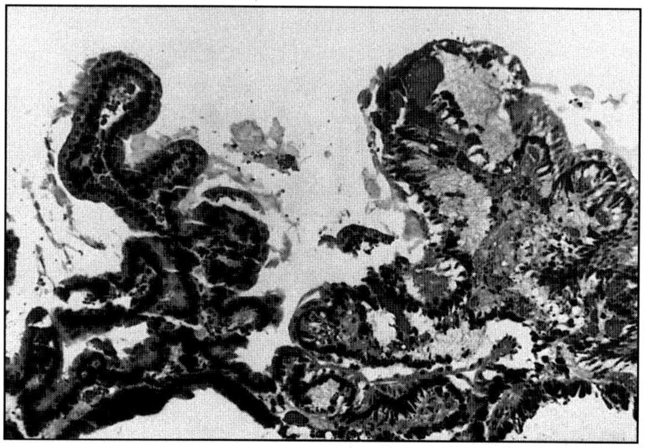

FIGURE 16-4. Light microscopic view of a monkey's eye, enucleated and fixed immediately after intraocular cyclophotocoagulation with endoscopic visualization. Note extensive disruption of ciliary epithelium and stroma in treated process on the right, compared with relatively normal structure of untreated process to the left. (hematoxylin and eosin; original magnification, × 125.) (*From* Shields [8]; with permission).

a moderate spot size between 100 and 200 µm. Two to five applications are usually sufficient to "paint" the visible (anterior) portion of a ciliary process. Up to 180° of the ciliary body may be treated at one time, with the remaining portion of the ciliary body available for further treatment. Topical steroids and cycloplegics are applied postoperatively. Therapy with miotic drops is generally to be avoided. Oral dosage of pain medication is prescribed as needed.

The long-term efficacy of the procedure has been disappointing [8]. In part, this may be due to the inability to treat both enough ciliary processes and enough of each ciliary process (*ie*, difficulty in reaching the posterior ciliary ridge) [9]. Even when most ciliary processes are photocoagulated by this technique, IOP often remains inadequately controlled.

Intraocular cyclophotocoagulation

Recent technologic developments have permitted construction of endolaser instruments consolidating three fiber groups—the image guide, the light guide, and the laser guide—into a single probe [10]. The separate equipment console houses the video camera, light source (175 W xenon), semiconductor diode laser (810 nm), video monitor, and videotape recorder. Probes come in both 18- and 20-gauge sizes, the larger size more suitable for the beginning endoscopist. Although endoscopic cyclophotocoagulation is an intraocular procedure, the surgeon does not peer through the operating microscope after the probe has been inserted into the eye. Rather, the progress of the surgical procedure is observed by viewing the video monitor while the probe is manipulated within the eye.

Early endoscopic cyclophotocoagulation procedures relied on a pars plana approach, usually performed by an experienced vitreoretinal surgeon using transpupillary viewing with independent light-source and laser probes. The pars plana entry could safely be performed only on pseudophakes, aphakes, or patients undergoing lensectomy, because the spherical shape of the natural lens caused it to be traumatized by the endoprobes.

The newest probes, which combine the light, imaging, and laser fibers, permit a limbal approach that is more familiar to the anterior segment surgeon. With slight modifications of technique, the ciliary processes may be accessed in phakic, aphakic, and pseudophakic eyes. The endoscopic cyclophotocoagulation procedure may be combined with cataract surgery and intraocular lens implantation. Most surgeons would, however, consider this a fairly invasive procedure in a phakic eye undergoing only endoscopic cyclophotocoagulation for glaucoma and without coincident cataract surgery.

The key to the technique in all situations is to use injected viscoelastic in order to separate anterior segment structures and visualize the ciliary processes most accurately. As with other cyclodestructive techniques, the ciliary processes are "whitened" and slightly shrunken. Gas bubbles, gross pigment dispersion, and audible "popping" are to be avoided. Again, 180° of the ciliary body may be treated, under direct visualization on the video monitor. Often, postoperative pressure spikes with endoscopic cyclophotocoagulation, and this should be treated aggressively. In addition to the patient's usual glaucoma medications (minus miotics), therapy with topical steroids, cycloplegics, and topical antibiotics is indicated, along with oral pain medications as needed.

Transscleral cyclophotocoagulation

Transscleral laser cyclophotocoagulation methods of cyclodestruction employ an external approach to the ciliary body. Laser energy is delivered through the scleral wall to photocoagulate a portion of the ciliary body without direct visualization of the ciliary processes. It is similar in this way to cyclocryotherapy. Two delivery systems are currently in use to provide laser energy. The noncontact Nd:YAG unit employs a modified slit lamp to transmit the laser energy, whereas contact systems use a fiberoptic and hand-held probe placed directly on the conjunctival surface.

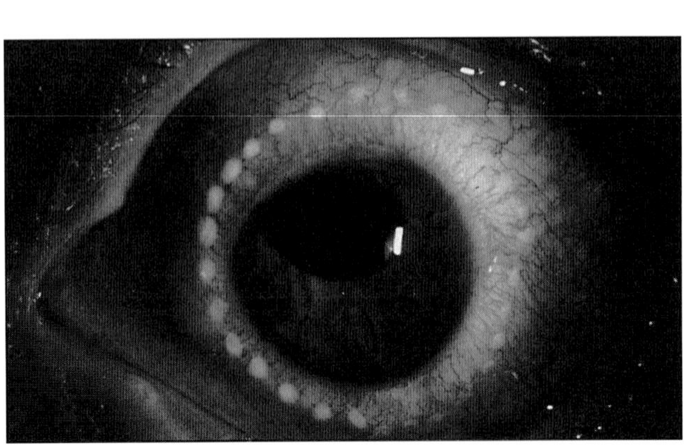

FIGURE 16-5. Slit lamp appearance of conjunctival burns, (*white spots*) immediately following noncontact pulsed transscleral neodymium:yttrium-aluminum-garnet cyclophotocoagulation. Note larger diameter of lesions on left side, treated without the contact lens, compared with lesions on right, treated with the lens. (*From* Shields [11]; with permission.)

Noncontact transscleral laser cyclophotocoagulation

The LASAG Microrupter II (HS Meridian, Mason, OH) is a noncontact, pulsed Nd:YAG laser. When operated in the free-running thermal (*ie*, nonphotodisruptive) mode, it delivers laser energy to the patient, who is seated at the slit lamp in the conventional way. The eye is anesthetized in the standard retrobulbar or peribulbar manner, with 4% lidocaine and 0.75% Marcaine (to permit several hours of pain control). Use of a lid speculum or contact lens is optional. The Microrupter II is set to 20-ms single pulses, with the maximum focus offset from the HeNe aiming beam and a setting of "9" on the instrument dial. This setting allows the Nd:YAG beam to penetrate the sclera about 2.7 mm. Laser applications are most effective when applied between 1 to 1.5 mm from the limbus. (A marking pencil may be used to ensure accuracy. Transillumination is used to localize the ciliary body for treatment.) The number of applications has varied in different studies, but generally 30 to 50 applications across three quadrants have been used. The 3- and 9-o'clock positions are avoided to prevent damage to the long posterior ciliary arteries (Fig. 16-5).

Contact transscleral cyclophotocoagulation

The LASAG Microrupter III employs a Nd:YAG laser in a continuous wave (nonpulsed) mode to deliver energy through a flexible contact probe delivery system. The energy can then be applied to the patient, who is placed in a supine position. The Microrupter III system is portable, which permits outpatient treatment as well as use in an operating room or hospital room. As with the noncontact system, the eye receives standard retrobulbar or peribulbar anesthesia. The lids are opened with a wire speculum, and 30 to 40 applications are placed perpendicular to the sclera between 0.5 and 3.0 mm from the limbus. The instrument is set to deliver 5 to 6 J of energy for each pulse.

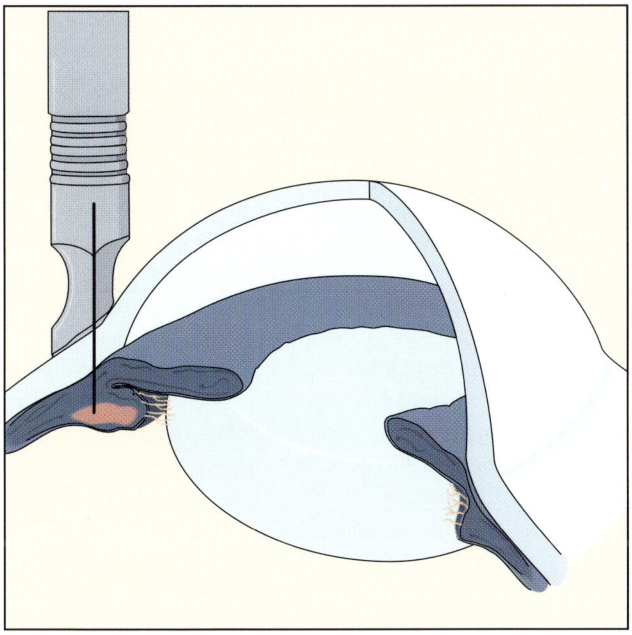

FIGURE 16-6. Treatment of ciliary body through sclera with contact G-probe and diode laser from Iris Medical (Mountain View, CA).

Surgical Laser Technologies' (Oaks, PA) continuous wave YAG lasers models CL60 and CL100 also have contact probe delivery systems. They use a sapphire tip for laser delivery that permits treatment in a manner similar to that of the LASAG Microrupter III. This device may also be used in urology, gynecology, and plastic surgery. With these systems, the power is generally set at 7 W (range, 4 to 8 W) with an exposure time of 0.7 seconds (0.5 to 0.7 seconds). The site of application is 1 to 3 mm from the limbus, involving 30 to 40 applications over 360°. Again, the 3- and 9-o'clock positions must be avoided to prevent damage to the long posterior ciliary arteries.

Recently, various solid-state laser systems have been used for contact transscleral laser cyclophotocoagulation. A popular commercial unit is the OcuLight Diode Laser System with the FDA-approved G-Probe (Iris Medical Instruments, Mountain View, CA) for transscleral ciliary body ablation. This 810-nm laser also may be used for laser trabeculoplasty and posterior segment pathology, including retinopathy of prematurity. The G-Probe orients the fiber about 1 mm behind the limbus while allowing for even spacing of 16 to 18 applications over 27° (omitting the 2-o'clock positions) (Fig. 16-6). Laser pulses begin at a power of 1750 mW, for durations of 2000 to 2500 ms. The surgeon listens for "popping" sounds. Laser power is increased in 250 mW increments until these "pops" are heard. The energy is applied at a level at or just below the power required for a "pop" to be audible. No external marks are produced by the laser application. The surgeon may use the temporary depression left by the G-Probe to guide the next application (Fig. 16-7). By aligning the edge of the probe with the indentation left by the fiber at the center of the last application, the clinician will produce appropriate separation of the burns over 270° (Fig. 16-8).

Postoperative treatments for transscleral laser cyclophotocoagulation modalities may include topical steroids, subconjunctival steroids, cycloplegics, and oral pain medications. Many patients will experience only minimal discomfort and can use a mild, nonsteroidal anti-inflammatory drug for pain relief. Iced compresses will often help decrease some postoperative discomfort. Patients should be maintained on their preoperative glaucoma medications, although avoiding the inflammatory effects of miotics if possible.

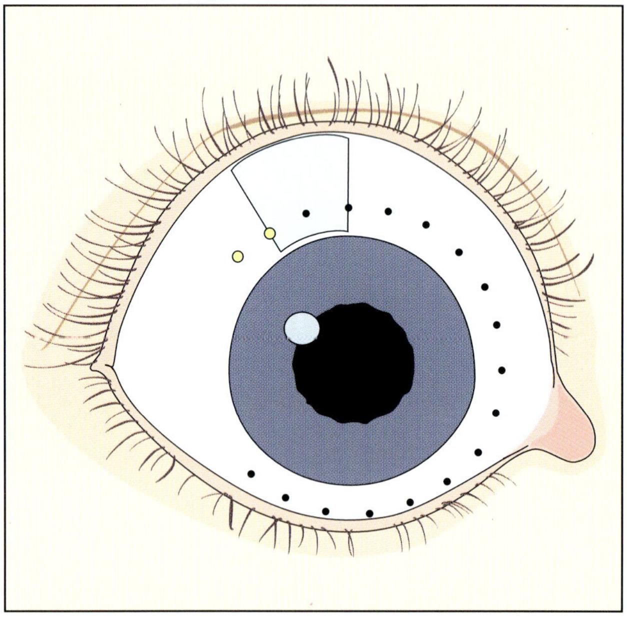

FIGURE 16-7. Imprint of G-probe (Iris Medical, Mountain View, CA) on conjunctiva showing spacing of laser lesions externally.

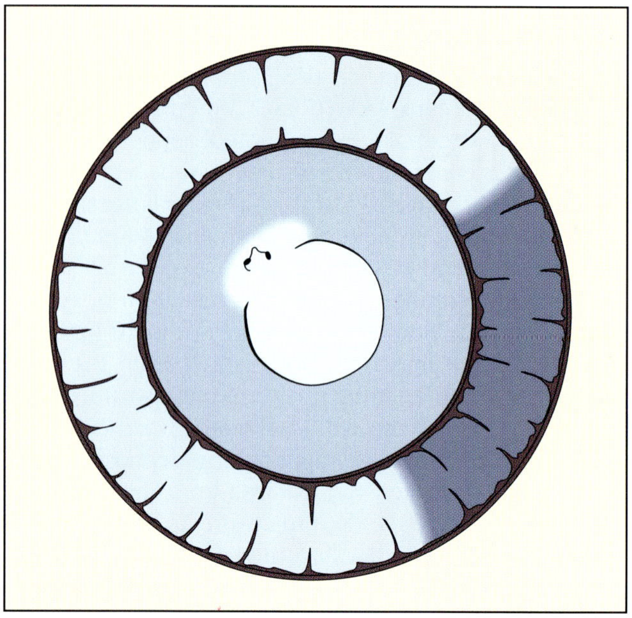

FIGURE 16-8. Internal view of ciliary body treatment after transscleral diode cyclophotocoagulation. (*Courtesy of* Iris Medical, Mountain View, CA.)

CLINICAL EXPERIENCE AND CHOICE OF TREATMENT MODALITIES

Choosing the "appropriate" laser for cyclodestructive procedures depends on both the availability of the instruments and the surgeon's preference [12]. The Nd:YAG units are larger, more expensive instruments most likely found in a hospital or university setting, whereas the solid-state diode devices are more portable and more affordable by private practitioners. Because the Nd:YAG equipment may be shared by several surgical specialties, ophthalmic capabilities may be had for the cost of adding the delivery system. Endoscopic procedures require an operating room setting and thus have the risks attendant in all intraocular surgeries. Trans-scleral procedures, however, are more easily mastered and may be performed in the surgeon's office.

All laser cyclodestructive techniques discussed have been used clinically and have been found to be effective at lowering IOP. The transscleral techniques are more easily mastered by the surgeon and allow for greater reproducibility of results with similar instrument settings. Some surgeons advocate an intraocular approach to ciliary destruction when combined with cataract surgery. Study has not been sufficient to endorse this approach at this time; however, some reports of good initial responses to this combined technique have been published [13].

After reviewing 63 of our cases over a 2.5-year period using the Iris Medical Diode laser and the G-Probe delivery handpiece, we determined that approximately 20% of patients needed re-treatment to obtain a therapeutic effect. Other studies have cited re-treatment rates of 11% to 20% [14,15]. Because damage is limited to local tissues, patient tolerance and acceptance of these procedures is far greater than of older cyclocryotherapy procedures. We have found that the diode laser seems to offer greater comfort in the postoperative period when compared with cyclocryotherapy and the noncontact laser procedures. Less postoperative inflammation and pain are seen in these patients. Usually, only small amounts of analgesic medication are needed. With these laser treatments, the maximal lowering of IOP should be expected at 4 to 6 weeks after surgery. Re-treatment should not be attempted before this time. The risk of complications increases with each laser attempt, and this should be considered before additional therapy is undertaken.

References and Recommended Reading

Recently published papers of particular interest have been highlighted as:

- • Of interest
- •• Of outstanding interest

1. Bechrakis NE, Muller-Stolenberg NW, Helbig H, *et al.*: Sympathetic ophthalmia following laser cyclocoagulation. *Arch Ophthalmol* 1994, 112:80–84.
2. Lam S, Tessler H, Lam B, *et al.*: High incidence of sympathetic ophthalmia after contact and noncontact neodymium YAG cyclotherapy. *Ophthalmology* 1992, 99:1818–1822.
3. Mastrobattista JM, Luntz M: Ciliary body ablation: where are we and how did we get here? *Surv Ophthalmol* 1996, 41:193–213.
4. Feldman RM, El-Harazi SM, LoRusso FJ: Histopathologic findings following contact transscleral semiconductor diode laser cyclophotocoagulation in human eye. *J Glaucoma* 1997, 6:139–140.
5. Marsh PBS, Wilson DJ, Samples JR: A clinicopathologic correlative study of noncontact transscleral Nd:YAG cyclophotocoagulation. *Am J Ophthalmol* 1993, 115:597–602.
6. Schubert HD: Non-contact and contact pars plana transscleral neodymium:YAG laser cyclophotocoagulation in postmortem eyes. *Ophthalmology* 1989, 96:1471.
7. Shields S, Stewart WV, Shields MB: Transpupillary argon laser cyclophotocoagulation in the treatment of glaucoma. *Ophthal Surg* 1988, 19:171.
8. Shields MB: Laser cyclophotocoagulation. In *Current Techniques in Ophthalmic Laser Surgery*, edn. 2. Edited by Benson WE, Coscas G, Katz LJ. Philadelphia: Current Medicine; 1994:167–173.
9. Shields MB: Cyclodestructive surgery for glaucoma: past present and future. *Trans Am Ophthalmol Soc* 1985, 83:283.
10. Uram M: Endoscopic cyclophotocoagulation in glaucoma management. *Curr Opin Ophthalmol* 1995, 6:19–29.
11. Shields MB: *Textbook of Glaucoma*, edn 3. Baltimore: Williams & Wilkins; 1992:622.
12. Gaasterland D: Glaucoma management: a surgical way to reduce aqueous production. *Rev Ophthalmol* 1995, 2:109–110.
13. Uram M: Combined phacoemulsification, endoscopic ciliary process photocoagulation and intraocular lens implantation in glaucoma management. *Ophthal Surg* 1995, 26:346–352.
14. Hille K, Waibel C, Weindleret J, *et al.*: Long-term results of diode laser cyclophotocoagulation in secondary angle block of glaucoma. *German J Ophthalmol* 1995, 1(Suppl):144.
15. Carassa RG, Brancato R, Bettin P, *et al.*: Contact transscleral cyclophotocoagulation with diode laser: a long-term follow-up study [ARVO abstract]. *Invest Ophthalmol Vis Sci* 1996, 37(Suppl):1193.

Index

Page numbers in *italic* indicate figures; page numbers followed by *t* indicate tables.

D

E

F

G

H

I

J

K

L

M

N

O

P

Q

R

S

T

U

V

W

X

Y